Lung Cancer 2021, Part 2

Editors

FARID M. SHAMJI

GILLES BEAUCHAMP

THORACIC SURGERY CLINICS

www.thoracic.theclinics.com

Consulting Editor
VIRGINIA R. LITLE

November 2021 • Volume 31 • Number 4

ELSEVIER

1600 John F. Kennedy Boulevard • Suite 1800 • Philadelphia, Pennsylvania, 19103-2899

http://www.thoracic.theclinics.com

THORACIC SURGERY CLINICS Volume 31, Number 4
November 2021 ISSN 1547-4127, ISBN-13: 978-0-323-79343-8

Editor: John Vassallo (j.vassallo@elsevier.com)
Developmental Editor: Jessica Nicole B. Cañaberal

Thoracic Surgery Clinics (ISSN 1547-4127) is published quarterly by Elsevier Inc., 360 Park Avenue South, New York, NY 10010-1710. Months of publication are February, May, August, and November. Business and editorial offices: 1600 John F. Kennedy Boulevard, Suite 1800, Philadelphia, PA 19103-2899. Periodicals postage paid at New York, NY, and additional mailing offices. Subscription prices are $397.00 per year (US individuals), $858.00 per year (US institutions), $100.00 per year (US students), $464.00 per year (Canadian individuals), $888.00 per year (Canadian institutions), $100.00 per year (Canadian students), $225.00 per year (international students), $485.00 per year (international individuals), and $888.00 per year (international institu-tions). Foreign air speed delivery is included in all Clinics' subscription prices. All prices are subject to change without notice. **POSTMASTER:** Send address changes to Thoracic Surgery Clinics, Elsevier Health Sciences Division, Subscription Customer Service, 3251 Riverport Lane, Maryland Heights, MO 63043. **Customer Service (orders, claims, online, change of address): Telephone: 1-800-654-2452 (U.S. and Canada); 314-447-8871 (outside U.S. and Canada). Fax: 314-447-8029. E-mail: jour-nalscustomerservice-usa@elsevier.com (for print support); journalsonlinesupport-usa@elsevier.com (for online support).**

Reprints. For copies of 100 or more, of articles in this publication, please contact Commercial Rights Department, Elsevier Inc., 360 Park Avenue South, New York, NY 10010-1710. Tel: 212-633-3874; Fax: 212-633-3820; E-mail: reprints@elsevier.com.

Thoracic Surgery Clinics is covered in *MEDLINE/PubMed (Index Medicus), EMBASE/Excerpta Medica, Science Citation Index Expanded (SciSearch®), Journal Citation Reports/Science Edition,* and *Current Contents®/Clinical Medicine.*

Contributors

CONSULTING EDITOR

VIRGINIA R. LITLE, MD
Section Chief of Thoracic Surgery,
Cardiovascular Surgery, Medical Director of
Thoracic Surgery, Intermountain Healthcare,
Murray, Utah, USA

EDITORS

FARID M. SHAMJI, MBBS, FRCSC, FACS
Adjunct Professor Surgery, University of
Ottawa, General Campus, The Ottawa
Hospital, Ottawa, Ontario, Canada

GILLES BEAUCHAMP, MD, FRCSC
Thoracic Surgery Unit, Department of Surgery,
Maisonneuve-Rosemount Hospital, University
of Montreal, Montreal, Quebec, Canada

AUTHORS

DANIEL ANKENY, MD, PhD
Department of Anesthesia, Critical Care and
Pain Management, Massachusetts General
Hospital, Boston, Massachusetts, USA

CAITLIN ANSTEE, BA
Database Manager and Software Developer,
Division of Thoracic Surgery, Department of
Surgery, The Ottawa Hospital, Ottawa, Ontario,
Canada

XIAODONG BAO, MD, PhD
Department of Anesthesia, Critical Care and
Pain Management, Massachusetts General
Hospital, Boston, Massachusetts, USA

GILLES BEAUCHAMP, MD, FRCSC
Thoracic Surgery Unit, Department of Surgery,
Maisonneuve-Rosemount Hospital, University
of Montreal, Montreal, Quebec, Canada

HOVIG CHITILIAN, MD
Department of Anesthesia, Critical Care and
Pain Management, Massachusetts General
Hospital, Boston, Massachusetts, USA

SE-IN CHOE, MD, FRCSC
Fellow, Division of Thoracic Surgery, McMaster
University, McMaster University and Service of
Thoracic Surgery, St. Joseph's Healthcare
Hamilton, Hamilton, Ontario, Canada

JOEL COOPER, MD, FACS, FRCSC
Hospital of the University of Pennsylvania,
Philadelphia, Pennsylvania, USA

**ROBERT JAMES CUSIMANO, MD, FRCSC,
FACS**
Professor of Surgery, University of Toronto,
Peter Munk Cardiac Centre, Toronto General
Hospital, Toronto, Ontario, Canada

MOLLY GINGRICH, H, BSc, MSc
Clinical Research Assistant, Ottawa, Ontario, Canada

MARCIO M. GOMES, MD, PhD, FRCPC
Department of Pathology and Laboratory Medicine, Ottawa Hospital Research Institute, University of Ottawa, Ottawa, Canada

SCOTT A. LAURIE, MD, FRCPC
Medical Oncologist, Division of Medical Oncology, The Ottawa Hospital Cancer Centre, Associate Professor, University of Ottawa, Ottawa, Ontario, Canada

BRYAN LO, MD, PhD, FRCPC
Medical Geneticist, Division of Pathology and Laboratory Medicine, The Ottawa Hospital Cancer Centre, Assistant Professor, University of Ottawa, Ottawa, Ontario, Canada

ROBERT MALCOLM MACRAE, MD, FRCPC
Radiation Oncologist/Assistant Professor, Division of Radiation Oncology and Radiation Medicine Program, The Ottawa Hospital, University of Ottawa, Ottawa, Ontario, Canada

DONNA E. MAZIAK, MDCM, MSc, FRCSC, FACS
Professor, University of Ottawa, Surgical Oncology, Division of Thoracic Surgery, General Campus, The Ottawa Hospital, Ottawa, Ontario, Canada

RAHUL NAYAK, MD, FRCSC
Consultant, Division of Thoracic Surgery, Director, Thoracic Surgery Research and Quality Improvement LHSC, Associate Scientist, Lawson Health Research Institute, Lecturer, Schulich School of Medicine and Dentistry, Western University, London, Ontario, Canada

G. ALEXANDER PATTERSON, MD
Division of Thoracic Surgery, Department of Surgery, Washington University School of Medicine in St. Louis, St Louis, Missouri, USA

SIMRAN RANDHAWA, MD
Division of Thoracic Surgery, Department of Surgery, Washington University School of Medicine in St. Louis, St Louis, Missouri, USA

ANDREW J.E. SEELY, MD, PhD, FRCSC
Vice-Chair Research, Department of Surgery, Division of Thoracic Surgery, Thoracic Surgery and Critical Care Medicine, The Ottawa Hospital, Professor, University of Ottawa, Scientist, Ottawa Hospital Research Institute, Ottawa, Ontario, Canada

HARMAN JATINDER S. SEKHON, MD, MSc, PhD
Full Professor, Department of Pathology and Laboratory Medicine, The Ottawa Hospital, Ottawa, Ontario, Canada

FARID M. SHAMJI, MBBS, FRCSC, FACS
Adjunct Professor Surgery, University of Ottawa, General Campus, The Ottawa Hospital, Ottawa, Ontario, Canada

YARON SHARGALL, MD, FRCSC
Professor, Surgery and Medicine, Head, Division of Thoracic Surgery, Juravinski Professor in Thoracic Surgery, MI-GMAC Chair in Thoracic Surgery, McMaster University, St. Joseph's Healthcare Hamilton, Hamilton, Ontario, Canada

CAROLINA A. SOUZA, MD, PhD, FRCPC
Division of Thoracic Imaging, Department of Medical Imaging, Ottawa Hospital Research Institute, University of Ottawa, Ottawa, Canada

NIKOLAOS TRIKALINOS, MD
Division of Medical Oncology, Department of Internal Medicine, Washington University School of Medicine in St. Louis, St Louis, Missouri, USA

KRISTIN WADDELL, BScN
Registered Nurse, General Campus, The Ottawa Hospital, Ottawa, Ontario, Canada

Contents

The objective of these notes is to stress the principles underlying the management of primary lung cancers and other types of malignancies in the thorax—diffuse malignant mesothelioma, invasive mediastinal tumors, chest wall sarcoma, and tracheal neoplasms—and from these considerations to outline a routine scheme for management, which can be followed easily by all staff. It is hoped that by adherence to this routine, adequate and efficient management of all cases will be obtained, both in the very important matter of preoperative preparation, as well in the postoperative management.

Lung cancer is a lethal disease, and chronic cigarette smoking is the most common cause. The selection of treatment is based on the histologic cell type, accurate staging, and adequacy of cardiopulmonary functional reserve. The risk for surgery is highest in patients over the age of 80 years.

Techniques for chest wall resection and reconstruction have evolved over the years. Chest wall resection in conjunction with pulmonary resection has several complications, including pulmonary and infectious. Risk factors for complications are related to the size of the defect, number of ribs resected, and the addition of a pulmonary resection. Material used for reconstruction does not impact the overall complication rate.

Increasingly, systemic treatment decisions in nonsmall cell lung cancer require the determination of predictive biomarkers on biopsy or surgical specimens. Although currently these have their major role in the advanced setting, these tumor-specific treatments are increasingly moving into earlier stage disease. As part of the multidisciplinary team managing those with nonsmall cell lung cancer, thoracic surgeons need to be aware of these biomarkers and in particular of the need for adequate biopsy specimens containing sufficient tissue to perform the necessary analyses that guide treatment selection.

Empyema may occur in the pleural space after pulmonary resection. Subsequent bacterial contamination results in infection and development of frank empyema. Pneumonectomy—surgical removal of the entire lung—is the treatment of choice for centrally located bronchogenic carcinoma, diffuse malignant mesothelioma, and chronic inflammatory lung diseases with destroyed lung from pulmonary tuberculosis, fungal infections, and bronchiectasis. In the uncomplicated case, on the pneumonectomy side, the diaphragm becomes elevated as the air–fluid level decreases with chest wall deformation and gradual disappearance of hydrothorax. The pneumonectomy space is at potential risk for getting infected from bacterial contamination and developing empyema.

Early diagnosis in lung cancer is desirable, because surgical resection offers the only hope of cure. In the face of suggestive symptoms, a normal plain chest radiograph does not exclude the diagnosis, and investigation is essential. The various imaging changes seen on computerized tomography and PET scan provide strong suggestive evidence of lung cancer, but proof of diagnosis rests on histologic examination, material that may be obtained by one of the following diagnostic procedures: bronchoscopy, mediastinoscopy, fine needle aspiration biopsy, thoracentesis and pleural biopsy, lymph node biopsy, and exploratory thoracotomy.

The knowledge of lymphatic spread of lung cancer permitted the study of anatomy of lymphatic drainage of the lungs. The history of anatomy of lymphatic drainage of the lungs began in the 15th century. In the human, pulmonary lymph flows to the lymph nodes around the lobar bronchi and thence to extrapulmonary lymph nodes located around the main bronchi and trachea and its bifurcation (tracheobronchial lymph nodes). These send their efferents to a right and left mediastinal lymph trunks, which may join the thoracic duct, but usually drain opening directly into the brachiocephalic vein of their own side.

There is great potential for standardized postoperative adverse events data collection to document, inform, audit, and feedback, all to optimize patient care. Adverse events, defined as any deviation from expected recovery from surgery, have harmful implications for patients, their families, and clinicians. Postoperative adverse events occur frequently in thoracic surgery, predominately due to the high-stakes (ie, high potential for cure) and high-risk (ie, vital physiology and anatomy and preexisting disease) nature of the surgery. As discussed, engaging surgeons in audit and feedback practices informed by standardized data collection would generate consensus recommendations to reduce adverse events and improve patient outcomes.

this article, existing knowledge on the pathogenesis, histology, imaging findings, and clinical and prognostic significance of these 2 entities is presented.

Farid M. Shamji

Lung cancer is the most common cause of cancer-related death worldwide among both men and women. Patients with lung cancer frequently have impaired pulmonary function, usually secondary to smoking-related chronic obstructive lung disease. Numerous techniques have been used to evaluate the postsurgical risk. These techniques include preoperative pulmonary function test, 6-minute walk test, stage 1 cardiopulmonary exercise test, 2D echocardiography, and quantitative ventilation-perfusion scintigraphy.

Farid M. Shamji, Joel Cooper, and Gilles Beauchamp

The purpose and conduct of medical audit is a means of quality control for medical practice by which the profession shall regulate its activities with the intention of improving overall patient care. The quality assurance depends on patient and physician satisfaction. The medical profession needs to be educated about the structure, process, and outcome. The structure equates to resources found within the hospital. The outcome is when quality of care becomes preeminent.

Daniel Ankeny, Hovig Chitilian, and Xiaodong Bao

Increasingly complex procedures are routinely performed using minimally invasive approaches, allowing cancers to be resected with short hospital stays, minimal postsurgical discomfort, and improved odds of cancer-free survival. Along with these changes, the focus of anesthetic management for lung resection surgery has expanded from the provision of ideal surgical conditions and safe intraoperative patient care to include preoperative patient training and optimization and postoperative pain management techniques that can impact pulmonary outcomes as well as patient lengths of stay.

Farid M. Shamji, Gilles Beauchamp, Donna E. Maziak, and Joel Cooper

Paraneoplastic syndromes are clinical entities associated with cancers and often overlap with metabolic and endocrine syndromes. The cell types of lung cancer involved are frequently small cell, squamous cell, adenocarcinoma, large cell, and carcinoid tumor. A number of neurologic paraneoplastic syndromes have been described for which the tumor product remains unknown. These include peripheral neuropathies, a myasthenia-like syndrome, and subacute cerebellar degeneration. Although all of these syndromes may improve with successful treatment of the primary tumor, complete resolution is rare.

THORACIC SURGERY CLINICS

SERIES OF RELATED INTEREST

Surgical Clinics
http://www.surgical.theclinics.com

Surgical Oncology Clinics
http://www.surgonc.theclinics.com

Advances in Surgery
http://www.advancessurgery.com

THE CLINICS ARE AVAILABLE ONLINE!
Access your subscription at:
www.theclinics.com

THORACIC SURGERY CLINICS

Foreword
Lung Cancer 2021, Part 2

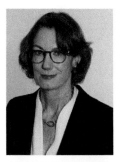

Virginia R. Litle, MD
Consulting Editor

We are excited to bring you the "Management of Lung Cancer: Part II" issue for the *Thoracic Surgery Clinics*. Invited guest editors, Drs Farid Shamji and Gilles Beauchamp, have brought together a diverse array of topics and invited authors to share their annotated reviews of topics relevant to lung cancer management. From soup to nuts, from presentation to adjuvant management, you will read about the role of biomarker assessment preoperatively, to optimizing clinical care through a fast-track program and to managing perioperative complications. Dr Shamji summarizes preoperative evaluation of the patient with compromised pulmonary function and the requisite testing for optimal triage of these high-risk individuals. In addition, our guest coeditors elaborate on the operative planning of all comers with lung cancer: when should we operate, when are we offering resection with true curative intent. Anesthesia colleagues from Mass General update us on risk scores and optimal ventilation strategies. Some useful out-of-the-box topics include the "medical audit" for improving thoracic patient care,

which is written by the guest editors and the legendary Dr Joel Cooper, who can provide seasoned advice about how to proceed with this quality improvement effort.

Thank you to *all* the contributors and to guest editors, Drs Shamji and Beauchamp. Enjoy the panoply of content, and please share with your trainees, who can anticipate a career of constant challenge and problem-solving. We hope you enjoy this issue!

Sincerely,

Virginia R. Litle, MD
Cardiovascular Surgery
Intermountain Healthcare
5169 South Cottonwood Street, Ste 640
Murray, UT 84107, USA

E-mail address:
Virginia.litle@imail.org

Twitter: @vlitlemd (V.R. Litle)

Thorac Surg Clin 31 (2021) xi
https://doi.org/10.1016/j.thorsurg.2021.09.003
1547-4127/21/© 2021 Published by Elsevier Inc.

Preface
Management of Lung Cancer in Part I and Part II

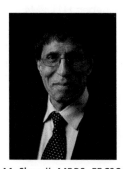

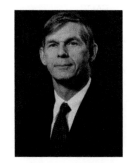

Farid M. Shamji, MBBS, FRCSC, FACS   Gilles Beauchamp, MD, FRCSC

Editors

The topic of lung cancer, both small cell and non–small cell, was prepared in two parts as a tribute to Dr Jean Deslauriers, a prominent Canadian Thoracic Surgeon, who died of lung cancer on September 13, 2019. The authors, who were selected to write their articles, were requested by Dr Farid Shamji (Ontario) and Dr Gilles Beauchamp (Quebec). In Part I, 16 articles were selected to be written by thoracic surgeons (N = 15), thoracic radiologists (N = 8), thoracic pathologists (N = 3), and thoracic oncologists (N = 5). In Part II, 16 articles were selected to be written by thoracic surgeons (N = 14), thoracic oncologists (N = 3), thoracic anesthetist (N = 1), thoracic pathologists (N = 4), thoracic radiologists (N = 2), cardiac surgeon (N = 1), thoracic research assistants (N = 2), and thoracic operating room senior nurse (N = 1).

The overall structure of the two parts of the issue, tried and tested as it is, remains the one that will be familiar to our readers, although every article has been completely rewritten and several new ones added; it will be a surprise to no one to find those on lung cancer, principles of thoracic treatment, postpneumonectomy sepsis lymphatic spread of lung cancer, postoperative adverse events, selection of thoracic surgical instruments, superior vena cava resection and reconstruction, neuroendocrine tumors of the lung, aerogenous metastases, thoracic surgical medical audit, anesthetic management of pulmonary resection, paraneoplastic syndromes, multidisciplinary thoracic oncology conferences, guiding principles in the management of synchronous and metachronous lung cancers, safety in lung cancer operations, management of air leaks postpulmonary resection, role of thoracic radiologists, management of acute and late complications of pneumonectomy, education and training of general thoracic surgeons, assessment and rehabilitation of the compromised thoracic surgical patient, oncologic management of small cell lung cancer, embolotherapy in bronchial hemorrhage, ethics for thoracic surgeon in the management of lung cancer, biology, science, and secondary growths in oligometastatic lung cancer, management of solitary fibrous tumors of the pleura, delays in managing lung cancer, and biological aggressiveness and metastatic potential of primary lung cancer.

The task of writing these two parts of the issue on lung cancer in a sufficiently short period to ensure that it is up-to-date at publication has been a taxing one, not least of all for our colleagues, to whom we owe a debt of gratitude we are unlikely to be able to repay. It has however been an educational experience, during which we have had an unusual opportunity of examining our own clinical practices in light of published evidence. We hope that the reader will find the issue in two parts as helpful as we have found the writing and the reading of the material written by colleagues. Having said this, we would not have been able to complete the work without the help of a number of friends and colleagues.

Thorac Surg Clin 31 (2021) xiii–xiv
https://doi.org/10.1016/j.thorsurg.2021.08.002
1547-4127/21/© 2021 Published by Elsevier Inc.

Finally, may we leave the reader with the words of Francis Bacon: "*Read not to contradict and confute, nor to believe and take for granted, nor to find talk and discourse, but to weigh and consider.*"

Farid M. Shamji, MBBS, FRCSC, FACS
Department of Surgery
University of Ottawa
Ottawa General Hospital
501 Smyth Road
Ottawa, K1H 8L6
Ontario, Canada

Gilles Beauchamp, MD, FRCSC
Thoracic Surgery Unit
Department of Surgery
Maisonneuve-Rosemount Hospital
University of Montreal
5415 L'Assomption Boulevard
Montreal, Quebec H1T 2M4, Canada

E-mail addresses:
faridmashamji@gmail.com (F.M. Shamji)
Gilles.d.beauchamp@sympatico.ca
(G. Beauchamp)

Guiding Principles on the Importance of Thoracic Surgical Education on Establishing Integrated Thoracic Surgery Program, Interdisciplinary Thoracic Oncology Conferences, and an Interdisciplinary Approach to Management of Thoracic Malignancies

Farid M. Shamji, MBBS, FRCSC, FACS[a],*,
Harman Jatinder S. Sekhon, MD, MSc, PhD[b],
Robert Malcolm MacRae, MD, FRCPC[c],
Donna E. Maziak, MDCM, MSc, FRCSC, FACS[d]

KEYWORDS

- Integrated thoracic surgery program • Requirements for thoracic surgical education • Fast tracking
- Surgical intuition

KEY POINTS

- Requirement for medical education is essential that begins with information and proceeds through knowledge, learning and understanding.
- The specifics on essential requirements for thoracic surgical education, beginning with knowledge of epidemiology of lung cancer, understanding pathogenesis of esophageal cancer, recognition of immediately life-threatening chest injuries and relatively life-threatening chest injuries, diagnosis of malignancies in the pleural space, management of pulmonary and pleural space complications of tuberculosis, fungal infections, and bacterial infections.
- Members of the integrated thoracic surgery program and thoracic team involved in fast tracking clinical care.
- Quotes by Claude Bernard and Walter Bradford Cannon.
- The life history of lung cancer: fast tracking of lung cancer.

Dr Maziak has nothing to disclose.
[a] University of Ottawa, General Campus, Ottawa Hospital, 501 Smyth Road, Ottawa, Ontario K1H 8L6, Canada; [b] Department of Pathology and Laboratory Medicine, The Ottawa Hospital, CCW, Room 4240, Box 117, 501 Smyth Road, Ottawa, Ontario K1H8L6, Canada; [c] Division of Radiation Oncology & Radiation Medicine Program, The Ottawa Hospital, The University of Ottawa, Box 903, 501 Smyth Road, Ottawa, Ontario K1H 8L6, Canada; [d] University of Ottawa, Surgical Oncology Division of Thoracic Surgery, Ottawa Hospital - General Division, 501 Smyth Road 6NW-6364, Ottawa, Ontario K1H 8L6, Canada
* Corresponding author.
E-mail address: faridmashamji@gmail.com

Thorac Surg Clin 31 (2021) 367–377
https://doi.org/10.1016/j.thorsurg.2021.07.007
1547-4127/21/© 2021 Elsevier Inc. All rights reserved.

INTRODUCTION
Establishing Integrated Thoracic Surgery Program

The objective of these notes is to stress the principles underlying the management of primary lung cancers and other types of malignancies in the thorax—diffuse malignant mesothelioma, invasive mediastinal tumors, chest wall sarcoma, and tracheal neoplasms—and from these considerations to outline a routine scheme for management, which can be followed easily by all staff. It is hoped that by adherence to this routine, adequate and efficient management of all cases will be obtained, both in the very important matter of preoperative preparation, as well in the postoperative management.

The system outlined has been the result of very careful study performed by self and by talented thoracic surgeons in both Canada and the United States and has been evolved over a considerable number of years, so that the modifications dictated by experience have been combined with the long-standing, traditional and well-established methods of management.

It is recognized that although the routine will be most suitable for most cases, there will in special circumstances be cases requiring different management. Such special instructions will be given only by the responsible thoracic surgeon and ought not to be embarked on without his or her specific instructions.

It is hoped that the routine outlined will be a sound basis for preoperative and postoperative care and as such will be of value to the surgical residents and fellows, nursing staff, medical students, physiotherapists, and allied health care workers in the routine management of thoracic surgical cases. It will also be of help to the nursing tutors in that it will provide a basis of consistent teaching in the School of Nursing, which will be put into practise when the student nurse leaves the school to take up ward duties.[1]

In order to develop a recognisable thoracic surgery program from a preexisting thoracic surgery service in an academic center, voluntary participation from other medical services is necessary to create integrated interdisciplinary thoracic surgery program; this promotes an academic environment, collegiality, collaboration, and medical professionalism; clinical research and participation in medical audit; a dedication to serving the interest of the patient; a sense of altruism contributing to the trust that is central to the physician-patient relationship; and international recognition. The quote by Robert Green written here reflects on the responsibility of the medical profession in promoting quality in medical education.

Requirement for Medical Education

I conceive that all education begins with information and

proceeds thence through knowledge, learning, and

understanding, to ultimate wisdom. Information may be

defined as the acquisition of factual data; knowledge is the

systematic organization of information; learning, the correlation

and integration of various bodies of knowledge and

understanding the perception of their significance. Finally,

wisdom is the fine art of applying all information, knowledge,

and learning, in light of understanding, to the problems of

human living. It is not enough that the physician should

"know the cause of every malady", the science of medicine.

He needs also the art, the understanding, and the wisdom to

apply that knowledge to his own life and to the lives of

others.

Robert Green

The essential requirements for thoracic surgical education
1. *Knowledge* of epidemiology of lung cancer, causative factors, clinical presentation, investigations for diagnosis, and invasive and noninvasive mediastinal staging; assessment of surgical operative risk from cardiopulmonary assessment; anatomy of the mediastinum and invasive mediastinal lymph node staging; fast tracking in the management of thoracic malignancies and decision for treatment from the multidisciplinary conference by a team approach of thoracic surgeons, pulmonary pathologists, thoracic radiologists, and nuclear medicine, radiation oncologists, and medical oncologists.[2–4]

2. *Understanding* pathogenesis of esophageal cancer, clinical presentation, and the need for early detection before clinical presentation from knowledge of causative factors, staging, and multidisciplinary approach to management that includes surgeons, gastroenterologists, radiology and nuclear medicine, and medical and radiation oncologists.
3. *Recognition* of immediately life-threatening chest injuries and relatively life-threatening chest injuries.
4. *Diagnosis* of malignancy in the pleural space, primary diffuse malignant mesothelioma, and metastatic tumor deposits from other primary malignancies; multidisciplinary management of mesothelioma.
5. *Management* of pulmonary and pleural space complications of tuberculosis, fungal infections, and bacterial infections.
6. *Precision* in the management of life-threatening massive airway hemorrhage.
7. *Recognition and diagnosis and urgent management* of proximal airway obstruction due to tumor or idiopathic tracheal stricture.
8. *Learning* thoracic anatomy and anatomic relationship in the mediastinum and classification and treatment of mediastinal tumors in different locations.
9. *Presentation and urgency* in the surgical management of life-threatening descending necrotizing mediastinitis, esophageal perforations and attendant mediastinal sepsis, and incarcerated giant hiatus hernias.

Surgery is an art as well as a science, whereas an operation is only a technique There is a far greater need for thorough understanding of the art of science in surgery, and learning only the surgical techniques is not considered sufficient in training. Learning only how to perform an operation is counter-productive. Learning how to perform an operation safely must be learned through an apprenticeship under an excellent teacher of surgery. The absolute requirement in surgical training is having in-depth knowledge in 3 basic sciences: gross anatomy and microanatomy, physiology and biochemistry, and surgical pathology. It is timely to remind the young doctor that although he or she can cure sometimes, and alleviate frequently, he or she must at all times be compassionate.

On October 1, 1823 the advice that Sir Astley Cooper (1768–1841), renowned and respected British surgeon, gave to upward of "four hundred medical students" attending his "introductory" surgery lecture, at St Thomas' Hospital, London, was as relevant then as it is today.[5] The real groundwork of all surgical science was proper *knowledge of anatomy*; Cooper had no doubts: "operations cannot be safely undertaken by any man, unless he possesses a thorough knowledge of anatomy"; the detailed knowledge that must be both *regional and applied anatomy*. A poor knowledge of anatomy caused what modern quality zealots would call an "adverse event." The students must understand that study of medicine is important to the surgeon; to be a good surgeon you must first become a good doctor; he should be able to prescribe with certainty—"should well understand the great influence of local disease on the constitution, as well as the origin of local disease from constitutional derangement". As well, understanding of *"physiologic knowledge"* is of the utmost importance to the profession of surgery ... "a knowledge of the healthy functions enables you to better understand the nature of diseased action." He advised the students that in "surgical science, hypothesis should be discarded, and sound theory derived from actual observation and experience ... experiments on living animals have been found of the greatest utility in directing us to a knowledge of the means by which Nature acts in the reparation of injuries." Surgery is a science that requires understanding of the disease with consequent pathologic changes in the tissues and organ resulting in disturbance of physiology and loss of function; the present descriptive terms used are *pathogenesis* and *pathophysiology*.

The four conditions necessary for the surgeon
First, he or she should be learned.
Second, he or she should be an expert.
Third, he or she should be ingenious.
Fourth, he or she should be able to adapt himself or herself.

It is required for the *FIRST* that the surgeon should know not only human anatomy and physiology but also pathophysiology—not only the principles of surgery but also those of medicine in theory and practice. To be a good surgeon, you must first aim to become a good doctor; for the *SECOND* that he or she should have seen others operate; for the *THIRD* that he or she should be ingenious, of judgment and memory to recognize conditions; and for the *FOURTH* that he or she be adaptable and able to accommodate himself or herself to circumstances.

Requirements for becoming a thoracic surgeon
1. Dedication and long-term commitment to the profession
2. Desire to be a life-long learner
3. Excellent knowledge in basic sciences of anatomy, physiology, histology, anatomic

pathology, biochemistry, chemical pathology, and microbiology
4. Looking after personal health and well-being of self and of the family
5. Expect to spend long hours at work
6. Acquire in-depth knowledge in thoracic oncology and application of this knowledge
7. Active participation in multidisciplinary thoracic oncology conferences to plan care for the patients with primary lung cancers, malignant mediastinal tumors, diffuse malignant mesothelioma, primary malignant chest wall tumors, and pulmonary metastases
8. Understand the requirements of becoming a thoracic surgical oncologist

Ignorance is lack of knowledge It must be understood and taught to the medical students and surgical trainees that the hospital exists for the sake of the patients. The very word "hospital" (Latin, *hospitium)* means a place where guests are received. Being a house of hospitality all patients within the walls of the hospital should therefore be treated as guests; this is a basic and changeless concept that has prevailed for centuries. The treating doctor must never display the arrogance of office. He or she should preserve a certain dignity. Bad language must never be used; evidence of haste and of indecision should be avoided. And lastly, never to make remarks in front of a patient or his or her relatives that might impugn the treatment given by an outside doctor.

Proper acquisition and application of knowledge in basic sciences is the most essential requirement for the training and practicing surgeons. The knowledge in anatomy, physiology, and pathology is the essential requirement for any doctor who wishes to train in surgery and equally important for training in medicine.

As *Edward Churchill (1895–1972)*, former professor of surgery at Harvard, once said, *"Surgery is not a single applied science; it is the application of many sciences to the management of disease and injury. Of these sciences, none outranks pathology in importance."* Learning surgical pathology is an absolute requirement during training to become a surgeon, and application of the knowledge of surgical pathology is essential in the surgical care of the patients. Dr Churchill was a Professor of Surgery at Harvard University. He performed the first pericardiectomy, mediastinal parathyroidectomy.

The Important Qualities of a Surgeon are as follows:

1. A good surgeon knows how to operate
2. A better surgeon knows when to operate
3. The best surgeon knows when not to operate

The presence of all 3 essential qualities is necessary in every surgeon. This famous saying surely applies right across medicine, whether it is surgical or medical. It takes wisdom, experience, strength, and courage not to intervene.

Selectivity *Selectivity* is the basis of *surgical treatment* for primary lung cancers. Surgical treatment offers the hope of cure to most of the patients with lung cancer; this requires careful clinical and pathologic staging in the selection of best therapeutic approach, with intent to cure. In selected patients with lung cancer, the treatment that completely eradicates the local growth gives the most appreciable survival both in terms of quality and duration. There is no role for palliative resection in lung cancer except in the infrequent cases of symptomatic hypertrophic pulmonary osteoarthropathy and infected lung from bronchial obstruction.

Selectivity is also the basis of surgical treatment of mediastinal tumors such as thymoma, germ cell tumors, and neurogenic tumors. Diffuse malignant mesothelioma is a difficult cancer to treat and difficult disease to cure, and surgical treatment is often for palliation rather than for cure. Mediastinal lymphoma is not a surgical disease for which the treatment with intent to cure is with chemotherapy. Neurogenic tumors in the posterior mediastinum that have intraspinal extension evident on MRI require combined thoracic and neurosurgical team for safe resection with intent to preserve spinal cord function.

Surgical intuition *Surgical intuition* becomes important when faced with having to make a surgical decision in the preoperative phase.[6] The surgeon must ask himself or herself the following questions before every operation, which must only be performed once each question has been answered satisfactorily:

1. HAS THE DIAGNOSIS BEEN FIRMLY ESTABLISHED?
   a. With modern techniques this can be done in most of the cases.
   b. Occasionally an exploratory operation is necessary if the possibility of serious disease cannot be confidently ruled out, but this must be an exception.
2. IS AN OPERATION NECESSARY?
   a. *Operations have Certain Indication* that must be present before an operation is justified.
   b. *Operation is potentially Dangerous* and is only indicated if the risks of the disease are

greater than the risks of the operation. For this one must know

    i. Natural history of the disease

    ii. Risk of the operation

  c. *Would You have the Operation* if you were in the patient's position?

  d. *If in Doubt*

    i. Seek a second opinion or

    ii. Reevaluate the case later

  e. *It is not Justifiable to perform an Operation merely on the Possibility that it may be Necessary*—there must be a reasonable probability or preferably certainty that it is required.

3. IS THE PATIENT FIT FOR THE OPERATION AND ANESTHETIC? If not, make him fit and examine and improve functions of the different body organ systems: heart, lung, kidneys, and liver before committing to an operation.

4. WHEN IS THE BEST TIME FOR OPERATION?

  a. In general, if an operation is well indicated, it should be done without undue delay.

  b. Reasons for postponing an operation

    i. to improve the patient's state of fitness—operate as soon as maximal improvement has taken place.

    ii. To allow inflammatory reaction to subside and so make operation easier—operate when maximal improvement has taken place.

    iii. The benefits of delay must be judged against the possible harm of progression of the disease—careful judgment and possible compromise required to balance out these 2 factors.

5. WHO SHOULD PERFORM THE OPERATION?

  a. Someone with the training to perform the operation competently

  b. In emergencies this may have to be compromised

Fast-tracking investigations and staging of patients with lung cancer

- *LIFE HISTORY OF LUNG CANCER*[7–9]: to determine whether fast-tracking investigations and clinical pathways are effective in reducing delays in the diagnosis, staging, and treatment of lung cancer, one must appreciate that there are 4 intervals in the life history of the disease (**Table 1**).

Interdisciplinary thoracic oncology team and conferences in fast tracking As frequently happens in other walks of life, investigation of a special problem leads to a solution of others (**Table 3**). The restructuring of health care delivery fostered creation of :integrated thoracic surgery program and

"interdisciplinary thoracic oncology team," resulting in a concerted team effort for promoting excellence of patient care by sharing knowledge at the weekly regular attendance of (**Fig. 1**):

> Thoracic surgeons
> Thoracic oncologists—radiation and medical oncologists for lung cancer, mediastinal tumors, chest wall sarcoma, and mesothelioma
> Thoracic radiologists
> Pulmonary pathologists
> Nuclear medicine physicians
> Social workers
> Residents and fellows in training
> Research assistants
> Thoracic nurses

What is a thoracic surgical oncologist? A thoracic surgical oncologist is defined as a surgeon who has acquired special skills and expertise in oncology and has made a commitment to treating patients who have developed malignancy in the lung, pleura, chest wall, and mediastinum. The thoracic surgical oncologist brings a body of knowledge that extends to all facets of cancer, including lung cancer screening and surveillance, cigarette smoking prevention, fast-tracking in diagnosis and treatment planning, and treatment. The thoracic surgical oncologist must be committed to dealing with all aspects of thoracic malignancies in a multidisciplinary manner interacting with thoracic radiologists, thoracic oncologists, and pulmonary pathologists.[10,11]

Responsibilities of a thoracic surgical oncologist:

1. Spends considerable amount of surgical practice time (>80%) looking after patients with different types of thoracic malignancies.

2. Is knowledgeable about the cancer biology of thoracic malignancies and appropriate treatment and the standard of care.

3. Is a competent technical surgeon with knowledge and judgment to provide safe surgical treatment.

4. Interacts and communicates effectively with the interdisciplinary thoracic oncology team.

5. Provides institutional leadership in the care of thoracic malignancies in screening, diagnosis, and prevention.

6. Maintains educational responsibilities, teaching medical students, surgery residents, and surgery oncology fellows.

7. Maintains active participation in the interdisciplinary cancer care team and involvement in cancer clinical trials including in translational research to foster molecular, biological, and

Table 1
Life history of lung cancer: fast tracking of lung cancer

Interval	Description	What Can be Done to Improve Care?
First	Preclinical asymptomatic phase	• Prevention of risks factors associated with lung cancer; smoking cessation education; lung cancer screening
Second	Symptomatic phase	• Education of general public and health providers
Third	Diagnosis and staging	• Use of standardized clinical care pathways • Multidisciplinary thoracic oncology clinic
Fourth	Treatment	• Improve supply—OR time and others for existing demand • Creation of formal surgical oncology divisions

Abbreviation: OR, operating room.

- *The first interval* is the preclinical asymptomatic phase, which begins with the first malignant changes in the bronchial epithelium. During that period, which can be quite long, not only does the tumor have the possibility to increase in size, but the lesion also has the potential for local invasion, lymphatic dissemination, and distant spread. During that preclinical phase, awareness of indicators of increased risk for developing lung cancer is important.
- *The second interval* is when patients recognize subtle changes in symptoms related to chronic obstructive lung disease or the onset of new symptoms, such as persistent cough or hemoptysis. The length of this interval is influenced by patients not seeking immediate medical attention or experiencing delays in getting a timely appointment with their family physician. This time is when educating the general public may have an impact by raising awareness for risk factors associated with lung cancer and symptoms that should be of concern. If health care providers, especially family physicians, are well aware of the early manifestations of lung cancer, this interval could be shortened, leading to a more rapid diagnosis and workup and increased resection rates.
- *The third interval* is between the time from suspicion of lung cancer by the family practitioner to patients being referred to a specialist for diagnosis, staging, and treatment planning. Ideally, all referrals should be triaged by a navigator nurse and investigations performed in an orderly fashion according to predetermined pathways, thus avoiding delays and fragmented care. During that interval, a treatment plan should be developed through a coordinated multidisciplinary approach. Shortening this interval may also be beneficial to the promotion of patients' mental and physical wellness as well as alleviating the mental distress associated with long delays.
- *The fourth interval* is between a confirmed diagnosis of lung cancer and treatment. Any significant delay encountered at this point is unacceptable and may have the counter-effect of decreasing chances of survival for some patients who would otherwise be potentially curable. This decreased chance of survival is likely a reflection of the biology of exponential tumor growth and metastatic potential observed in the form of stage migration becoming more rapid with increasing tumor size and early nodal spread. The British Thoracic Society (**Table 2**) recommends that there should be a maximum of 8 weeks between the first consultation with a specialist (respirologist or thoracic surgeon) and surgery in an uncomplicated case, and surgery should be performed within 4 weeks of surgical evaluation unless patients have to receive induction therapy. Similarly, the Canadian Association of Thoracic Surgeons recommends that this delay be 4 weeks but in reality it has been delayed for as long as 6 to 8 weeks. The creation of formal surgical oncology divisions with accountability for timely care may also be a good option to help decreasing waiting times during this interval.

Table 2
Time-line standards for patient flow during the investigation and staging of lung cancer

Patient Profile	British Thoracic Society Guidelines	Canadian Society for Surgical Oncology and Canadian Association of Thoracic Surgery Guidelines
Referral of patient	1 wk	2 wk
Initial visit	2 wk	1 wk
Diagnostic and staging techniques	3 wk	2–3 wk
Treatment	2 wk	1 wk
Total	8 wk	6–8 wk

Data from The Lung Cancer Working Party of the British Thoracic Society Standards of Care Committee. BTS recommendations to respiratory physicians for organizing the care of patients with lung cancer. Thorax 1998;53(Suppl 1): S1–8; and Darling GE, Maziak DE, Clifton JC, et al. The practice of thoracic surgery in Canada. Can J Surg 2004; 47:438–44.

other basic science concepts in the therapeutic scheme.

8. Provides timely surgical care to the patients with thoracic malignancies following the requirements of fast-tracking.
9. Maintains long-term follow-up care for detection of recurrences and second primary cancer.
10. Demonstrates willingness to participate in the implementation of clinical protocols.
11. Maintains clinical responsibility and willingly coordinates all thoracic oncology-related aspects of patient care and communicates effectively and competently with the medical and radiation oncologists.
12. Has specific surgical expertise in the management of patients with cancer.

The concept of integrated thoracic surgery program in academic setting: the history A modern hospital is a highly complex organization made up of administration and bureaucracy, physicians from different disciplines of medicine and surgery, oncology, pathology department medical laboratories, nurses, allied health care personnel, and support staff. Within this environment, necessity is the mother of invention, and the medical staff must believe in providing the best possible care for the patients. The process takes time, and it is known that "The journey of thousand miles begins with a single step" ascribed to Laozi in China.

It was with this commitment that Dr Farid M Shamji embarked on this journey of changing the face of thoracic surgery at The Ottawa Hospital from a long-standing hospital-based thoracic surgery service to a university and hospital-based academic thoracic program. The journey took 19 years, and this was the lesson learnt during training from the most successful thoracic surgery program at the Toronto General Hospital under the leaderships of the late Dr Frederick G. Pearson, the late Dr Robert J. Ginsberg, and Dr Joel D. Cooper.

To be successful in this journey, the thoracic surgeon had to assume "Leadership," just as it happened in North America when the Lung Cancer Study Group conducted several clinical trials in the management of lung cancer. To do so, the thoracic surgeon must first become an "Organizer and a Leader" and establish a thoracic program working in cohort with pulmonologists, thoracic radiologists, thoracic anesthetists, thoracic oncologists, pulmonary pathologists, and intensivists. These are the "Essential Ingredients" necessary for success. The thoracic surgeon must remain a committed "Guide and Counselor" and provide an unfailing source of information to his or her colleagues, operating room nurses, intensive care nurses, and paramedical personnel on all aspects of treatment in the thoracic surgery program. It is about "Preparedness and Team Effort" that are essential in achieving good results in all aspects of thoracic surgical care. A basic concept intelligently used in the planning of medical audit and applicable in the setting up an integrated thoracic surgery program is by having a *"structure (defined), process (commitment),* and *output (measurable outcome)."*

The "Essential Elements" that have been put into place to foster an academic Thoracic Surgery Program are as follows:

1. A group of dedicated and collaborative thoracic surgeons to share the workload
2. Weekly Multidisciplinary Thoracic Oncology Conference attended by thoracic surgeons,

Table 3
Members of the integrated thoracic surgery program and thoracic team involved in fast tracking and standardized clinical care pathways for lung cancer

Team	Responsibilties
Thoracic surgeons	Expertise with knowledge and ability to perform safe invasive and noninvasive staging procedures for lung cancers and all types of lung resectional procedures
Medical oncologists	Expertise in principles and indications of induction and adjuvant chemotherapy treatments
Radiation oncologists	Expertise with latest radiation treatment indications, techniques, and results
Respirologist	Expertise in the evaluation of cardiopulmonary function and operative risk
Dedicated thoracic radiologists	Expertise with imaging techniques used for evaluation of the patients, staging of lung cancer, and diagnostic needle aspiration biopsy MRI Thorax and Head
Dedicated pulmonary pathologists	Expertise with new histologic classification of lung cancers Ability to correctly interpret small biopsy specimens and cytology Molecular markers and mutations
Allied health care personnel	Psychologists, nutritionists, specialized thoracic nurses, physiotherapists, social workers, occupational therapists, residents in training, and research assistants
Palliative care specialists	Expertise with palliative care for patients with advanced disease
Residents in training in all the aforementioned disciplines	Education and training in thoracic oncology
Nuclear medicine	PET, quantitative pulmonary ventilation/perfusion, nuclear bone scan

thoracic medical and radiation oncologists (for lung, mediastinum, pleura, and chest wall), pulmonary pathologists, chest radiologists, nuclear medicine, residents and fellows from respective services, cancer assessment center nurses, and social workers. There is a separate group of gastrointestinal (GI) pathologists who conduct weekly GI pathology rounds, and thoracic surgeon attends to discuss his/her cases for management.

3. Academic teaching rounds to be held jointly every 6 weeks by thoracic surgeon, chest radiologists, and pulmonary pathologist and residents from 3 respective specialties. The cases selection (n = 4) for discussion is by one thoracic surgeon, Dr Farid Shamji who initiated these rounds in 1983.

4. Thoracic Oncology Retreats for Continuing Professional Development and Lung Pathology Rounds have been the recent initiative of pulmonary pathologist Dr Marcio Gomes in the last 2 years. These retreats have been key and ongoing annual event after formally taken over by Dr Marcio Gomes. Before 2 years ago, the retreats were intermittent beginning in early 2000.

5 Monthly morbidity and mortality rounds for audit and documented for point deviance and changing practices by thoracic surgeon, Dr Andrew Seely.

6 Monthly Thoracic Surgery Research rounds (Dr Andrew Seely).

7. Cancer Assessment Center and Communities of Practice (CoP) coordinated by thoracic surgeon Dr Donna E. Maziak and radiation oncologist Dr Jason Pantarotto. The Communities of Practice is intended to involve not only the thoracic surgeons and thoracic oncologists

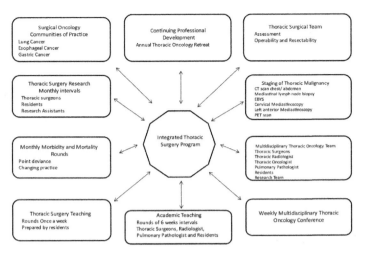

Fig. 1. Integrated thoracic surgery program for lung cancer care.

but also thoracic nurses, administrative representation, and family doctors.

8. Endobronchial Ultrasound Biopsy of mediastinal lymph nodes for diagnosis when needed and for mediastinal staging of lymph nodes in lung cancer.

9. PET scan for staging lung cancer, mediastinal tumors, esophageal cancer, and stomach cancer.

SUMMARY

Surgery is an art as well as a science. Surgery has been defined as that part of the art of medicine that deals with the treatment of disease and injury mainly by operative methods. Although this may define the end product, the modern surgeon must build his knowledge on a sound foundation of the basic sciences, especially Surgical Physiology, Human Anatomy, and Surgical Pathology, and as well on abroad understanding of General Medicine. The word "surgeon" is derived from 2 Greek Words: "working or done by hand" — "*Cheir*" a *hand*, and "*Ergon*," *work*.

It is no longer possible for a surgeon merely to be craftsman. He or she must know about the metabolic response to surgical or accidental trauma, essential for survival, in order to maintain patient in normal nitrogen balance, physiology, and biochemistry of the body fluids if he or she is to maintain the patient in good fluid balance before, during, and after operation. The responsible surgeon must be familiar with the neuroendocrine response to trauma and the intricacies of the metabolism of fats, carbohydrates, and proteins and the mechanism of hemostasis and maintenance of homeostasis. A detailed knowledge of microbiology, surgical infections, cross-infections, opportunistic infections, and nosocomial infections has become necessary.

Surgery is an art as well as a science. And it is timely to remind all the surgeons that although the responsibility is to cure often, and alleviate suffering frequently, compassion must always be maintained. The practice of surgery is one of the best examples of such integrated knowledge where anatomy, physiology, biochemistry, pharmacology, pathology, and microbiology are applied to the understanding and treatment of disease processes in surgical patients; this is the Basis of Surgical Education. The factors governing normal circulation and respiration are thus essential to life and cell function by restoring gas exchange, oxygen delivery, and stable normal blood sugar level and maintaining vital enzyme function, which requires normal arterial blood pH. Normal neurologic function is essential to life as is the renal function. Trauma, surgical and injury, results in the physiologic neuroendocrine response to metabolic response to trauma in order to restore cell normality and maintain life.

Uneventful postoperative recovery, without development of adverse events, is essential to life by maintaining stable arterial pH at 7.40 (7.35–7.45), normal gas exchange (arterial PO_2 95–98 mm Hg) and oxygen transport, and normal blood sugar level; this requires restoring normal physiologic function in all the organs of the body.

This concept is in keeping with Claude Bernard (1813–1878) who described about the regulation of the continuous constancy of the internal environment ("*milieu intérieur*"); he called the interstitial fluid (which bathes the cells) and the plasma (with which it carries out continuous exchanges), the internal environment.[11,12] As a French physiologist he was regarded "one of the greatest of all men of science."

Later on, Walter Cannon coined the word "homeostasis," reflecting on Claude Bernard about the constancy of the internal environment, to describe the "various physiologic arrangements which serve to restore normal state, once it has been disturbed." The actual internal environment ("*milieu intérieur*") of the cells of the body is the interstitial component of the extracellular fluid and plasma.[13–15]

QUOTES BY CLAUDE BERNARD

- Man can learn nothing except by going from the known to the unknown.
- It is what we know already that often prevents us from learning.
- A fact in itself is nothing. It is valuable only for the idea attached to it or for the proof that it furnishes.

QUOTE BY WALTER BRADFORD CANNON (1871–1945)

Chance throws peculiar conditions in everyone's way. If we apply; intelligence, patience and special; vision, we are rewarded with new; creative breakthroughs.

These changes described by Walter Cannon—the more rapid pulse, the deeper breathing, the increase of sugar in the blood, the secretion from the adrenal glands—were very diverse and seemed unrelated. Then, one wakeful night, after a considerable collection of these changes had been disclosed, the idea flashed through my mind that they could be nicely integrated if conceived as bodily preparations for supreme effort in flight or in fighting. Further investigation added to the collection and confirmed the general scheme suggested by the hunch.

The factors governing normal circulation and respiration are thus essential to life and cell function by restoring gas exchange, oxygen delivery, stable normal blood sugar level, and maintaining vital enzyme function, which requires normal arterial blood pH. Normal neurologic function is essential to life as is the renal function. Trauma, surgical and injury, results in the physiologic neuroendocrine response to metabolic response to trauma in order to restore cell normality and maintain life.

There should be early recognition and prompt treatment of postoperative complications, which frequently are wound infection, urosepsis, infected pulmonary atelectasis, venous thrombosis with pulmonary embolism, electrolyte imbalance, threatening myocardial ischemia and cardiac arrhythmias, specific complications after tracheal resection, mediastinal tumor resection, pulmonary resection and esophagectomy, and sudden postoperative collapse:

a. Complications of the operation:
   i. hemorrhage
   ii. infection—septicemia and sepsis syndrome with septic shock
   iii. fluid and electrolyte disturbances
   iv. massive pulmonary embolism
   v. acute coronary thrombosis
   vi. metabolic disturbances—hypocalcaemia, hypokalemia, hypoglycemia
b. Cerebrovascular accident

CLINICS CARE POINTS

- The essential requirements for thoracic surgical education about knowledge, diagnosis and recognition, malignancies in the thorax, life-threatening massive airway hemorrhage.
- The four conditions necessary for the surgeon and the requirements for becoming a thoracic surgeon.
- The importance of surgical intuition.
- Fast-tracking investigations and staging of patients with lung cancer.
- What are the defining qualities of a thoracic surgical oncologists?
- Life history of lung cancer: fast-tracking of lung cancer.

REFERENCES

1. McKeown KC. Surgical management. Darlington Memorial Hospital; 1970. p. 1–35.
2. Allison PR, Temple LJ. The future of thoracic surgery. Thorax 1966;21:99–103.
3. Henry Ellis F. Education of thoracic surgeon. Thorax 1980;35:405–14.

4. Alexander J. The training of a surgeon who expects to specialize in thoracic surgery. J Thorac Surg 1936;5(6):579–82.

5. Coote W. Is sir astley cooper's 1823 advice to medical students still relevant? Med J Aust 2006;185(11):664–6.

6. Du Plessis DJ. Principles of surgery. 2nd edition. Bristol: John Wright & Sons LTD; 1976. p. 92–9. Chapters XXII and XXIII.

7. Shamji FM, Deslauriers J. Fast-tracking investigations and staging of patients with lung cancer. In: Thoracic surgery clinics, part I: screening, diagnosis, and staging. Canada: Elsevier; 2013. p. 187–91.

8. Moody A, Muers M, Forman D. Delays in managing lung cancer. Thorax 2004;59:1–3.

9. Myrdal G, Lambe M, Hillerdal G, et al. Effect of delays on prognosis in patients with non-small cell lung cancer. Thorax 2004;59:45–9.

10. Balch CM, Bland KI, Brennan MF, et al. Editorial: what is a surgical oncologist? Ann Surg Oncol 1994;1:2–4.

11. Cohen IB. Foreword. In: Claude B, editor. An introduction to the study of experimental medicine. Dover edition; 1957. Introduction to the study of experimental medicine (originally published in 1865 first English translation by Henry copley Greene Macmillan & Co, Ltd, 1927).

12. Olmsted JM, Harris E. Claude bernard and the experimental method in medicine. New York: Henry Schuman; 1952.

13. Cannon WB. Bodily changes in pain, hunger, fear and rage. New York, NY: D. Appleton & Company; 1915.

14. Cannon WB. The way of an investigator: a scientist's experiences in medical research. New York, NY: W. W. Norton; 1945. p. 130–45.

15. Cannon WB. The role of emotions in disease. Ann Intern Med 1936;9:1453–65.

Assessment of Operability and Resectability in Lung Cancer

Farid M. Shamji, MBBS, FRCSC, FACS[a],*, Gilles Beauchamp, MD, FRCSC[b]

KEYWORDS

- Lung cancer • Operability • Resectability • Mediastinal node map

KEY POINTS

- Factors to consider in operability and resectability.
- Patient-related factors and tumor-related factors and surgery-related factors to consider.
- Attention to details on operability and resectability necessary in the preoperative care of the patients.
- Mediastinal lymphatic staging.

INTRODUCTION

Distinction is made between operability and resectability. The terms are not synonymous and should not be confused. A resectable tumor is one in which there is no technical barrier to surgical excision. An operable tumor is one in which various parameters identify surgical excision as the most appropriate treatment. A tumor may be considered technically resectable, yet deemed inoperable because of other criteria, such as the extent of lymph node involvement, cell type, distant metastases, prohibitively high surgical risk in a compromised patient, distant metastases, and so forth. In many cases, operability implies that resection offers some prospect for cure. The opinion is shared by many that there are rarely indications for deliberate, palliative resection in patients with bronchial carcinoma. In an occasional case, benefit may follow a palliative resection for obstructed or infected lung, or for relief of disabling hypertrophic pulmonary osteoarthropathy.[1–3] Troublesome hemoptysis is almost always controlled by radiotherapy.

OPERABILITY AND RESECTABILITY

In the Introduction to *Surgery and Basic Surgical Principles*, the terms operability and resectability are not synonymous.[1] The patient may be operable on the basis of treatable disease, operative risk, and surgical diagnosis. The disease may be resectable on the basis of cure rate and risk factors.

Surgical diagnosis is based on a sound knowledge of anatomy, physiology, and pathology, a specific clinical history and examination with confirmation by imaging and operative surgery. It is unnecessary to learn what can be deduced, and thus, surgery concerns defining the basic facts on which the consequences of a disease process can be built. The actual operation in surgery is but one part of the process of surgical care: diagnosis, preoperative care and postoperative management being of equal importance in differing circumstances. No matter how good the operation, if it is performed for the wrong diagnosis, the benefit to the patient will be limited or void. In other situations, such as the patient who

[a] University of Ottawa, General Campus, Ottawa Hospital, 501 Smyth Road, Ottawa, Ontario K1H 8L6, Canada;
[b] Thoracic Surgery Unit, Department of Surgery, Maisonneuve-Rosemount Hospital, University of Montreal, 5415 L'Assomption Boulevard, Montreal, Quebec H1T 2M4, Canada
* Corresponding author.
E-mail address: faridshamji@hotmail.com

Thorac Surg Clin 31 (2021) 379–391
https://doi.org/10.1016/j.thorsurg.2021.07.008
1547-4127/21/© 2021 Elsevier Inc. All rights reserved.

presents as a surgical emergency in association with severe illness, a common occurrence in this era of the elderly patient, skilled preoperative resuscitation and management can turn a high-risk procedure into a routine operation. Similarly, the very ill patient can be salvaged by expert post-operative management.

Operability

Assessment

The assessment of operability requires consideration of the following factors:

1. Exclusion of detectable extrathoracic and distant metastases
2. Determination of the presence or absence of superior mediastinal lymph node metastases
3. Definition of the histologic or cell type, whenever possible
4. Evaluation of operative risk

Distant metastases History and physical examination may alert the physician to the presence of hematogenous metastases, particularly to brain, bone, and skin. Liver metastases are common and, unfortunately, are frequently "silent." Computed tomography (CT) and PET are sensitive in detecting metastases to the liver, adrenal glands, and bone. There is less reliance on serum alkaline phosphatase level for detecting liver metastases. There is now rarely a need for small laparotomy or laparoscopy for direct examination of the liver. Metastatic spread to the brain is best detected by CT or MRI.

Lymphatic spread There is accumulating evidence that superior mediastinal lymph node involvement influences prognosis profoundly and adversely in most cases. Paulson and Urschel[2] reported a 6% 5-year survival in 251 patients with superior mediastinal lymph node involvement managed by resection. Bergh and Schersten[4] reported similar survival statistics in such cases and make an important observation relating prognosis to the extent of lymph node involvement observed: if tumor had invaded the capsule of the node (perinodal spread), then 5-year survival following resection is limited to 4%. If this type of perinodal spread occurs in the superior mediastinum, the 5-year survival is less than 2%. It is recognized that patients with superior mediastinal lymph node involvement show a very high incidence of hematogenous spread, and although the intrathoracic tumor may be eradicated by surgical excision, the majority succumb to distant metastases. The exceptions to this observation are cases with limited, ipsilateral intranodal mediastinal node involvement associated with a favorable cell type (squamous cell carcinoma) in which more favorable survival statistics are achieved following resection, sometimes combined with radiotherapy.

Cell type The histologic or cell type profoundly affects the prognosis, with well-differentiated squamous cell tumors at the favorable end of the scale, adenocarcinoma in an intermediate position, and small cell carcinoma with such an unfavorable prognosis that many surgeons will not recommend resection if this cell type is identified on needle biopsy. In a randomized, multicenter trial conducted by the British Medical Research Council, it was clearly shown that chemotherapy and radiotherapy were preferable to surgical excision in cases of small cell carcinoma: there were no 2-year survivors following resection in this series, and the mean survival in resected cases was 7 months.

It may be difficult, however, to identify the cell type with certainty before thoracotomy. The pathologist may have difficulty in precisely defining the cell type from sputum analysis or from material obtained by percutaneous needle aspiration lung biopsy. If doubt exists, it is preferable to operate on such patients provided there is no involvement of superior mediastinal lymph nodes. If, however, the pathologist states that the biopsy material shows unequivocal small cell carcinoma, it is then recommended to treat with radiotherapy or chemotherapy as primary treatment. If the primary tumor is, in fact, small and of the small cell type, it will respond favorably to the treatment and disappear radiologically within 4 to 6 weeks of completing irradiation.

Operative risk There has been a relatively greater increase in the incidence of lung cancer in patients in the sixth, seventh, and eighth decades during recent years, and there is an increasing trend to resect bronchogenic carcinoma in the elderly. At 1 time, it was suggested that no patient over the age of 70 was likely to tolerate pulmonary resection, but this approach is no longer accepted. With careful preoperative selection, patients in the seventh and even in the eighth decades may be operated on with reasonably low levels of morbidity and mortality. This attitude has been favorably affected by the increasing preference for lobectomy (rather than pneumonectomy) and lung-saving bronchoplastic procedures in the management of lung cancer.

It is clear from the report by Golebiowski[5] that careful selection of patients over the age of 70 years requiring pulmonary resection should be assessed for coexisting disease with the particular risks of postoperative gastrointestinal hemorrhage, cardiac arrhythmias, heart failure, and venous thrombosis with pulmonary embolism. It is clear that the decision to operate on the elderly may be a difficult judgment requiring a more extensive preoperative assessment, and ultimate selection will vary with differing rates at which individuals age and deteriorate.

Pulmonary functional reserve Resection must not result in a "pulmonary cripple" or fatal postoperative failure. Pulmonary function tests are increasingly precise and sophisticated, but there is little practical information reported that will help the surgeon with his decision about management in the patient with marginal respiratory reserves. A recent study by Legge and Palmer[6] analyzes the results of a variety of preoperative pulmonary function tests in relation to the incidence of postoperative respiratory failure in 225 patients with bronchial carcinoma undergoing thoracotomy. In this series, 13 developed postoperative respiratory failure, and 6 of the 13 died of this complication. The following function tests were significantly related to the incidence of respiratory failure: a higher incidence of airway obstruction with low forced expiratory volume in first 1 second (FEV_1)/forced vital capacity ratio less than 1.0, higher mean levels of $PaCO_2$, higher respiratory rate and lower tidal volumes, low arterial oxygenation, and low maximum oxygen consumption (MVO_2) less than 10 mL/kg/min.

Mediastinoscopy The influence of superior mediastinal lymph node involvement on prognosis in patients with bronchogenic carcinoma has already been discussed. Cervical mediastinoscopy provides reasonably precise information about the site and degree of superior mediastinal lymph node involvement. The experience with this procedure at the Toronto General Hospital began in 1961. The information obtained has been so useful that mediastinoscopy is adopted as a routine part of the preoperative assessment in patients with presumably operable lung cancer in 1963. The only exceptions to such routine application are in patients with early occult tumors or peripheral tumors less than 1.5 cm in diameter.

Technique for mediastinoscopy Mediastinoscopy is done under general anesthesia with endotracheal intubation and is combined with bronchoscopy. The useful application of cervical mediastinoscopy requires considerable experience and a clear understanding and familiarity with the lymphatic drainage of the lung. In general,

the procedure should be done by the surgeon who will subsequently do the resection.

Anterior subcarinal (station 7), tracheobronchial (station 10), and paratracheal nodes (station 4) are accessible for biopsy at mediastinoscopy. Some superior mediastinal nodes are inaccessible in this operation: anterior mediastinal nodes, which lie in front of the aortic arch and its major branches (station 5) and subaortic lymph nodes lying inferolateral to the subaortic window and low, posterior subcarinal nodes (station 7). Tumors in the left upper lobe or left hilum may spread through the anterior mediastinal lymphatic chain, and cervical mediastinoscopy is least useful in assessing lymphatic spread for tumors in this location. This is of particular importance because the left upper lobe is the largest of all pulmonary lobes, and approximately 35% of the primary tumors arise in this location. For these reasons, additional exploration may be indicated in patients with left hilar or left upper lobe tumors when the cervical mediastinoscopy is negative. With the cervical mediastinoscopy incision still open (previous biopsies having been assessed by frozen section), left anterior mediastinotomy is added to access the anterior mediastinal nodes, identified by palpation and biopsied using the mediastinoscope for access.

Complications of mediastinoscopy
1. Right pneumothorax
2. Left recurrent nerve palsy
3. Significant bleeding
4. Bronchomediastinal fistula
5. Postoperative death

Results Most patients with "positive" mediastinoscopy are considered inoperable. These include small cell carcinoma and non–small cell carcinoma with perinodal and extranodal extension of tumor with fixation to the surrounding mediastinal structures, high right paratracheal nodes and subcarinal nodes, and subinnominate and preaortic lymph nodes. There are reports in the literature that indicate a favorable prognosis in patients managed by resection of squamous cell carcinoma with ipsilateral superior mediastinal node involvement. It is frequently stated that mediastinal node involvement can be determined using the noninvasive technique of CT and PET.

Comparison of mediastinoscopy and computed tomography It is frequently stated that superior mediastinal lymph node involvement can be determined using the noninvasive technique of CT. The criterion for positive CT is a lymph node that is larger in size by more than 1.5 cm supported by finding of a hypermetabolic "hot" lymph node. These findings permit targeted lymph node biopsy at mediastinoscopy or by needle aspiration at ultrasound bronchoscopy or enlarged cervical lymph node at ultrasound.

Resectability

The hospital exists for the sake of the patients. The very word "*hospital*" (Latin, *hospitium*) means a place where guests are received. As a hospital is a house of hospitality, all patients within the walls of a hospital should therefore be treated as guests; this is a basic and changeless concept that has prevailed for centuries. In the Introduction by the late Hamilton Bailey on *Pye's Surgical Handicraft*, one of the first medical books published by John Wright & Sons Ltd, Mr Pye had put into the hands of the profession a work of exceptional merit.[7]

Selectivity is the basis of surgical treatment for bronchogenic carcinoma in order to avoid unwarranted, injudicious exploratory thoracotomy and resection, both of which carry significant operative risks without benefit to the patient's survival.[2] Distinction should be made between *operability* (patient factors) and *resectability* (tumor factors). *Preoperative clinical staging* reflects in prognosis, facilitates the choice of treatment, correlates well with survival after resection, and clarifies the results of selected treatment. *Postoperative pathologic staging* is precise after detailed analysis of the resected lung and lymph node specimens and is used to determine prognosis, likely cure rate, and the need for adjuvant therapy.

The *4 treatment options* are as follows: (a) Surgery with or without induction chemoradiotherapy in the operable patients with limited and potentially curable disease; (b) Definitive combined chemotherapy and radiotherapy in patients with locally advanced but treatable and controllable disease even if it is incurable; (c) Palliative radiotherapy or chemotherapy alone in patients with advanced incurable disease; and (d) Targeted immunotherapy on the basis of molecular markers.

Major advances have been made in resectability of lung cancer by complete pretreatment assessment of the patient and classification of the lesion according to the cell type and extent and stage of lymph node involvement, systemic staging, attention to details in the international pathologic classification of lung cancer into small cell or non–small cell types, mutation and molecular staging of lung cancer, accuracy in the histologic assessment by pulmonary pathologists, thorough preoperative and intraoperative lymphatic staging in the mediastinum by the surgeon, and safe conduct of the operation. By the means of advances made over time, a decision can be made with better than 90% accuracy regarding resectability with benefit

and to the extent of resection necessary. The use of all available means of preoperative assessment has increased surgical salvage and with moderate increase in 5 years.

Resectability in lung cancer surgery needs careful attention, taking into consideration the following: attention to details, surgical skills and knowledge, diagnosis, precision in surgical techniques, and precision in the operation.

Surgical treatment

There are clinical situations in which patients stand to benefit by resection when the preoperative cardiopulmonary assessment is favorable, and the tumor is localized and resectable with intent to cure with acceptable operative risk. However, there are situations with a concomitant reduction in the number of useless resections or unnecessary thoracotomies for inoperable tumors.

Non–small cell lung cancer with resectable extrathoracic metastases

There are limited situations in lung cancer in which resection of primary tumor and metastases is feasible. One of these is the presence of solitary brain metastasis with absence of lymphatic spread in the thorax and the primary tumor that is technically resectable. Another situation that arises is when solitary adrenal gland metastasis becomes evident after the primary tumor has been surgically controlled. Lung cancer that has resulted in metastases to the bone, liver, and lung are not amenable to surgical treatment.

Mediastinoscopy

Mediastinoscopy may occasionally be useful in determining resectability of the primary lesion for tumors in 2 locations. Superior sulcus tumors may be examined directly on either the right or the left side at the time of mediastinoscopy by deliberately breaching the mediastinal pleura and entering the pleural space lateral to the trachea. It is then possible to palpate or directly observe the gross extent of involvement of vertebral bodies by tumor. Second, bulky tumors in the right upper lobe may fix and distort the right lateral wall of the trachea and be considered inoperable on the basis of radiography and bronchography.

Preoperative angiography

Evaluation of the pulmonary arteries is obtainable by preoperative angiography. Pulmonary angiography may be in determining resectability and is useful for tumors in the right superior mediastinum, left hilum, and lobar arteries. It provides less precise information about pulmonary veins and heart. Such information may clearly obviate an unnecessary thoracotomy, or it may indicate the feasibility of lobectomy, lobectomy with sleeve resection of the bronchus, or even lobectomy with sleeve resection of both bronchus and pulmonary artery. Involvement of the superior vena cava with proximity to the large tumor mass in the right upper lobe may be evident on contrast-enhanced CT or on angiogram precluding operation and pulmonary resection.

Thoracic spine invasion

Superior sulcus cancer extending within the confines of the thoracic inlet may directly extend into vertebral bodies of the upper thoracic spine, precluding surgical intervention. Similarly, lung cancer arising in the paravertebral gutter may invade the chest wall and extend into the extrathoracic muscles, preventing tumor resection with intent to cure.

Factors to Consider in Operability and Resectability

Operability and resectability in bronchial carcinoma require attention to details before making surgical decision with respect to the following[1]:

1. *Patient-related factors*: patient characteristics, functional status and general heath, and operative risk factors for specific treatment.
2. *Tumor-related factors*: tumor characteristics, classification of the tumor according to the histologic type, and extent and stage of the disease at presentation.
3. *Surgery-related factors*: the type of surgical procedure, extended or limited pulmonary resection; standard lobectomy or sleeve lobectomy, standard pneumonectomy or sleeve pneumonectomy or carinal pneumonectomy; segmentectomy; en bloc chest wall resection with pulmonary resection; resection of superior sulcus tumor with or without subclavian vascular reconstruction, en bloc partial or total superior vena cava resection with pulmonary resection and reconstruction, whether the operation is elective or emergent; surgical skills and experience of the operating surgeon; and the skills of the anesthetist.[8]

From the above thoughtful considerations, patients are classified into the 4 following groups regarding management:

i. The patient may be considered to be *medically operable* and localized lung *cancer resectable* with intent to cure by an operation.
ii. The patient may be considered to be *medically inoperable*, but the lung cancer found to be localized and *potentially resectable* and yet the treatment recommended would have to be nonsurgical with intent to control and cure

with concurrent chemotherapy and radiotherapy.
iii. The patient may be considered to be *medically operable*, but lung cancer is found to be *locally advanced and unresectable*, but still treatable, and the recommended treatment would have to be with concurrent chemotherapy and radiotherapy with intent to control and cure.
iv. The patient may be deemed to be *medically inoperable* and lung *cancer unresectable* in which case only palliative treatment is feasible.

PREPARATION AND PLANNING OF OPERATION FOR LUNG CANCER

The objectives of these notes are to stress the principles underlying the management of lung cancer and other thoracic malignancies, and from these considerations to outline a routine scheme for management, which will be followed easily by all staff. It is hoped that by adherence to this routine, adequate and efficient management of all cases will be obtained, in the very important matter of preoperative preparation as well as in the postoperative management.

It is recognized that although the routine will be most suitable for most cases, there will in special circumstances be cases requiring different management. Such special instructions will be given only by the surgeon in charge and should not be embarked upon without his or her specific instructions. It is hoped that the routine outlined will be a sound basis for preoperative and postoperative care and as such will be of value to the surgical and nursing staff in the routine management of thoracic surgical cases. It will also be of help in teaching the young doctors who wish to embark on a surgical career.

The guiding principle that must be followed is outlined in **Table 1**. *Selectivity is the basis of surgical treatment* for bronchogenic carcinoma in order to avoid unwarranted, injudicious exploratory thoracotomy and resection, both of which carry significant operative risks, without benefit to the patient's survival.[2] Selection is based on complete pretreatment evaluation of the patient's functional status, general medical condition, perioperative cardiac risk, pulmonary function tests, and medical condition; when thoughtfully used, resection rates, adverse events, perioperative morbidity and mortality rates, survival figures, and total salvage should improve.

Attention to Details on Operability and Resectability Necessary in the Preoperative Care of the Patients

Surgical intuition becomes important when faced with having to make a surgical decision in the

Table 1
Clinical predictors of risk for lung surgery

Predictors	Clinical Determinants
A. Major risk factors	*Worrisome*
"Major"	Increasing age >80 y
	Reduced functional capacity by cardiopulmonary exercise testing (CPET): MVO_2 < 10 mL·kg·min[6]
	Low FEV_1 < 1.2 L
	Calculated postoperative (ppo) FEV_1 < 0.8 L
	Low diffusion capacity (diffusing capacity of the lungs for carbon monoxide [DLCO]) at rest <25 mL·min·mm Hg (<75%); as low as 5 mL·min·mm Hg in pulmonary fibrosis
	Modified Medical Research Council *dyspnea scale*: 0–4
	Grade 3: Breathlessness stops walking after ~100 m or a few minutes
	Grade 4: Breathless when dressing or not able to leave the house
	Type of elective operation
	Standard pneumonectomy
	Carinal pneumonectomy
	Tracheal carinal resection
	En bloc lung and chest wall resection
	En bloc superior vena cava resection with pulmonary resection
	Continuous supplemental O_2
	Unstable coronary artery syndrome
	Low ejection fraction <35 (normal from 55% to 80%)
	Decompensated congestive heart failure
	Severe valvular aortic stenosis usual definition criteria:
	■ Mean transvalvular gradient >40 mm Hg.
	■ Aortic valve area (AVA) <1 cm^2
	■ Peak aortic jet velocity >4.0 m/s
	Critical valvular aortic stenosis usual definition criteria:
	■ High fixed cardiac output
	■ Mean transvalvular gradient >80 mm Hg.
	■ AVA < 0.5 cm^2
	Assessment of aortic stenosis severity should integrate the flow-gradient pattern to the classic measurement of AVA:
	Normal flow/high gradient and AVA < 1 cm^2: benefit from aortic valve replacement (AVR)
	Low flow/high gradient and AVA <1 cm^2 benefit from AVR
	Pulmonary arterial hypertension: mean PAP > 24 mm Hg
	BMI > 30
	Low arterial blood gases PaO_2 < 70 mm Hg
	Low oxygen saturation <70%
B. Intermediate risk factors	*Cautious*

(continued on next page)

Table 1
(continued)

Predictors	Clinical Determinants
"Intermediate"	Chronic lung disease: Panacinar emphysema, interstitial pulmonary fibrosis, pulmonary sarcoidosis, asbestosis, silicosis, recurrent pneumonia, fibrosing alveolitis Diffuse bronchiectasis Age 70–79 y Active cigarette smoker $\geq$1 ppo for 20 y Reduced functional capacity by cardiopulmonary exercise test (CPET): $MVO_2 < 15$ mL·kg·min[6] FEV_1 1.2–1.5 L Ejection fraction <50 BMI 25–29.9 Significant cardiac arrhythmias: >5 PVCs documented before the operation, bundle branch block, uncontrolled atrial fibrillation
C. Minor risk factors	*Acceptable*
"Minor"	Modified Medical Research Council *dyspnea scale*: 0–4 *Grade 0:* No breathlessness *Grade 1:* Breathless when hurrying or walking up a hill Age 60–69 y Ex-smoker Normal functional capacity $MVO_2 > 20$ mL·kg·min[6] $FEV_1 > 1.5$ L for lobectomy $FEV_1 > 2.0$ L for pneumonectomy BMI 18.5–24.9 Ejection fraction >55% (55%–80%) and mean 67% Diffusion capacity (DLCO) at rest 25–30 mL·min·mm Hg (>90%) *Type of elective operation:* Standard lobectomy Sleeve lobectomy Segmental resection Wedge resection Normal pulmonary artery pressure: 25/8 mm Hg and mean pulmonary arterial pressure 15 mm Hg

Abbreviation: ppo, predicted postoperative pulmonary function; PVCs, premature ventricular contractions.

preoperative care.[8] The clinician must ask himself or herself the following questions before every operation, which must only be performed once each question has been answered satisfactorily:

A. HAS THE DIAGNOSIS BEEN FIRMLY ESTABLISHED?
   a. With modern techniques of imaging and tissue biopsy, this can be done in the vast majority of cases.
   b. Occasionally, an exploratory operation is necessary if the possibility of serious disease cannot be confidently ruled out, but this must be an exception.
B. IS AN OPERATION NECESSARY?
   1. *Operations have certain indications*, which must be present before an operation is justified.

   2. *Operation is potentially dangerous* and is only indicated if the risks of the disease are greater than the risks of the operation. For this, one must know the following:
      1. Natural history of the disease
      2. Risk of the operation
   3. *Would you have the operation* if you were in the patient's position?
   4. *If in doubt:*
      a. Seek a second opinion
      b. Reevaluate the case later
   5. It is not justifiable to perform an operation merely on the possibility that it may be necessary: there must be a reasonable probability, or preferably certainty that it is required.
C. IS THE PATIENT FIT FOR THE OPERATION AND ANESTHETIC? IF NOT, MAKE HIM FIT and examine and improve functions of the different body organ systems: heart, lung, kidneys, and liver before committing to an operation.

a. Heart: normalize cardiac function after appropriate cardiac investigations

b. Lungs: improve lung function after investigations to minimize risk for postoperative atelectasis, bronchitis, and pneumonia

c. Kidneys: restore renal function

d. Liver: investigate and prepare liver function if required

e. Bladder-neck obstruction: if significant, this must be treated before operation

f. Hemoglobin level: restore adequate hemoglobin level before operation if low

g. Serum proteins: estimate and rule out protein deficiency

h. Serum electrolytes: should be corrected before an operation

i. Control sepsis: clear up infection before operation

j. Colon preparation: must be done before operation on the colon to reduce risk

k. Previous cortisone therapy: cortisone replacement to sustain the patient during and after the operation

l. Reduce risk for postoperative deep vein thrombosis by prophylaxis anticoagulation

D. WHEN IS THE BEST TIME FOR OPERATION?

a. In general, if an operation is well indicated, it should be done without undue delay

b. Reasons for postponing an operation

1. To improve the patient's state of fitness: operate as soon as maximal improvement has taken place.

2. To allow inflammatory reaction to subside and so make operation easier: operate when maximal improvement has taken place.

3. The benefits of delay must be judged against the possible harm of progression of the disease: careful judgment and possible compromise required to balance out these 2 factors.

E. WHEN IS THE BEST TIME FOR OPERATION?

a. In general, if an operation is well indicated, it should be done without undue delay.

b. Reasons for postponing an operation

1. To improve the patient's state of fitness: operate as soon as maximal improvement has taken place.

2. To allow inflammatory reaction to subside and so make operation easier: operate when maximal improvement has taken place.

3. The benefits of delay must be judged against the possible harm of progression of the disease: careful judgment and possible compromise required to balance out these 2 factors.

F. WHO SHOULD PERFORM THE OPERATION?

1. Someone with the training to perform the operation competently.

2. In emergencies, this may have to be compromised.

NECESSARY POSTOPERATIVE CARE

A. MAINTAIN PATIENT DURING RECOVERY[8]:

1. Immediate postoperative period in the post-anesthesia care unit

a. Until recovered from respiratory and circulatory disturbances of the anesthetic and operation

b. Maintain open airway

c. Maintain circulation

2. Intermediate postoperative period in the ward

B. PREVENT COMPLICATIONS:

1. Abdominal distension

2. Pulmonary complications

3. Deep vein thrombosis

4. Fluid and electrolyte imbalance

5. Wound infection

6. Urinary retention

C. EARLY RECOGNITION AND PROMPT TREATMENT OF COMPLICATIONS:

1. Postoperative fever

2. Pulmonary atelectasis

3. Deep vein thrombosis

4. Fluid and electrolyte imbalance

5. Wound infection

6. Coronary thrombosis

7. Urinary retention

8. Sudden postoperative collapse may be due to the following:

a. Complications of the operation:

i. Hemorrhage

ii. Infection (septicemia)

iii. Fluid and electrolyte disturbances

iv. Massive tissue damage and metabolic disturbances

b. Major organ failure

i. Heart (coronary thrombosis)

ii. Lungs (atelectasis, pneumonia, or pulmonary thromboembolism)

iii. Adrenal gland insufficiency (hypoadrenal response)

iv. Kidneys (uremia)

v. Liver failure

vi. Brain (cerebrovascular accident)

OPERABILITY
Assessment

The assessment of operability requires consideration of the following factors:

1. Exclusion of detectable extrathoracic and distant metastases
2. Determination of the presence or absence of superior mediastinal lymph node involvement
3. Definition of the histologic or cell type, whenever possible
4. Evaluation of operative risk
5. Determination of the local extent of the tumor growth within the lung and direct invasion within the chest involving the bony chest wall, mediastinal structures, phrenic nerve on the pericardium and the brachial plexus in the thoracic inlet, and central extension through the intervertebral foramen and produce epidural compression of the spinal cord

Distant metastases

History and physical examination may alert the physician to the presence of hematogenous metastases, particularly to brain, bone, and skin. Liver metastases are common and, unfortunately, are frequently "silent." Metastatic liver involvement no longer requires laparoscopy or a small laparotomy for direct examination of the liver in equivocal cases now because PET is available for systemic staging at all distant sites except for the brain. PET is a noninvasive method for systemic staging of cancer, and it provides more reliable and accurate information about staging and planning of treatment for lung cancer. MRI of the head is most frequently required for completeness of staging of primary lung cancer for determining presence of intracranial metastases if the patient has suggestive neurologic symptoms and signs, if the cancer appears to be at an advanced unresectable stage in the lung, and in the high-surgical-risk patient in the absence of neurologic symptoms in order to plan for the most appropriate treatment.

Lymphatic spread

There is now accumulated evidence that superior mediastinal lymph node involvement by lung cancer influences prognosis profoundly and adversely in most cases.[9] The 5-year survival rate in patients with documented preoperative superior mediastinal lymph node metastases managed by resection has been reported to be as low as 6% (4% to 9%), and even worse at 4% following resection if tumor has invaded the capsule of the lymph node (perinodal spread). If this type of perinodal spread occurs in the superior mediastinum, the 5-year survival is less than 2%. When the preoperative staging cervical mediastinoscopy is normal and the presence of lymphatic metastases are discovered in the mediastinal lymph nodes during pulmonary resection, the 5-year cure rate is no higher than 25% to 30%.

Cell type and histologic grading

The histologic or cell type and the degree of differentiation, defined in 3 grades: well differentiated, poorly differentiated, and undifferentiated, profoundly affect the prognosis; with well-differentiated squamous cell tumors at the favorable end of the scale; adenocarcinoma in an intermediate position; and small cell carcinoma at the most unfavorable end of the scale. Small cell lung cancer is frequently described in 3 stages: very limited truly stage I disease (potentially surgical), limited intrathoracic disease within the ipsilateral hemithorax (nonsurgical), and extensive advanced disease (nonsurgical) associated with such an unfavorable prognosis and outcome, that it is not recommended for surgical resection if this cell type is identified. There is 1 exception to the rule in small cell lung cancer when surgery is considered for treatment when it is a true very limited stage I disease and complete staging is favorable, including normal brain MRI, normal mediastinal nodal staging, and normal systemic staging with PET scan.

The recommended treatment for localized primary non–small cell lung cancer is surgery; for small cell cancer, it is chemotherapy for extensive systemic disease and chemotherapy combined with radiotherapy for limited intrathoracic disease.

Operative risk

There has been a relatively greater increase in the incidence of lung cancer in patients in the fourth to eighth decades of life during recent years, and there is an increasing trend to resect bronchial carcinoma in the elderly patients in the sixth, seventh, and eighth decades. The increase in the incidence is due to change in the distribution of the 2 cell types with adenocarcinoma spectrum disorder with variable cure rate in this heterogeneous group of 4 descriptors becoming more common than the squamous cell cancer.

The factors that have been identified to be associated with increased surgical risk are advanced age older than 80 years, in those with compromised pulmonary function owing to diffuse emphysematous lung disease, interstitial pulmonary fibrosis, and pulmonary artery hypertension, and in those with marginal heart function from congestive heart failure owing to coronary artery disease, valvular heart disease, and cardiomyopathy.

Although limited pulmonary resections may be well tolerated in elderly patients even over the age of 80 years with low operative mortality, the risk will be increased if more extensive pulmonary resection is undertaken, including standard and sleeve pneumonectomy and pulmonary resection with en bloc chest wall resection.

With careful preoperative selection, patients in the seventh and even in the eighth decades may be operated on with reasonably low levels of morbidity and mortality. This attitude has been favorably affected by the increasing preference for limited resections with wedge, segment, standard lobectomy, and lung-saving sleeve lobectomy rather than performing high-risk pneumonectomy in the management of lung cancer; pneumonectomy in itself is considered to be a disease from loss of a significant amount of lung function.

It is clear that the decision to operate on the elderly patient may be a difficult judgment requiring a more extensive preoperative assessment and preparation, and ultimate selection will vary with the differing rates at which individuals age with reduction in physiologic function and deteriorate.

The postoperative complications are prolonged air leak, empyema, significant hemothorax, deep vein thrombosis and pulmonary embolism, cardiac arrhythmias, respiratory failure, pneumonia, bronchopleural fistula, and wound infection.

Pulmonary functional reserve

Pulmonary resection must *not* result in a "pulmonary cripple" or suffer fatal postoperative respiratory failure. The risk is the highest with pneumonectomy, which compromises half of the total lung capacity. The adequacy of lung function before operation should be established before subjecting the patient to lung resection. Pulmonary function tests have become increasingly precise and sophisticated now with the ability to determine more accurately the postoperative exercise capacity from cardiopulmonary exercise test measuring MVO_2 and the acceptable low risk is when it is greater than 20 mL/kg/min.[10] However, there is little practical information that will help the surgeon with the decision about management in the patient with compromised lung function and marginal respiratory reserve. The following pulmonary function test results are significantly related to high incidence of postoperative respiratory failure and morbidity and mortality: a higher incidence of airway obstruction, higher mean levels of arterial $PaCO_2$ greater than 45 mm Hg, higher resting respiratory rate and lower tidal volumes, and reduced calculated postoperative $FEV_1 < 1$ L, higher Vd/Vt ratio on exercise, and reduced $MVO_2 < 15$ mL/kg/min on exercise testing.

Mediastinal lymph node biopsy for staging lung cancer

This surgical procedure to advance surgical care of the patients with lung cancer was the brainchild of late *Dr Frederick Griffith Pearson* of the Toronto General Hospital in Canada. He recognized the value of this procedure, to be diligently learned by a thoracic surgeon, after his visit to the Karolinska Institute in Sweden in 1961 as a visiting postgraduate surgical fellow where he witnessed the procedure and assisted *Dr Eric Carlens*, who was performing *cervical mediastinoscopy*.[11]

Further advances in managing lung cancer came from Japan by *Dr T. Naruke*, who put forward a map of thoracic lymph nodes, deservedly called the internationally accepted Naruke Map, to guide standard nomenclature of the mediastinal lymph nodes to be sampled at cervical mediastinoscopy and to maintain consistency in biopsy of the named lymph nodes.[12]

Then came the most remarkable publication by *Dr H.C. Nohl Oser*[13] in 1972, Consultant Thoracic Surgeon to Harefield, Hillingdon, and West Middlesex Hospitals in London on "An investigation of the anatomy of the lymphatic drainage of the lungs as shown by the lymphatic spread of bronchial carcinoma."[13] This profoundly increased the understanding of the diverse lymph flow in the thoracic region from each lung and from each pulmonary lobe, resulting in advancing mediastinal lymph node staging for lung cancer. The staging-diagnostic value of left anterior mediastinotomy for lymphatic staging of cancer in the left upper lobe and left hilum became accepted.

Cervical mediastinoscopy became the gold standard in the staging of lung cancer on either side in the thorax. Later in time, after publication on the pattern of mediastinal lymphatic drainage by Dr H.C. Nohl Oser[13] in 1972, it was recognized, from this publication, that the different pathway of lymph flow from the left upper lobe and left hilum was different from the rest of the lungs, and this resulted in addition of *left anterior mediastinotomy* to cervical mediastinoscopy for staging left lung cancer in these 2 sites. Diagnostic anterior mediastinotomy was first reported by *Dr Thomas M McNeill and Dr J Maxwell Chamberlain* in 1966 and came to be known as the *Chamberlain Procedure*.[14]

In order to perform safe mediastinal staging by cervical mediastinoscopy and left anterior mediastinotomy requires considerable surgical experience and knowledge of the mediastinal anatomy, and a clear understanding and familiarity with the lymphatic drainage of the lung as described by *Nohl Oser*.[13] In general, the procedure should be done by the experienced senior surgeon who will subsequently perform the pulmonary resection.

Cervical mediastinoscopy and/or left anterior mediastinotomy The adverse influence of superior mediastinal lymph node metastases on prognosis in patients with bronchial carcinoma is now well recognized. Cervical mediastinoscopy is performed for cancer in the right and left lung, and to which is added, left anterior mediastinotomy when the cancer is in the left upper lobe or left hilum to provide reasonably precise information about the site and extent of superior mediastinal lymph node involvement.[9,15–18] The only exception to routine application of the procedure was when the lung tumor is small in size measuring less than 1.5 cm in diameter and peripherally placed in the lung and there is an absence of enlarged mediastinal lymph nodes (<1.5 cm in size) on CT scan of the chest. The accuracy of staging lung cancer was advanced further in recent times with the advent of the metabolic scan with PET, but it has not eliminated the need for surgical staging of lung cancer, which remains the gold standard for mediastinal nodal staging. PET has been shown to benefit, not only by directing mediastinal lymph node biopsy but also for intrathoracic assessment of the primary lung cancer and for extrathoracic staging at all sites except the brain, for which MRI is necessary.

The standard for precise identification and biopsy of the mediastinal and bronchopulmonary lymph nodes was first described by T. Naruke in Japan (*Naruke Mediastinal Lymph Node Map*)[12] and much later by the *International Association for Staging of Lung Cancer* (IASLC).[15,16] These are now uniformly accepted in the mediastinal lymph node staging, providing accurate information on the number and location of the normal and metastatic superior mediastinal lymph nodes. The fundamental difference is that the Naruke Map is preoperative for guiding mediastinal nodal staging whereas the IASLC Map is for surgical-pathologic staging of the primary tumor and the lymph nodes after pulmonary resection.

Cervical mediastinoscopy Cervical mediastinoscopy is performed under general anesthesia with endotracheal intubation for mediastinal lymph node staging for right and left lung cancers in all of the pulmonary lobes and is combined with bronchoscopy. Lymph flow from the right lung is ipsilateral to the right side in 96% and to the contralateral left side in 4%. Lymph flow from the left lung is not the same as from the right lung. It differs in that the lymph flow is to the contralateral side from the left lower lobe in 25% and from the left hilum and upper lobe in 12%. For left lung cancer, left anterior mediastinotomy is added to the cervical mediastinoscopy, with negative lymph node biopsies, when the cancer is in the left upper lobe or in the left hilum because of a different lymphatic drainage pathway through the anterior lymphatic chain in stations 5 and 6 lymph nodes. In this situation, lymphatic spread to the contralateral mediastinal lymph nodes must be determined first by cervical mediastinoscopy by sampling paratracheal lymph nodes. Contralateral lymphatic spread from the left lung occurs through subcarinal station 7 lymph node and pretracheal station 3 lymph nodes, particularly from the left lower lobe (25%) and left upper lobe (12%).[9,17–23]

Anterior subcarinal (station 7, N2), tracheobronchial lymph node (station 10, N1), paratracheal lymph nodes (ipsilateral N2 stations 4 and 2 and contralateral N3 stations 4 and 2), and pretracheal lymph node (station 3) are *accessible* for biopsy at cervical mediastinoscopy. The superior mediastinal lymph nodes, which are *not accessible* for biopsy at cervical mediastinoscopy include the anterior mediastinal nodes, which lie in front of the aortic arch and its major branches (station 6) and the subaortic lymph nodes lying inferolateral to the subaortic window (station 5). Access to these specific lymph nodes for sampling will require left anterior mediastinotomy. The low, posterior subcarinal nodes (station 7) are *not accessible* by either of the procedures and will require video-assisted thoracoscopic surgical technique for sampling.

Left anterior mediastinotomy Left anterior mediastinotomy is performed for mediastinal lymphatic staging for bronchial cancer in the left upper lobe or left hilum after cervical mediastinoscopy and frozen section analysis of the mediastinal lymph nodes has ruled out ipsilateral and contralateral lymphatic spread of cancer. Diagnostic anterior mediastinotomy was introduced in 1966 by *Thomas McNeill and J. Maxwell Chamberlain.*[14] The lymphatic drainage from these 2 sites in the left lung takes a different route through the anterior mediastinal lymphatic vessels; first into the subaortic (station 5) lymph node in the aortopulmonary window and from station 5 lymph nodes into the lymph nodes located along the inferior phrenic nerve (station 6) in front of the transverse aortic arch. Cervical mediastinoscopy does not permit access to these 2 lymph node stations and is least useful in assessing lymphatic spread for cancer in these locations. There is an increased tendency for cancer in these locations to spread to the contralateral mediastinal lymph nodes through a different lymphatic route passing through the subcarinal station 7 and pretracheal station 3 lymph nodes; cervical mediastinoscopy should always be performed first with frozen-section analysis of the contralateral sampled lymph nodes (stations 7, 10R, 4R, 3, 2R) and ipsilateral lymph nodes (10L, 4L). It is important to remember that 10R and 10L once were considered mediastinal N2 stations, and now these nodes are considered N1 stations. If there is no evidence of cancer spread at cervical mediastinoscopy, then left anterior mediastinotomy[16] should be added for sampling anterior mediastinal lymph nodes in stations 5 and 6.

For these reasons, additional mediastinal exploration is indicated in patients when the lung cancer is in the left hilum or left upper lobe. There is a higher incidence of contralateral lymphatic spread of primary lung cancer from these 2 sites in the left lung. In this case, left anterior mediastinotomy should be combined with cervical mediastinoscopy. With the cervical mediastinoscopy incision still open, and the sampled mediastinal lymph node biopsies proven to be negative for metastases by frozen section, this rules out N3 lymphatic spread.

Cervical mediastinoscopy became the gold standard in the staging of lung cancer on either side. Later in time, after publication on the pattern of mediastinal lymphatic drainage by Dr Nohl Oser in 1972, it was recognized that the pathway of lymph flow from the left upper lobe and left hilum was different from the rest of the lungs, and this resulted in adding left anterior mediastinotomy concomitantly to cervical mediastinoscopy for staging left lung cancer in these 2 sites.

Mediastinoscopy by cervical approach and left anterior mediastinotomy were reported in the International Association for the Study of Lung Cancer (IASLC)[9,10] and Clinical predictors of risk for Lung Cancer Surgery.[5,18,20]

SUMMARY

Lung cancer is a lethal disease, and chronic cigarette smoking is the most common cause. The selection of treatment is based on the histologic cell type, accurate staging, and adequacy of cardiopulmonary functional reserve. The risk for surgery is highest in patients over the age of 80 years.

The *TNM Cancer Staging System* was introduced in France by *Pierre Denoix* in 1940.[24] It describes the *extent of cancer anatomically* and it is globally accepted as

- TUMOR: local
- NODE: regional
- METASTASES: distant

Cancer staging is important in the patient care because

- It determines *Treatment*
- It determines *Prognosis*
- It is an important component of *Cancer Research* and *Advances in Treatment*

CLINICAL CARE POINTS

- Factors to consider in assessment of operability: exclusion of detectable extrathoracic and distant metastases; determination of the presence of superior mediastinal lymph node metastases; definition of the histologic cell type, evaluation of operative risk.
- Pulmonary functional reserve.
- Complications of mediastinoscopy.
- Factors to consider in resectability: non-small cell lung cancer, mediastinoscopy, preoperative angiography, thoracic spine invasion, mediastinoscopy, preoperative angiography, patient-related factors, tumor-related factors, surgery-related factors.
- Attention to details in the preoperative patient care.
- Clinical predictors of risk for lung surgery.

REFERENCES

1. Assessment of Resectability and Operability in Bronchial Carcinoma. Cancer of the Lung. 8th Annual Symposium on Malignant Disease, Chapel Hill, North Carolina 1974; 67–83; FG Pearson.
2. Paulson DL, Urschel HC Jr. Selectivity in the surgical treatment of bronchogenic carcinoma. J Thorac Cardiovasc Surg 1971;62(4):554–62.
3. Gould G, Pearce. Assessment of suitability for lung resection. Contin Educ Anaesth Crit Care Pain 2006;6(3):97–100.
4. Bergh NP, Rydberg B, Schersten T. Mediastinal exploration by the technique of carlens. Dis Chest 1964;46:399–410.
5. Golebiowski A. Pulmonary resection in patients over 70 years of age. J Thorac Cardiovasc Surg 1971 Feb;61(2):265–70.
6. Legge JS, Palmer KNV. Pulmonary function in bronchogenic carcinoma. Thorax 1973;28(5):588–91.
7. Kyle J. Pye's surgical Handicraft. Bristol (England): John Wright & Sons Ltd; 1969.
8. Du Plessis DJ. Principles of surgery. Bristol (England): Publisher John Wright & Sons; 1976. p. 92–9. Part I Chapters XXII AND XXIII.
9. Pearson FG, Nelems JM, Henderson RD, et al. The role of mediastinoscopy in the selection of treatment for bronchial carcinoma with involvement of superior mediastinal lymph nodes. J Thorac Cardiovasc Surg 1972;64:382–90.
10. Nha V. Physiology and clinical applications of cardiopulmonary exercise testing in lung surgery. Thorac Surg Clin 2013;23:233–45.

11. Carlens E. Mediastinoscopy: a method for inspection and tissue biopsy in the superior mediastinum. Dis Chest 1959;4:343–52.

12. Naruke T, Suemasu, Ishikawa S. Lymph node mapping and curability at various levels of metastasis in resected lung cancer. J Thorac Cardiovasc Surg 1978;76:832–9.

13. Nohl-Oser HC. An investigation of the lymphatic drainage of the lungs. Ann Roy Coll Surg Engl 1972;51:157–76.

14. McNeill TM, Maxwell Chamberlain J. Diagnostic anterior mediastinotomy. Ann Thorac Surg 1966; 2(4):532–9.

15. International Association for the Study of Lung Cancer. Staging Handbook in Thoracic Oncology 2016 edited by Dr. Ramon Rami-Porta.

16. Goldstraw P, Chansky K, Crowley J, et al. The IASLC Lung Cancer Staging project. J Thorac Oncol 2015; 11:39–51.

17. Pearson FG. An evaluation of mediastinoscopy in the management of presumably operable bronchial carcinoma. J Thorac Cardiovasc Surg 1968;55:617–25.

18. Pearson FG, Delarue NC, Ilves R, et al. Significance of positive superior mediastinal nodes identified at mediastinoscopy in patients with resectable cancer of the lung. J Thorac Cardiovasc Surg 1982;83:1–11.

19. Ginsberg RJ, Hill LD, Eagen RT. Modern thirty-day operative mortality for surgical resections in lung cancer. J Thorac Cardiovasc Surg 1983;86:654–6.

20. Patterson GA, Piazza D, Pearson FG, et al. Significance of metastatic disease in the subaortic lymph nodes. Ann Thorac Surg 1987;43:155.

21. Goldman L, Caldera DL, Nussbaum SR, et al. Multifactorial index of cardiac risk in noncardiac surgical procedures. N Engl J Med 1977;297:845–50.

22. Wynands JE. Anesthesia for cardiac patients having non-cardiac operations. Can Anaesth Soc J 1982; 29(4):341–8.

23. Armstrong P, Congleton J, Fountain SW, et al. Guidelines on the selection of patients with lung cancer for surgery. Thorax 2001;56:89–108.

24. Denoix PF. Nomenclature des cancers. Bull Inst Nat Hyg 1944;1:52–82.

Complications of Chest Wall Resection in Conjunction with Pulmonary Resection

Rahul Nayak, MD, FRCSC[a], Se-In Choe, MD, FRCSC[b],
Yaron Shargall, MD, FRCSC[c],*

KEYWORDS

- Chest wall resection • Chest wall reconstruction • Lung resection
- Complications of chest wall resection

KEY POINTS

- Chest wall reconstruction is typically required for anterolateral defects and some larger posterior defects
- Risk factors for developing complications after chest wall resection are related to the size of the defect and the addition of a pulmonary resection, as well as patient-specific factors
- The material used for reconstruction does not significantly impact the complication rate
- Performing a rigid reconstruction in patients who will be left with large flail segments after resection may benefit from decreased pulmonary complications

OVERVIEW OF CHEST WALL RESECTION

Components of the Chest Wall

The chest wall is a cylindrical cage that serves to protect the heart, lungs, and great vessels of the thorax; it also helps protect the diaphragm, liver, and spleen. The chest wall assists with respiratory dynamics and can help augment the work of the diaphragm. In addition, it helps with movement of the upper limbs and shoulder. The chest wall is composed of both bone and soft tissue components. The bony component consists of ribs 1 to 7, which form a complete circumference with attachments to the corresponding thoracic vertebra posteriorly and the sternum anteriorly. Ribs 8 to 10 have posterior thoracic attachments but fuse with the cartilaginous components of ribs 7 anteriorly and are labeled "false ribs." Ribs 11 to 12 have no anterior attachments and are thus labeled "floating ribs." Although they are not considered part of the chest wall, the scapula and clavicle are bony structures that can come into play when planning chest wall resections and reconstructions. These bony structures can be thought of as a collar and cape attached to the upper portion of the chest wall. These bones also serve as attachments for several of the chest wall muscles.

The external, internal, and innermost intercostal muscles connect the individual ribs to one another and allow for coordinated movement of the chest wall. The muscles overlying the bony rib cage are the serratus anterior and posterior, latissimus dorsi, pectoralis major and minor, trapezius, sacrospinalis, and rhomboids. These muscles assist with movement of the upper limbs and shoulders; they can also be harvested as vascularized pedicled flaps for coverage of large chest wall defects.

[a] Division of Thoracic Surgery, Thoracic Surgery Research & Quality Improvement LHSC Schulich School of Medicine and Dentistry – Western University, Lawson Health Research Institute, 800 Commissioners Road East, Suite E2-124, London, Ontario N6A 5W9, Canada; [b] Division of Thoracic Surgery, McMaster University, and Service of Thoracic Surgery, St. Joseph's Healthcare Hamilton, 50 Charlton Avenue East, T-2105, Hamilton, Ontario L8N 4A6, Canada; [c] Surgery and Medicine, Division of Thoracic Surgery, McMaster University, McMaster University and Service of Thoracic Surgery, St. Joseph's Healthcare Hamilton, 50 Charlton Avenue East, T-2105, Hamilton, Ontario L8N 4A6, Canada
* Corresponding author.
E-mail address: shargal@mcmaster.ca

Thorac Surg Clin 31 (2021) 393–398
https://doi.org/10.1016/j.thorsurg.2021.07.010
1547-4127/21/© 2021 Elsevier Inc. All rights reserved.

Indications for chest wall resection in malignancies

Chest wall resections are indicated in locally advanced non–small cell lung cancer (NSCLC) and primary malignancies of the chest wall.[1] In rare instances, isolated oligometastatic disease of the chest wall may also be treated with resection.[2] However, NSCLC is the most common reason for resection of the chest wall in conjunction with a pulmonary resection. The eighth edition of the American Joint Committee on Cancer defines NSCLC involving the chest wall as a T3 lesion.[3,4]

Determining the need for reconstruction

Following chest wall resection, the need for reconstruction is predicated on the need to support respiratory dynamics and also to prevent herniation of and/or damage to underlying structures and to prevent entrapment of the overlying structures (eg, tip of the scapula). In general, resection of 3 or more ribs or greater than 5 cm of anterolateral chest wall, defects greater than 10 cm on the posterior chest wall, and defects at risk of scapular tip impingement all require reconstruction.[5]

Materials for reconstruction

The ideal material for chest wall reconstruction would have similar rigidity and plasticity as the native chest wall. The material should be easily incorporated into tissue, thereby making it more resistant to infection, and it should also be easy to work with and moldable to fit any defect or contour required.[6] Whenever a material shows superior properties in one domain, it typically compromises on another aspect. The following are the common materials used for chest wall reconstruction along with their advantages and disadvantages.

Nonabsorbable mesh Polytetrafluoroethylene (PTFE) and polypropylene (PP) meshes are the most common materials available for reconstruction. These meshes are mostly used in the repair of abdominal wall hernias. PTFE and PP meshes are highly malleable and come in a variety of sizes. Multiple meshes can be sewn together to cover larger defects. These meshes can be easily cut to fit any configuration of a defect. However, owing to their pliable nature, they do not provide rigid fixation in the early postoperative period; this is particularly true if the mesh fixation is not tight. As such, patients who undergo reconstruction with a nonabsorbable mesh alone will experience flail physiology and be at increased risk of pulmonary complications until tissue incorporation and a more rigid fibrous shell develops. In animal models for hiatal hernia repair, PP has been shown to have better performance characteristics than PTFE.[7] PP has an increased rate of tissue incorporation and is less prone to shrinkage over time.

Methyl methacrylate Methyl methacrylate is an organic polymer that is primarily used to produce acrylic plastics. In medicine, its most common use is to act as bone cement for the fixation of joint replacement. To provide more rigidity to a mesh reconstruction, methyl methacrylate can be sandwiched between 2 mesh sheets; it is applied in liquid form and allowed to harden as it cools. During the cooling phase, the operator can mold the cast to fit the defect at hand. However, the addition of methyl methacrylate reduces tissue incorporation, and as a consequence, infectious complications can be seen in up to 20% of patients. In other instances, the chest wall reconstruction can become too rigid and can become prone to fracturing.

Metallic prosthesis There are multiple rib fixation systems available on the market. These systems use titanium-based components that anchor to each end of a rib. These rib fixation systems can be molded to some degree to create a natural contour seen with a native chest wall. They are prone to fracturing and displacement, particularly in osteoporotic bone and are also at risk for acquired hardware infections.

Autologous tissue The main advantage of autologous tissue for reconstruction is avoidance of alloplastic implantable materials.[8] The disadvantages, however, include donor site morbidity and limited quantity of tissue available to cover larger defects.[8] For defects that do not require stabilization, pedicled muscle, myocutaneous, fasciocutaneous, perforator, and omental flaps are common options of reconstruction.[8] Free-tissue transfer, however, may be needed in areas that are difficult to reach with pedicled flaps or when local flaps are compromised and when a regional flap is insufficient to cover the total defect.[8]

Risk factors for complications with chest wall resection

Complications after a chest wall resection are not uncommon and have been reported to occur in 37% to 46% of patients.[9] Furthermore, mortality rates after chest wall resection can range from 3% to 7% based on the largest published series.[9–13] There have been multiple attempts to determine risk factors for developing complications. A study from Memorial Sloan Kettering examining outcomes after chest wall resection demonstrated that 33% of the 262 patients with chest wall resections experienced a complication.[9] In this series, 34% of patients had a concomitant lung resection. After performing multivariate analysis, patient age, concomitant lobectomy or pneumonectomy, and size of the chest wall defect were found to have increased odds ratios for a complication. A larger series from the MD Anderson Cancer Center examining 1096 patients who underwent chest wall resection also found concomitant lobectomy and number of ribs resected to be associated with an increased risk of complications on multivariate analysis.[14] In both these series, pulmonary and wound-related issues made up the largest proportion of complications. These complications are discussed further in the following sections.

COMMON COMPLICATIONS AFTER CHEST WALL RESECTION
Pulmonary Complications

Pulmonary complications encompass the greatest proportion of postoperative complications after lung and chest wall resection. The rate of postoperative pulmonary complications can be as high as 24%.[11] The reasons for this are multifactorial. However, there are specific mechanisms of postoperative pulmonary failure as a direct result of a chest wall resection. The disruption of the normal anatomic chest cage results in a flail type physiology. The loss of rigidity after bony resection causes paradoxic movement in the region of the chest wall resection during inspiration; this is mostly pronounced with anterolateral and more inferior resections. Subsequently, the flail type physiology results in the patient having impaired cough, poor pulmonary toilet, and thereby increased risk of atelectasis, pneumonia, and respiratory failure. In the series from Memorial Sloan Kettering, 70% of the mortalities were attributed to a pulmonary complication.[9] In this study, the investigators comment on a lower overall pulmonary complication rate of 11% when compared with the literature and attribute it to the routine use of rigid reconstruction with a methyl methacrylate mesh sandwich. There are no randomized trials comparing types of reconstruction; however, a single-center retrospective study comparing methyl methacrylate to PTFE mesh alone does support this postulate.[15] In this study, patients who underwent rigid reconstruction experienced a lower mortality rate (0% vs 4.5%), lower complication rate (5.2% vs 24%), and decreased length of hospital stay (10 days vs 13.3 days). As such, consideration should be given for rigid reconstruction if a large flail segment after resection is anticipated. However, the materials used for rigid reconstruction are prone to other complications (see later discussion).

In a retrospective cohort study, on multivariate analysis, the investigators found a relationship between the number of ribs resected and the incidence of postoperative respiratory complications in patients undergoing lobectomy with en bloc chest wall resection for NSCLC.[16]

Prosthesis-Related Complications

Infectious complications after chest wall resection and reconstruction pose a particularly difficult challenge. Wound complications after chest wall resection and reconstruction can be seen in up to 20% of patients. The use of omentum for reconstruction and the presence of an ulceration on the chest wall have been demonstrated to be risk factors for wound complications specifically after chest wall resection. The size of the defect to be reconstructed also seems to increase the rate of infectious wound complications. In a study comparing reconstruction of small defects (<60 cm^2) and large defects (>60 cm^2), infectious complications were seen in 0% and 7% of patients, respectively. The use of prosthetic material, such as polytetrafluoroethylene (Gore-Tex and Gore-Dualmesh, W.L. Gore& Associates, Inc, Flagstaff. AZ), when compared with a myocutaneous flap for reconstruction did not seem to have an impact.[17]

In the setting of chest wall resection in NSCLC, the overlying soft tissue is rarely involved to the point of requiring pedicled myocutaneous flaps. In most instances, a local advancement or rotational flap will suffice to cover the prosthetic reconstruction. As such, a discussion involving pedicled flap-related complications is beyond the scope of this article.

RARE COMPLICATIONS AFTER CHEST WALL RESECTION
Subarachnoid-Pleural Fistula

Subarachnoid-pleural fistula (SPF) is an abnormal fistulous connection that develops between subarachnoid and pleural spaces, from a traumatic injury or as a complication of chest operations, such as lung or chest wall resection, closure of patent ductus arteriosus, transthoracic discectomy, vertebral tumor removal, or spinal fusion.[18,19] Most often, this complication arises when techniques like extrapleural dissection, excessive rib retraction, or costotransverse joint disarticulation are required as tumor extends to the costovertebral angle.[18] Incidence is reported as less than 1% in patients undergoing en bloc resection of lung with chest wall invasion into costovertebral angle.[18] In addition, the use of preoperative and intraoperative radiotherapy can predispose patients to fistula formation due to poor wound healing. Patients can experience accumulation of pleural fluid, decreased volume of cerebrospinal fluid (CSF), presence of intracranial air, or development of meningitis.[18] More specifically, neurologic symptoms include headache, altered mental status, and deteriorating level of consciousness. Life-threatening complications can occur if SPF is not recognized and treated, such as tension pneumocephalus, cerebellar infarction and bleeding, meningitis, and large pleural effusion.[18]

Therefore, prompt recognition of SPF is necessary for operative repair. Computed tomography (CT) myelography or radionuclide cisternography are diagnostic methods used to confirm SPF.[20] Chest tube drainage of pleural effusion via watertight seal can provide both diagnostic and therapeutic advantage for symptomatic patients. Definitive operative repair involves dural defect closure with fine nonabsorbable suture and tissue patch buttressing.

Spinal Cord Ischemic Injury

Intraoperative spinal cord ischemic injury can be caused by several mechanisms, such as perioperative hypotension, acute thromboembolic events, need for aortic cross-clamping during the surgery, increased CSF pressure, and compression or disruption of intercostal arterial supply.[21] Although spinal hypoperfusion during aortic repairs is the most cited cause of spinal cord ischemic injury in the literature, other thoracic procedures involving dissection of the posterior mediastinum have also been documented to contribute to ischemic injury.

Manifestations of spinal cord ischemia are variable; they can present as transient ischemic attacks, autonomic dysfunction, or even motor or sensory deficits.[21] Moreover, the mechanism of ischemic injury is also highly variable: prolonged hypoxia during rib retraction during thoracotomy, posterior sectioning of intercostal vessels for chest wall resection, direct reduction of perfusion during aortic cross-clamping, injury to artery of Adamkiewicz or other tributaries during resection of tumor, or dissection and routine ligation of intercostal vessels.[21]

Prompt evaluation of a postoperative patient with neurologic deficit with emergent CT or (preferably) MRI and neurosurgical consult is necessary. The role of preoperative identification and preservation of the artery of Adamkiewicz as well as recognition of watershed areas in the spinal cord circulation may be beneficial but needs further investigation in that context.[21]

COMPLICATIONS OF CHEST WALL RESECTIONS SPECIFIC TO SUPERIOR SULCUS TUMORS

Superior sulcus tumors are rare and only represent 3% to 5% of all lung carcinomas. Apicoposterior chest wall resections for superior sulcus or Pancoast tumors present with their own unique set of complications. The resection of these tumors does not create the same degree of flail physiology as seen with anterolateral defects. Moreover, the resection of these tumors is quite complex and

often requires multidisciplinary interventions including neoadjuvant chemoradiation followed by neurosurgical and thoracic instrumentation and resection. Complications with the treatment of these tumors pertain more to the resection than the reconstruction performed.

Osteomyelitis

For Pancoast tumors affecting the spine, multilevel unilateral laminectomy, nerve root division inside spinal canal, and vertebral body division can be done using a posterior midline incision. Tumor is removed en bloc with lung, ribs, and vessels, and spine fixation is then mandatory.[22,23]

In general, spinal instrumentation is associated with a 2% to 20% infection rate.[24] Spinal instrumentation infection is associated with long hospitalizations, poor long-term patient outcomes, morbidity, and increased health care costs.[24] At present, there are no universally accepted protocols for treating deep wound infections from spinal instrumentation.

Several risk factors exist for surgical site infections after adult spine surgery: type of spinal surgery, age, male sex, use of steroid therapy, diabetes, smoking, American Society of Anesthesiology score (ASA), obesity, malnutrition, previous surgery, and comorbidities.[24] Risk of intraoperative/postoperative infection rate is increased using posterior surgical approach, applying instrumentation, using allograft, requiring blood transfusion, and conducting longer operations.[24]

Posterior spinal instrumentation is associated with high risk of infection, due to dissection and retraction of the posterior musculature that devascularizes paraspinal muscles, increases potential for blood loss, and results in larger dead spaces.

There are 2 types of postoperative spinal infections: early and delayed.[24] Early infection is defined as infection that occurs within a month from surgery. Signs and symptoms include pain, fever, erythema, swelling, warmth, tenderness, and wound drainage. Associated microorganisms are usually virulent pathogens: *Staphylococcus aureus*, beta-hemolytic streptococci, and aerobic gram-negative bacilli. In addition, methicillin-sensitive *S aureus* infection is common, but methicillin-resistant *S aureus* incidence is increasing. Polymicrobial infections may involve 10% to 50% of cases. Delayed infections occur 3 to 9 months postoperatively. Signs and symptoms include chronic pain, implant failure, or lack of adequate spinal fusion. Cultures are often negative because delayed infections are frequently caused by less virulent pathogens (*Propionibacterium acnes*, coagulase-negative *Staphylococcus epidermidis*, and *Bacillus* and *Micrococcus* species).

Biofilm is an important defense mechanism that is produced by certain bacteria to grow on the surface of implants, providing protection against antibiotics and immune defenses, including phagocytes and cellular or humoral responses.[24] Common organisms are *S aureus*, coagulase-negative *Staphylococcus*, and *Propionibacterium*. Several studies have demonstrated that certain materials are more prone to biofilm production. In addition, titanium has been shown to have lower infection rates than other materials like stainless steel.[25,26] Polyethyletherketone, a polymer widely used for spinal surgery, has a relatively high tendency for biofilm formation and therefore increased risk of infection.[24]

Management of infection after spinal instrumentation remains controversial. Two important factors that need to be considered are the total duration of antibiotic therapy and the need for instrumentation removal. Removal of underlying spinal instrumentation is recommended in the presence of biofilm. Delayed wound infections require removal or replacement of instrumentation when compared with surgical debridement/irrigation and antibiotic therapy for acute infections.

Cerebrospinal Fluid Leak

Leakage of CSF after a superior sulcus tumor resection is a relatively rare event. Care must be taken during the resection to ensure that an inadvertent dural puncture does not occur. Small punctures that are identified intraoperatively can be repaired primarily. In the postoperative period, they manifest as ongoing pleural drainage, postural headache, or with symptoms of meningeal irritation, such as neck stiffness and high fevers. In most instances, this complication can be managed conservatively with bed rest, elevation of the head of the bed, and diligent avoidance of hypertension to reduce CSF pressures. Similarly, coughing, sneezing, and any Valsalva maneuvers are preferably avoided, to prevent spikes in CSF pressures. This management is attempted for 7 to 10 days before declaring failure of conservative management. Most CSF leaks will subside with a conservative approach. Management of a CSF leak that fails conservative management involves CSF diversion via the use of lumbar drains with surgery reserved as a last resort.

One of the main concerns with the presence of a CSF leak is the development of pneumocephalus and meningitis. The risk of this occurring is increased substantially in the presence of a concomitant pneumothorax. By extrapolating from the trauma literature regarding the management of CSF leaks, there does not seem to be any benefit to administering prophylactic antibiotics to reduce the risk of developing meningitis.[27]

Intradural Hematoma

Intradural spinal hematomas refer to subdural, subarachnoid, or mixed hematoma. These entities are rare. Common causes include issues with coagulopathy (use of aspirin, thrombocytopenia, coagulopathy, or complication of anticoagulation use), iatrogenic injury, trauma, or tumors.[28] The pathophysiology of subdural hematoma in the thoracic spine is unclear. Spinal subdural hematomas should be included in the differential diagnosis in patients presenting with paraplegia following spinal surgery. Similarly, patients undergoing chest wall resection with disarticulation of the ribs off the spine, and those who will have spine resection as part of their surgery, might develop intradural hematoma as a result of a bleeding vessel retracting into the spinal canal. Prompt recognition and treatment, including decompression and evacuation, are needed for favorable patient outcome.

The cause of spinal hematoma is still unknown. There is a hypothesis that multilevel spinal procedures increase the risk of rupture of the internal vertebral venous plexus of Batson, which can increase the risk of development of a spinal compressive hematoma.[29] There are also several case reports on spontaneous spinal epidural hematoma associated with use of anticoagulant therapy.

CLINICS CARE POINTS

- Choice of material for reconstruction does not significantly impact the complication rate.
- Common complications after chest wall resection include infectious/prosthetic and pulmonary complications.
- Complications like subarachnoid-pleural fistula and spinal cord ischemic injury can occur rarely but are important to recognize and evaluate promptly.

SUMMARY

Our techniques and ability to perform chest wall resections and reconstructions have improved over the years. Chest wall resection in conjunction with pulmonary resections presents with many challenges. There are significant complications, such as pulmonary and prosthetic/infectious, that present a substantial risk of morbidity to the patients.[30] Risk factors for complications are related to the size of the defect, number of ribs resected, and the addition of a pulmonary resection. Rigid reconstruction for large flail segments postresection may provide decreased pulmonary complication rates. There are numerous materials that are used for reconstruction, but there is no clear superior material. More future studies are warranted for comparative analysis of different materials and methods of reconstruction.

REFERENCES

1. Scarnecchia E, Liparulo V, Capozzi R, et al. Chest wall resection and reconstruction for tutors: analysis of oncological and functional outcome. J Thorac Dis 2018;10(Suppl 16):S1855–63.

2. Plönes T, Osei-Agyemang T, Krohn A, et al. Surgical treatment of extrapulmonary oligometastatic non-small cell lung cancer. Indian J Surg 2015; 77(Suppl 2):216–20.

3. Detterbeck FC. The eighth edition TNM stage classification for lung cancer: what does it mean on main street? J Thorac Cardiovasc Surg 2018;155:356–9.

4. Lim W, Ridge CA, Nicholson AG, et al. The 8th lung cancer TNM classification and clinical staging system: review of the changes and clinical implications. Quant Imaging Med Surg 2018;8(7):709–18.

5. Sanna S, Brandolini J, Pardolesi A, et al. Materials and techniques in chest wall reconstruction: a review. J Vis Surg 2017;3:95.

6. Le Roux BT, Shama DM. Resection of tumors of the chest wall. Curr Probl Surg 1983;20(6):345–86.

7. Müller-Stich BP, Senft JD, Lasitschka F, et al. Polypropylene, polyester or polytetrafluorothylene- is there an ideal material for mesh augmentation at the esophageal hiatus? Results from an experimental study in a porcine model. Hernia 2014;18(6):873–81.

8. Mahabir RC, Butler CE. Stabilization of the chest wall: autologous and alloplastic reconstructions. Semin Plast Surg 2011;25(1):34–42.

9. Weyant MJ, Bains MS, Venkatraman E, et al. Results of chest wall resection and reconstruction with and without rigid prosthesis. Ann Thorac Surg 2006; 81(1):279–85.

10. Mansour KA, Thourani VH, Losken A, et al. Chest wall resections and reconstruction: a 25-year experience. Ann Thorac Surg 2002;73:1720–6.

11. Deschamps C, Tinrnaksiz BM, Darbandi R, et al. Early and long-term results of prosthetic chest wall reconstruction. J Thorac Cardiovasc Surg 1999;117:588–92.

12. Pairolero PC, Arnold PG. Chest wall tumors: experience with 100 consecutive patients. J Thorac Cardiovasc Surg 1985;90(3):367–72.

13. McKenna RJ Jr, Mountain CF, McMurtrey MJ, et al. Current techniques for chest wall reconstruction: expanded possibilities for treatment. Ann Thorac Surg 1988;46:508–12.

14. Spicer JD, Shewale JB, Antonoff MB, et al. The influence of reconstructive technique on perioperative pulmonary and infectious outcomes following chest wall resection. Ann Thorac Surg 2016;102(5):1653–9.

15. Kilic D, Gungor A, Kavukcu S, et al. Comparison of mersilene mesh-methyl metacrylate sandwich and polytetrafluoroethylene grafts for chest wall reconstruction. J Invest Surg 2006;19(6):353–60.

16. Geissen NM, Medairos R, Davila E, et al. Number of ribs resected is associated with respiratory complications following lobectomy with en bloc chest wall resection. Lung 2016;194:619–24.

17. Hanna WC, Ferri LE, McKendy KM, et al. Reconstruction after major chest wall resection: can rigid fixation be avoided? Surgery 2011;150(4):590–7.

18. Shamji MF, Sundaresan S, Da Silva V, et al. Subarachnoid-pleural fistula: applied anatomy of the thoracic spinal nerve root. ISRN Surg 2011;2011:168959.

19. Hentschel SJ, Rhines LD, Wong FC, et al. Subarachnoid-pleural fistula after resection of thoracic tumors. J Neurosurg 2004;100:332–6.

20. Ozgen S, Boran BO, Elmaci I, et al. Treatment of the subarachnoid-pleural fistula. Neurosurg Focus 2000;9(1):1–4.

21. Shamji MF, Maziak DE, Shamji FM, et al. Circulation of the spinal cord: an important consideration for thoracic surgeons. Ann Thor Surg 2003;76(1):315–21.

22. Parissis H, Young V. Treatment of Pancoast tutors from the surgeons prospective: re-appraisal of the anterior-manurial sternal approach. J Cardiothorac Surg 2010;5:102.

23. Fadel E, Missenard G, Chapelier A, et al. En bloc resection of non-small cell lung cancer invading the thoracic inlet and intervertebral foramina. J Thorac Cardiovasc Surg 2002;123(4):676–85.

24. Kasliwal MK, Tan LA, Traynelis VC. Infection with spinal instrumentation: review of pathogenesis, diagnosis, prevention and management. Surg Neurol Int 2013;4(Suppl 5):S392–403.

25. Schildhauer TA, Robie B, Muhr G, et al. Bacterial adherence to tantalum versus commonly used orthopedic metallic implant materials. J Orthop Trauma 2006;20(7):476–84.

26. Soultanis K, Pyrovolou N, Karamitros A, et al. Instrumentation loosening and material of implants as predisposal factors for late postoperative infections in operated idiopathic scoliosis. Stud Health Technol Inform 2006;123:559–64.

27. Prosser JD, Vender JR, Arturo Solares C. Traumatic cerebrospinal fluid leaks. Otolaryngol Clin North Am 2011;44(4):857–73.

28. Al Ani AH, Alhuarrat MAD, Al kasabreh MA, et al. Traumatic cervical spine intradural hematoma: a case report and review of literature. Interdiscip Neurosurg 2020;20(10):100779.

29. Awad JN, Kebaish KM, Donigan J, et al. Analysis of the risk factors for the development of postoperative spinal epidural hematoma. J Bone Joint Surg Br 2005;87(9):1248–52.

30. Hazel K, Weyant MJ. Chest wall resection and reconstruction: management of complications. Thorac Surg Clin 2015;25:517–21.

Systemic Therapy in Nonsmall Cell Lung Cancer and the Role of Biomarkers in Selection of Treatment

Bryan Lo, MD, PhD, FRCPC[a], Scott A. Laurie, MD, FRCPC[b],*

KEYWORDS

- Biomarkers • Systemic therapy • Next-generation sequencing • Nonsmall cell lung cancer

KEY POINTS

- An increasing number of molecular alterations are being discovered in nonsmall cell lung cancer (NSCLC).
- Many of the molecular alterations are actionable, in that there are targeted agents that are highly effective as treatment.
- Together with PD-L1 staining on tumor specimens, these predictive biomarkers are used for systemic treatment selection for patients with advanced NSCLC, and, increasingly, in earlier stage patients also.
- Adequate biopsy material is required at workup of a patient with suspected NSCLC to perform these necessary tests.

Lung cancer is a leading cause of cancer-related mortality and can be divided into 2 broad categories, small cell lung cancer and non-small cell lung cancer (NSCLC). NSCLC represents 85% of all lung cancers and can be subdivided into histologic subtypes, primary adenocarcinoma (60%) and squamous cell carcinoma (35%). In recent years, there has been significant improvement in NSCLC treatment algorithms and outcomes because of the identification of targetable driver mutations.[1,2] Otherwise known as predictive biomarkers, these mutations help identify which treatment the patient is most likely to respond to or benefit from. Although the original clinical trials ascertained these driver mutations using traditional molecular approaches, the use of next-generation sequencing (NGS) is being used increasingly by clinical laboratories to perform molecular profiling of NSCLC. As this trend to NGS continues, together with advancements in understanding the molecular

mechanisms underlying lung cancer, there are clearly important opportunities to expand the clinical utility of molecular profiling beyond predictive biomarkers for NSCLC.

CLINICALLY ACTIONABLE MUTATIONS IN NONSMALL CELL LUNG CANCER

A mutation is a permanent change in the nucleotide sequence of DNA. Currently, targetable driver mutations in NSCLC are mutations in oncogenes that fall into 5 mutation categories: base substitutions, deletions, insertions, gene fusions, and copy number gains.[3] Base substitutions most often are single base substitutions, but can also involve multiple bases, and can lead to an amino acid substitution that produces a gain of function in the protein (eg, EGFR L858R). Small deletions and insertions that keep the reading frame intact can lead to a loss or gain of a small sequence of amino

a Division of Medical Oncology, The Ottawa Hospital Cancer Centre, University of Ottawa, 501 Smyth Road, Ottawa, Ontario K1H8L6, Canada; b Division of Pathology and Laboratory Medicine, The Ottawa Hospital Cancer Centre, The University of Ottawa, 501 Smyth Road, Ottawa, Ontario K1H8L6, Canada
* Corresponding author.
E-mail address: slaurie@toh.ca

Thorac Surg Clin 31 (2021) 399–406
https://doi.org/10.1016/j.thorsurg.2021.05.004
1547-4127/21/© 2021 Elsevier Inc. All rights reserved.

acids that also produces a gain of function in the protein (eg, *EGFR* exon 19 deletion). Gene fusions or translocations are made by joining parts of 2 different genes, and the resulting fusion protein can have altered functional properties (ex. *ALK-EML4*). Copy number gains refer to an increase in the number of copies of a gene and can result in increased or dysregulated gene expression (eg, *MET* amplification). Of note, mutations falling into several different mutation categories can cause altered gene splicing, leading to a mutant protein that is abnormally activated because of an altered domain structure (eg, *MET* exon 14 skipping mutation).

In addition to somatic mutations in oncogenes, lung cancers also harbor somatic mutations in tumor suppressors. At risk of oversimplification, these mutations in tumor suppressors are loss of function mutations. Because there are many more ways to knock out a protein than there are ways to enhance its activity, loss of function mutations tend to be more diverse and include DNA variations that are more challenging to detect and interpret. For instance, large rearrangements, in addition to small insertions and deletions, can lead to loss of function in the protein, and copy number loss and epigenetic changes can result in significant decreased protein expression. Moreover, a significant proportion of loss of function tumor suppressor mutations resides in genomic locations that are difficult to analyze because of segmental duplications or low sequence complexity.[4–6] Presently, loss of function mutations in tumor suppressors have not yet emerged as clinically actionable predictive biomarkers in NSCLC, although preclinical and translational research suggests that this will likely change in the future.

DETECTING TARGETABLE DRIVER MUTATIONS IN NONSMALL CELL LUNG CANCER

Targetable driver mutations in NSCLC have traditionally been detected by molecular techniques that are essentially single gene assays. For instance, real-time quantitative polymerase chain reaction (PCR) approaches have been widely employed to analyze *EGFR*, whereas immunohistochemistry and fluorescence in situ hybridization (FISH) have been used to detect *ALK* and *ROS1* translocations.[7] However, as the list of targetable driver genes in NSCLC has grown, so has the recognition that next-generation sequencing (NGS) assays that simultaneously analyze multiple gene targets are ultimately more cost-effective and achieve better turnaround times.[8]

NGS is the sequencing of millions of small fragments of DNA in a massively parallel fashion.[9] The remarkable capacity of NGS technology can be applied broadly, to sequence, for example, an entire genome, or deeply, to sequence mixtures of DNA to detect mutations found at low frequencies. For NSCLC, most clinical laboratories are using targeted NGS gene panels and sequencing at sufficient depth to overcome the technical challenges imposed by clinical specimens.[10] These technical challenges result from the fact that formalin fixed paraffin embedded (FFPE) tumor specimens are the mainstay of pathologic diagnosis, and DNA samples extracted from FFPE tissues are fragmented, poor quality and contain deamination artifacts. In addition, patient specimens may contain a low percentage of tumor cells compared with normal cells, and NGS assays need to have the sensitivity to detect tumor mutations against a high background of non-tumor DNA. Although there are caveats to this, the most straightforward way to increase the sensitivity of an NGS test is to increase the sequencing depth in order to increase the number of observables in the assay.

The size of targeted NGS gene panels can vary significantly in size from a small number of regions of interest within actionable genes (hotspot panels) to more comprehensive profiling of hundreds of genes. Larger panels might better characterize the genetic profile of a cancer, provide mutational signatures, and include the calculation of tumor mutation burden (TMB), but at the expense of decreased throughput, increased cost, and need for greater bioinformatics support.[11,12] Smaller panels might be simpler to validate, analyze and report, and have a higher throughput and lower cost, but sacrifice the detection of variants that lie outside the regions being targeted.

Both small and large NGS commercial panels have been developed to detect targetable driver mutations in all the main mutation categories (eg, base substitutions, deletions, insertions, copy number gains, or gene fusions). It should be noted that while a DNA-based assay can detect gene fusions, there are technical challenges to designing robust assays when breakpoints are ill-defined and occur in large intronic regions. Therefore, in many targeted NGS panels, gene fusion detection is accomplished by detecting RNA fusion transcripts.[13] Similarly, altered gene splicing (eg, *Met* exon 14 skipping) detection may require the sequencing of RNA transcripts to achieve adequate performance.

LIQUID BIOPSY IN NONSMALL CELL LUNG CANCER

Circulating tumor DNA (ctDNA) is tumor-derived DNA in the blood that has emerged as an important alternative and complementary method to invasive tumor biopsies. The liquid biopsy is especially important in NSCLC because of the substantial number of fragile patients and lesions that are not easily accessible to a tissue biopsy. In addition, NSCLC tumor biopsies are sometimes insufficient for molecular analysis, and the liquid biopsy can efficiently substitute for an expensive and invasive repeat biopsy that is often difficult to obtain and which inevitably introduces significant treatment delays. A simple blood draw can also be performed repeatedly over time and thus, ctDNA can provide a means to monitor tumor evolution, treatment response and development of resistance mutations.

Despite its advantages, ctDNA does have drawbacks. The concentrations of ctDNA are typically very low, and ctDNA assays have to have, at least, an order of magnitude higher level of analytical sensitivity. Unlike tissue biopsy, there is no equivalent to a pathology review for a liquid biopsy to assess for tumor content, and this can result in ambiguity over whether negative results are simply caused by an absence of ctDNA. More recently, there is also an increasing recognition that clonal hematopoeisis, where WBC lineages can harbor and contribute mutations to DNA in the blood, can confound the interpretation of ctDNA assays.[14]

Analogous to tissue biopsies, liquid biopsies can be analyzed by single gene assays (real-time quantitative PCR, digital droplet PCR) or by NGS. NGS analysis of ctDNA has made use of high sequencing depth, specialized bioinformatics and unique, molecular indexing tags to increase the analytical sensitivity required by ctDNA. Proof of principle studies have also explored ways to preanalytically enrich the ctDNA fraction. With respect the NSCLC, ctDNA assays are an acceptable means to profile a tumor for targetable driver mutations,[15] and there have been many studies establishing the clinical utility and cost-effectiveness of detecting EGFR T790M resistance mutation in ctDNA in patients relapsing on EGFR TKI therapy.[16]

NEXT-GENERATION SEQUENCING APPLICATIONS BEYOND PREDICTIVE BIOMARKERS FOR NONSMALL CELL LUNG CANCER

Because lung cancer is often diagnosed after it has progressed to advanced and metastatic stages and beyond the early stages where surgery can be curative, the development of a cost-effective screening assay that can detect localized lung cancer would be extremely desirable. Several proof of concept studies have explored the application of NGS to blood-based screening strategies. Some combine an NGS assay to detect mutations with other cancer biomarkers.[17] Others use NGS to profile methylation patterns that are specific to cancer.[18] Recently, NGS has also been used to analyze whole genome sequences of circulating cell-free DNA on the basis that tumor DNA exhibits distinct fragmentation patterns.[19] Although it remains to be seen whether any of these approaches have sufficient sensitivity and specificity to be applied to the general population or even at-risk subpopulations, recent history suggests that continued technological advancements in NGS will drive innovation toward transformative diagnostics.

SYSTEMIC THERAPY OF NONSMALL CELL LUNG CANCER

The term systemic therapy encompasses a broad spectrum of classes of medications used in the treatment of cancer, and not only includes cytotoxic chemotherapy, but also hormonal therapy, targeted agents, biologic agents such as oncolytic viruses, and immunotherapy. The role of these various classes in NSCLC beyond cytotoxic chemotherapy has expanded dramatically in the last decade, particularly in the palliative metastatic setting, but also increasingly in earlier stage disease as both adjuvant and neoadjuvant treatments.

METASTATIC NONSMALL CELL LUNG CANCER

It has been known for over 25 years that palliative platinum-based doublet chemotherapy in fit patients with a good performance status offers a modest prolongation of survival in those with metastatic disease.[20] Furthermore, despite the potential toxicities of chemotherapy, in general, patients who receive chemotherapy have a better quality of life than those who receive only best supportive care; this reflects the fact that a progressive, uncontrolled cancer has a major detrimental effect on symptoms and thus quality of life. In 2000, randomized trials then showed that single-agent docetaxel was superior to best supportive care in those patients whose cancer had progressed despite platinum-based chemotherapy.[21]

The differential effect of the agent pemetrexed on squamous compared with nonsquamous histology caused a shift to the use of platinum-pemetrexed as the preferred first-line doublet in patients with nonsquamous histology the mid-2000s,[22] with the continued use of pemetrexed as an ongoing maintenance treatment in those without disease progression after 4 cycles of the doublet.[23] The addition of the antiangiogenic agent bevazicumab, a monoclonal antibody against the vascular endothelial growth factor (VEGF), to first-line platinum-doublet chemotherapy was also found to offer a modest benefit in those with nonsquamous histology,[24] while being contraindicated in those with squamous histology because of the increased risk of fatal hemoptysis. These differential effects require that pathologists adequately characterize the subtype of NSCLC.

Overexpression, relative to what is seen in normal lung, of the epidermal growth factor receptor (EGFR), which is involved in a signal cascade that promotes cell growth and survival, is common in NSCLC. The EGFR is a transmembrane receptor with an extracellular domain that, when bound by the ligand EGF, causes activation of the intracellular tyrosine kinase domain that initiates the signal cascade that sends growth signals to the cell nucleus. The activity of EGFR can be inhibited by monoclonal antibodies that block the extracellular domain and prevent ligand binding (used in colorectal cancer), or by small molecule inhibitors of the tyrosine kinase domain (used in NSCLC). The Canadian Cancer Trials Group study BR21 enrolled patients with advanced NSCLC of any histology whose disease had progressed following platinum-doublet chemotherapy to either erlotinib, a small molecule inhibitor of EGFR, or placebo.[25] This trial revealed a modest benefit to the use of erlotinib in terms of survival and quality of life, and led to this becoming a standard therapy for patients following failure of cytotoxic chemotherapy in the mid-2000s.

With increased use of EGFR tyrosine kinase inhibitors (TKIs) it became clear that responses were much more likely and significant in certain types of patients, namely those with adenocarcinoma, those of East Asian ethnicity, and never smokers or light smokers, and it was determined that mutations in the tyrosine kinase domain that occurred in such patients conferred sensitivity to these TKIs.[26] These EGFR mutations lead to a receptor that is continuously active independent of ligand binding. Mutated EGFR functions as an oncogenic driver, and adenocarcinomas with these mutations are a distinct subtype. Randomized trials have shown that in patients whose tumors harbor an EGFR mutation, these agents are more effective and lead to a better quality of life than chemotherapy when used as the first treatment in newly diagnosed patients.[27,28] With this discovery, the use of EGFR TKIs in those without such mutations has fallen out of favor, as it is felt that the benefits, if any, are minimal.

As previously discussed, an increasing number of oncogenic drivers beyond EGFR has been discovered in adenocarcinomas, along with agents that target the oncogenic proteins that arise (**Table 1**). In those subtypes that are sufficiently common, such as ALK translocations, randomized trials have confirmed that targeted agents are superior to chemotherapy and are now the first-line treatment of choice.[29] In other, rarer, subtypes, it is more difficult to conduct randomized trials, and although it is clear that targeted agents are effective, it is not clear at what point in the treatment trajectory they should be used. Mechanisms of resistance to these agents can develop after their use, and can include the appearance of secondary mutations, which in turn can be successfully inhibited by newer TKIs.[30] Thus it is common that patients with some oncogenic drivers will be treated with

Table 1
Targeted therapies in nonsmall cell lung cancer

Molecular Alteration	Frequency of Occurrence in Non-squamous NSCLC	Agents Available?
EGFR mutations	40%–50% of East Asian patients 12%–15% of all other patients	Marketed
ALK translocations	4%	Marketed
ROS1 translocations	<1%	Marketed
NTRK translocations	<1%	Marketed
RET translocations	1%–2%	Marketed
BRAF mutations	1%	Marketed
MET exon 14 skip mutations	<1%	Marketed
KRAS G12C mutation	10%–15%	In clinical trials

sequential targeted agents before having to move on to chemotherapy. These oral agents are generally well tolerated, particularly compared with cytotoxic chemotherapy, and suitable for long-term administration. It is important to realize that patients with metastatic NSCLC and EGFR or ALK alterations can survive for many years. The number of oncogenic drivers discovered for NSCLC continues to increase, as does the number of targeted agents available to treat each specific molecular alteration, thus highlighting the importance of adequate genomic examination of each patient's tumor.

The most common molecular alterations in NSCLC are mutations in *KRAS*, a downstream member of the EGFR pathway, seen in up to 30% of adenocarcinomas and a smaller proportion of squamous lung cancers. Although mutations in *KRAS* in NSCLC have been known for many years, attempts to target these alterations were unsuccessful, leading some to speculate that it was undruggable. More recently, however, significant anti-tumor activity has been observed with sotorasib, which can inhibit a specific *KRAS* mutation (G12 C), which is the most common variant of mutation seen in NSCLC, accounting for up to 15% of cases.[31] Other pan-*KRAS* inhibitors are in early clinical trials. If these inhibitors prove to be effective in larger trials, *KRAS* mutations will join the list of actionable targets in NSCLC. Given the frequency of these mutations, this has the potential to impact a very large number of patients.

Attempts to harness the patient's own immune system to fight cancer have a decades-long history and include the use of nonspecific stimulation with interferon and interleukins, attenuated infectious agents, and vaccines targeting antigens found preferentially on the surface of cancer cells. As an example, in lung cancer, this includes a trial conducted many years ago investigating BCG instilled into the pleura at the time of resection.[32] However, none of these early investigations led to improved outcomes in patients with NSCLC.

With a greater understanding of the complexity of the immune response comes the knowledge that there are many checkpoints, or inhibitory signals, that suppress the activation of T cells. Cancers co-opt these checkpoints to evade immune detection. The use of monoclonal antibodies which impede these negative signals help to permit T cell activation and subsequent recognition of the cancer as foreign by the immune system. Monoclonal antibodies that target the programmed death ligand 1 pathway (PD-1/PD-L1) and the cytotoxic T lymphocyte antigen 4 (CTLA-4) pathway are now approved for use in

various malignancies, including lung cancer. These agents upregulate the immune system, and although generally well-tolerated, they can lead to a variety of autoimmune adverse effects on any organ system. Examples of potential toxicities include rash, pneumonitis, colitis with diarrhea, arthritis, and endocrinopathies including altered thyroid function, panhypopituitarism, and type 1 diabetes.

In the metastatic setting, PD-(L)1 agents can be used alone,[33,34] in combination with chemotherapy,[35] or in combination with a CTLA-4 agent.[36] In those patients with high PD-L1 expression by immunohistochemistry, an anti-PD-(L)1 inhibitor alone has been shown to be superior to standard cytotoxic chemotherapy in patients with advanced NSCLC without an known oncogenic driver such as EGFR mutations or ALK translocations. In those with low or intermediate PD-L1 expression, the addition of such an inhibitor to standard, histology appropriate cytotoxic chemotherapy has been shown to be superior to chemotherapy alone. Thus all patients with advanced NSCLC without an oncogenic driver now receive immunotherapy, either alone or in combination with chemotherapy, as a standard first-line treatment, provided they do not have a contraindication to their use, such as an underlying autoimmune disorder. What is particularly exciting about immunotherapy for NSCLC is that several trials appear to have a tail on the Kaplan-Meier survival curves that the suggest the possibility of long-term survival (cure) in a proportion of patients with metastatic disease who receive these agents. However, there are still many patients who do not respond to these agents, even if they have high PD-L1 expression. Clearly more research is needed to understand which patients ultimately benefit from immunotherapy.

EARLY STAGE RESECTED AND RESECTABLE NONSMALL CELL LUNG CANCER

Adjuvant chemotherapy has been established as standard of care for fit patients who can tolerate cisplatin-based chemotherapy after complete resection of stage II and IIIA, and selected stage IB (those node negative tumors >4 cm) NSCLC. This is based on several trials reported in the early 2000s that consistently demonstrated an improvement in overall survival in those patients randomized to receive postoperative chemotherapy compared with those who were observed. A meta-analysis confirms an absolute improvement in 5-year survival of 5%[37]; given the sheer numbers of patients with NSCLC, this represents a large number of lives saved with adjuvant chemotherapy. All patients who undergo resection and are node-positive, and those node negative patients with a primary tumor size of greater than 4 cm should be referred to a medical oncologist for an assessment regarding adjuvant chemotherapy.

Trials of the addition of bevacizumab to chemotherapy[38] or of vaccines[39] did not lead to improved outcomes in the adjuvant setting. Despite the success in the metastatic setting of targeted agents in those with molecular drivers, until recently there were no data on their use as adjuvant treatment. However, in a phase III trial, patients with stage IB-IIIA completely resected EGFR mutation-positive NSCLC, who may or may not have received standard postoperative cisplatin-based chemotherapy, were randomized to receive the third-generation EGFR inhibitor osimertinib or placebo for 3 years.[40] This trial revealed a remarkable improvement in disease-free survival in those randomized to osimertinib, regardless of stage of disease or the receipt of adjuvant chemotherapy; what remains to be determined is whether its use will improve overall survival. Clinical trials of targeted agents as adjuvant therapy following resection of tumors with other molecular drivers are either planned or ongoing. The same is true for the use of immunotherapy; multiple trials of adjuvant use of these agents have completed accrual, and their results are eagerly awaited.

The use of preoperative chemoradiation in those with resectable Pancoast tumors is routine. In those patients with resectable stage IIIA disease, many centers opt for a trimodality approach of induction chemoradiation followed by surgery.[41] However, up-front resection followed by adjuvant therapy is also an acceptable option for these patients. It must be emphasized that these patients must be resectable at their initial assessment by the thoracic surgeon; the use of induction treatment attempting to render an unresectable patient resectable is not supported by evidence. Multiple trials are evaluating preoperative treatment with immunotherapy agents. These trials show that their use is safe in the preoperative setting, and associated with high rates of response.[42] It remains to be determined, however, whether routine preoperative use will improve cure rates of early stage NSCLC.

LOCALLY ADVANCED, UNRESECTABLE NONSMALL CELL LUNG CANCER

Standard therapy for patients with unresectable stage III NSCLC has been concurrent chemoradiation since trials showed that the addition of chemotherapy to radiation improves survival. More recently a randomized trial of the PD-L1 agent durvalumab, given as adjuvant therapy for 1 year in those patients whose disease did not progress at the completion of chemoradiation, has been shown to improve survival, and is now the standard of care.[43] Trials are ongoing evaluating the addition of immunotherapy from the commencement of chemoradiation. With respect to targeted therapy, clinical trials are evaluating the addition of these agents in the postchemoradiation setting.

SUMMARY

Systemic therapy has an ever-increasing role to play in NSCLC, including in the adjuvant and neo-adjuvant setting. Management of these patients requires a multidisciplinary team that includes thoracic surgeons, medical and radiation oncologist, radiologists, and pathologists. Surgeons need to be aware of which patients to refer for consideration of (neo) adjuvant therapy. They also need to be aware of the importance of obtaining sufficient tissue in those patients with locally advanced or metastatic disease in order for there to be adequate assessment of all the biomarkers required to determine the most appropriate systemic therapy. Finally, clinical trials of systemic therapies in earlier stage NSCLC are important to improve outcomes in these patients, and surgeons should consider referring such patients for participation.

CLINICS CARE POINTS

- Biomarkers are essential for selection of appropriate treatment.
- Biomarker results should ideally be available at the time of initial consultation with a medical oncologist.
- New predictive biomarkers are continuously being discovered, and laboratory techniques used to detect them are evolving rapidly.

DISCLOSURE

S.A. Laurie reports consulting fees/honoraria from Roche, Eli Lilly, Novartis, Pfizer. Bryan Lo - (consulting / honoraria): AstraZeneca, Amgen, Pfizer.

REFERENCES

1. Chen R, Manochakian R, James L, et al. Emerging therapeutic agents for advanced non-small cell lung cancer. J Hematol Oncol 2000;13:58.

2. Lindeman NI, Cagle PT, Aisner DL, et al. Updated molecular testing guideline for the selection of lung cancer patients for treatment with targeted tyrosine kinase inhibitors: guideline from the College of American Pathologists, the International Association for the Study of Lung Cancer, and the Association for Molecular Pathology. J Mol Diagn 2018;20:129–59.

3. Sondka Z, Bamford S, Cole CG, et al. The COSMIC Cancer Gene Census: describing genetic dysfunction across all human cancers. Nat Rev Cancer 2018;18:696–705.

4. Ebbert MTW, Jensen TD, Jansen-West K, et al. Systematic analysis of dark and camouflaged genes reveals disease-relevant genes hiding in plain sight. Genome Biol 2019;20(1):97.

5. Freeman TM, Genomics England Research, Wang D, et al. Genomic loci susceptible to systematic sequencing bias in clinical whole genomes. Genome Res 2020;30(3):415–26.

6. Goldfeder RL, Priest JR, Zook JM, et al. Medical implications of technical accuracy in genome sequencing. Genome Med 2016;8(1):24.

7. Vanderlaan PA, Roy-Chowdhuri S. Current and future trends in non-small cell lung cancer biomarker testing: the American experience. Cancer Cytopathol 2020;128(9):629–36.

8. Mosele F, Remon J, Mateo J, et al. Recommendations for the use of next-generation sequencing (NGS) for patients with metastatic cancers: a report from the ESMO Precision Medicine Working Group. Ann Oncol 2020;31:1491–505.

9. Gao G, Smith DI. Clinical massively parallel sequencing. Clin Chem 2020;66(1):77–88.

10. Yip S, Christofides A, Banerji S, et al. A Canadian guideline on the use of next-generation sequencing in oncology. Curr Oncol 2019;26(2):e241–54.

11. Karimnezhad A, Palidwor GA, Thavorn K, et al. Accuracy and reproducibility of somatic point mutation calling in clinical-type targeted sequencing data. BMC Med Genomics 2020;13(1):156.

12. Li MM, Datto M, Duncavage EJ, et al. Standards and guidelines for the interpretation and reporting of sequence variants in cancer: a joint consensus recommendation of the association for molecular pathology, American Society of Clinical Oncology, and College of American Pathologists. J Mol Diagn 2017;19(1):4–23.

13. Cohen D, Hondelink LM, Solleveld-Westerink N, et al. Optimizing mutation and fusion detection in NSCLC by sequential DNA and RNA sequencing. J Thorac Oncol 2020;15(6):1000–14.

14. Chan HT, Chin YM, Nakamura Y, et al. Clonal hematopoiesis in liquid biopsy: from biological noise to valuable clinical implications. Cancers (Basel) 2020;12(8):2277.

15. Mezquita L, Swalduz A, Jovelet C, et al. Clinical relevance of an amplicon-based liquid biopsy for detecting ALK and ROS1 fusion and resistance mutations in patients with non-small-cell lung cancer. JCO Precis Oncol 2020;4. https://doi.org/10.1200/PO.19.00281.

16. Remon J, Caramella C, Jovelet C, et al. Osimertinib benefit in EGFR-mutant NSCLC patients with T790M-mutation detected by circulating tumour DNA. Ann Oncol 2017;28(4):784–90.

17. Cohen JD, Li L, Wang Y, et al. Detection and localization of surgically resectable cancers with a multianalyte blood test. Science 2018;359(6378):926–30.

18. Shen SY, Singhania R, Fehringer G, et al. Sensitive tumour detection and classification using plasma cell-free DNA methylomes. Nature 2018;563(7732):579–83.

19. Cristiano S, Leal A, Phallen J, et al. Genome-wide cell-free DNA fragmentation in patients with cancer. Nature 2019;570(7761):385–9.

20. Non-small Cell Lung Cancer Collaborative Group. Chemotherapy in non-small cell lung cancer: a meta-analysis using updated data on individual patients from 52 randomised clinical trials. BMJ 1995;311:899–909.

21. Shepherd FA, Dancey J, Ramlau R, et al. Prospective randomized trial of docetaxel versus best supportive care in patients with non-small-cell lung cancer previously treated with platinum-based chemotherapy. J Clin Oncol 2000;18:2095–103.

22. Scagliotti GV, Parikh P, von Pawel J, et al. Phase III study comparing cisplatin plus gemcitabine with cisplatin plus pemetrexed in chemotherapy-naive patients with advanced-stage non-small-cell lung cancer. J Clin Oncol 2008;26:3543–51.

23. Paz-Ares L, de Marinis F, Dediu M, et al. Maintenance therapy with pemetrexed plus best supportive care versus placebo plus best supportive care after induction therapy with pemetrexed plus cisplatin for advanced non-squamous non-small-cell lung cancer (PARAMOUNT): a double-blind, phase 3, randomised controlled trial. Lancet Oncol 2012;13:247–55.

24. Sandler A, Gray R, Perry MC, et al. Paclitaxel-carboplatin alone or with bevacizumab for non-small-cell lung cancer. N Engl J Med 2006;355:2542–50.

25. Shepherd FA, Pereira JR, Ciuleanu T, et al. Erlotinib in previously treated non-small cell lung cancer. N Engl J Med 2005;353:123–32.

26. Paez JG, Jänne PA, Lee JC, et al. EGFR mutations in lung cancer: correlation with clinical response to gefitinib therapy. Science 2004;304:1497–500.

27. Yang JC, Wu YL, Schuler M, et al. Afatinib versus cisplatin-based chemotherapy for EGFR mutation-positive lung adenocarcinoma (LUX-Lung 3 and LUX-Lung 6): analysis of overall survival data from two randomised, phase 3 trials. Lancet Oncol 2015;16:141–51.

28. Mok TS, Wu Y-L, Thongprasert S, et al. Gefitinib or carboplatin-paclitaxel in pulmonary adenocarcinoma. N Engl J Med 2009;361:947–57.

29. Solomon BJ, Mok T, Kim DW, et al. First-line crizotinib versus chemotherapy in ALK-positive lung cancer. N Engl J Med 2014;371:2167–77.

30. Mok TS, Wu Y-L, Ahn M-J, et al. Osimertinib or platinum–pemetrexed in *EGFR* T790M–positive lung cancer. N Engl J Med 2017;376:629–40.

31. Hong DS, Fakih MG, Strickler JH, et al. KRAS(G12C) inhibition with sotorasib in advanced solid tumors. N Engl J Med 2020;383:1207–17.

32. The Ludwig Lung Cancer Study Group (LLCSG). Immunostimulation with intrapleural BCG as adjuvant therapy in resected non-small cell lung cancer. Cancer 1986;58:2411–6.

33. Reck RM, Rodríguez-Abreu D, Robinson AG, et al. Pembrolizumab versus chemotherapy for PD-L1–positive non–small-cell lung cancer. N Engl J Med 2016;375:1823–33.

34. Herbst R, Giaccone G, de Marinis F, et al. Atezolizumab for first-line treatment of PD-L1-selected patients with non-small cell lung cancer. N Engl J Med 2020;383:1328–39.

35. Gandhi L, Rodríguez-Abreu D, Gadgeel S, et al. Pembrolizumab plus chemotherapy in metastatic non-small cell lung cancer. N Engl J Med 2018; 378:2078–92.

36. Hellman MD, Paz-Ares L, Caro RB, et al. Nivolumab plus ipilimumab in advanced non-small cell lung cancer. N Engl J Med 2019;381:2020–31.

37. Pignon JP, Tribodet H, Scagliotti GV, et al. Lung adjuvant cisplatin evaluation: a pooled analysis by the LACE Collaborative Group. J Clin Oncol 2008; 26:3552–9.

38. Wakelee HA, Dahlberg SE, Keller SM, et al. Adjuvant chemotherapy with or without bevacizumab in patients with resected non-small-cell lung cancer (E1505): an open-label, multicentre, randomised, phase 3 trial. Lancet Oncol 2017;18:1610–23.

39. Vansteenkiste JF, Cho BC, Vanakesa T, et al. Efficacy of the MAGE-A3 cancer immunotherapeutic as adjuvant therapy in patients with resected MAGE-A3-positive non-small-cell lung cancer (MAGRIT): a randomised, double-blind, placebo-controlled, phase 3 trial. Lancet Oncol 2016;17: 822–35.

40. Wu YL, Tsuboi M, He J, et al. Osimertinib in resected EGFR-mutated non-small-cell lung cancer. N Engl J Med 2020;383:1711–23.

41. Albain KS, Swann RS, Rusch VW, et al. Radiotherapy plus chemotherapy with or without surgical resection for stage III non-small-cell lung cancer: a phase III randomised controlled trial. Lancet 2009; 374:379–86.

42. Forde PM, Chaft JE, Smith KN, et al. Neoadjuvant PD-1 blockade in resectable lung cancer. N Engl J Med 2018;378:1976–86.

43. Antonia SJ, Villegas A, Daniel D, et al. Overall survival with durvalumab after chemoradiotherapy in stage III NSCLC. N Engl J Med 2018;379:2342–50.

Sepsis in the Postpneumonectomy Space
Pathogenesis, Recognition, and Management

Farid M. Shamji, MBBS, FRCSC, FACS

KEYWORDS

- Postpneumonectomy sepsis • Empyema • Microbiology • Aerobic and anaerobic bacteria
- Bronchopleural fistula • Esophagopleural fistula

KEY POINTS

- Factors predisposing to the formation of bronchopleural fistula and subsequent empyema.
- Bacteriology in postpneumonectomy empyema due to aerobic and anaerobic infection.
- Factors that are incriminated in the development of postpneumonectomy bronchopleural fistula.
- Investigations necessary in the management.
- Three phases in the pathogenesis of empyema and clinical findings in each phase.

INTRODUCTION

Empyema may occur in the pleural space after pulmonary resection in the presence of bronchopleural fistula. This also is usually the result of a dead space within the pleural cavity after pneumonectomy, which is filled with blood or serosanguinous fluid. Subsequent bacterial contamination results in infection and the development of a frank empyema. It may be associated with a transient bronchopleural fistula that closed spontaneously and may occur any time after surgery, even years after a pneumonectomy.[1]

Pneumonectomy is the surgical removal of the entire lung.[2] Pneumonectomy is the treatment of choice for centrally located bronchogenic carcinoma, diffuse malignant mesothelioma, and chronic inflammatory lung diseases with destroyed lung from pulmonary tuberculosis, fungal infections, and bronchiectasis. It is considered to be a major chest operation, often elective and sometimes urgent. Uncomplicated, the postpneumonectomy space must be radiologically monitored with chest radiographs at 3-day intervals as it gradually fills up with serosanguinous fluid over 3 to 6 weeks.

The mediastinum shifts gradually toward the operated side as it decreases in volume from the expected physiologic changes. These changes are expected, compensatory expansion of the contralateral lung and decrease in the pneumonectomy space owing to the absorption of air and the gradual accumulation of pleural fluid, as well as the gradual development of pleural thickening and fibrosis from inflammatory organization. In the uncomplicated case, on the pneumonectomy side, the diaphragm becomes elevated as the air–fluid level decreases, there is chest wall deformation, and the hydrothorax gradually disappears.

The pneumonectomy space is at potential risk for getting infected from bacterial contamination and developing empyema. The accumulating serosanguinous fluid is a good bacterial culture medium. Bronchopleural fistula and esophagopleural fistula are the 2 major sources of infection in the in the postpneumonectomy space in the surgical patient. Another source of space infection is direct extension from infected thoracotomy incision or septicemia from urosepsis, subdiaphragmatic abscess, or peritonitis.[3–9]

University of Ottawa, General Campus, Ottawa Hospital, 501 Smyth Road, Ottawa, Ontario K1H 8L6, Canada
E-mail address: faridshamji@hotmail.com

Thorac Surg Clin 31 (2021) 407–416
https://doi.org/10.1016/j.thorsurg.2021.08.001
1547-4127/21/

UNCOMPLICATED POSTOPERATIVE COURSE AFTER PNEUMONECTOMY

As soon as the operation is completed and the diseased lung is removed, the integrity of the closed bronchial stump must be confirmed. Surgical division and closure of the bronchial stump must be tested for unexpected air leak. To do so, it requires that the pleural space be partially filed with normal saline solution and the anesthesiologist exerts a tracheal airway pressure of up to 45 cm H_2O by manual "bagging" to identify any bronchial stump air leaks. After ensuring that the bronchial stump is completely secure and intact, thereafter the bronchial stump is covered and protected, and reinforced with viable tissue such as pedicled pericardial fat pad, a pedicled flap of the pericardium, intercostal muscle pedicled flap, proximal and distal ligation, and division of azygous–superior vena cava junction and filleted azygous vein pedicle surrounded by parietal pleura flap, or anterior transdiaphragmatic retrosternal route for omentum. After satisfactory bronchial stump reinforcement, the bronchial stump must be tested again for an air leak under positive pressure ventilation with an airway pressure of up to 45 cm H_2O while submerged under saline solution. Without evidence of bronchial stump air leak, the integrity of the bronchial stump is now confirmed and the chest tube must then be clamped after the mediastinum is properly balanced by the responsible thoracic surgeon, permitting some shift of the mediastinum toward the pneumonectomy side by partial hyperinflation of the contralateral lung without excessive ipsilateral mediastinal shift. The chest tube must be left clamped overnight; it is removed the following day after radiologic assessment is confirmed to be satisfactory and the mediastinum is well-balanced with minor shift to the operated side.[10]

Postoperatively, the fluid balance must be maintained. Cardiac function and rhythm must be monitored. Daily body temperature and white blood cell count should be recorded. Daily chest radiographs are required to monitor the integrity of the postpneumonectomy space until the patient is ready to be discharged from the hospital. The white blood cell count is monitored daily for 7 days for leukocytosis. The thoracotomy incision is examined every day for unexpected infection.

PATHOGENESIS OF SEPSIS IN THE POSTPNEUMONECTOMY SPACE

Pathophysiological changes that occur in the postpneumonectomy space are related to the following factors.

1. Infection in the thoracotomy incision with subsequent extension into the dead pleural space within the pleural cavity resulting in empyema. This finding is particularly worrisome in the postpneumonectomy patient, and the infecting micro-organism is frequently *Staphylococcus aureus.* The other pathogenic bacterial infections causing empyema may be pneumococci (*Streptococcus pneumoniae*), beta-hemolytic streptococci (*S pyogenes*), gram-negative enteric bacilli such as *Escherichia coli*, *Pseudomonas aeruginosa*, *Proteus spp.*, *Klebsiella pneumoniae*, and *S milleri* (of the viridans streptococci group). Anaerobic infections (usually peptostreptococci, *Bacteroides fragilis*, and fusobacteria) are probably more common than is often reported. Mixed infections may occur, and microbiological study may record both aerobic and anaerobic organisms.

2. The postpneumonectomy space gradually fills up with a serosanguinous fluid. Bacterial contamination of the pleural fluid is harmful. The fluid is a good culture medium for contaminating bacteria resulting in empyema.

3. There are several causes of postpneumonectomy bronchopleural fistula resulting from impaired healing of the bronchial stump. The main causes of this complication are technical errors in the closure of the bronchus, closure of a diseased bronchus, and leaving an excessively long bronchial stump, technical factors caused by increased rigidity of the bronchial cartilaginous rings affecting satisfactory bronchial stump closure, increased tension and dehiscence of the bronchial staple line when the division of the closed main bronchus is too close to the rigid cartilaginous tracheal carina, residual cancer in the divided bronchus impairing healing process, preoperative lung and bronchial infection, preoperative radiation therapy resulting in bronchial ischemia owing to endarteritis obliterans, excessive devascularization of the bronchus owing to overzealous dissection, and intraoperative bacterial contamination. The bronchopleural fistula may be small in size, resulting in infection of the postpneumonectomy serosanguinous fluid and empyema, or it may be large in size resulting in transbronchial aspiration of postpneumonectomy fluid into the contralateral lung and infection, leading to respiratory failure. The diagnosis should be suspected by unsuspected decrease in the air–fluid level in the pneumonectomy space, by the presence of aspiration pneumonia in the contralateral lung, and by documentation of multiple loculated air pockets in the accumulating pleural fluid. The diagnosis of bronchopleural fistula should be suspected from clinical examination and

radiologic examination with chest radiographs and computed tomography scans. It may be confirmed by bronchoscopic visualization of the bronchial stump or by the instillation of contrast material (Omnipaque) into the appropriate bronchus and sinogram demonstration of communication with the pleural space. Sepsis developing in the postpneumonectomy space is a major serious complication and threat to life. Bronchopleural fistula occurring after pneumonectomy presents a significantly greater hazard than that following a lesser pulmonary resection with lobectomy, segmentectomy, or wedge resection.[11,12]

4. The postpneumonectomy space may change in configuration with the presence of multiple loculated air pockets and a decreasing air–fluid level owing to the bronchopleural fistula.

5. Gram-negative enteric bacilli such as *E coli*, *P aeruginosa*, *Proteus spp.*, and *K pneumoniae* are found most commonly in empyema complicating esophagopleural fistula caused by esophageal injury during pulmonary resection.

6. An esophagopleural fistula is an uncommon postoperative problem.[4] It is the result of esophageal injury at the time of pneumonectomy. Extensive extrapleural dissection, especially on the right, and extensive mediastinal lymph node dissection are probably the precipitating factors. Dumont and DeGraef[8] pointed out that the blood supply to the esophagus is segmental and that the part of the esophagus just below the carina has the poorest blood supply; this site of fistula formation is the commonest. The majority of fistulas after pneumonectomy occur on the right.[12]

The development of esophagopleural fistula were described by Dumont and De Graef in 1961,[8] by Takaro and colleagues in 1960,[6] and by Erikson[7] in 1964. Takaro reported 24 cases occurring after pneumonectomy for tuberculosis or suppurative pulmonary disease and the mortality rate was 49%; the cure rate was 21%.[4] Erikson reported 3 cases of esophagopleural fistula occurring after right pneumonectomy for carcinoma of the lung.[5] Benjamin and colleagues[9] reported 3 cases of esophagopleural fistula after right pneumonectomy for carcinoma. Two cases occurred early in the postoperative period, and one occurred 8 months later. They pointed out that the clinical picture may be confused with that of bronchopleural fistula and empyema, but that a diatrizoate (Gastrografin) radiographic study is diagnostic. Esophagoscopy and bronchoscopy were performed in each case to rule out the presence of tumor.

Benjamin and colleagues[9] recommended empyema drainage followed by direct closure of the fistula with protection by a flap of pleura. After the fistula healed, the empyema was treated by the Clagett method: making an open window thoracostomy, pleural cavity irrigation with antibiotic solution, and finally closing the window after complete secure healing of the fistula.[13–15] Engelman and associates[10] reported a case of postpneumonectomy esophagopleural fistula successfully treated with a 1-stage procedure of intercostal muscle pedicle flap closure of the fistula with thoracoplasty. The collapsed empyema space was then continuously irrigated with antibiotic solution.

The best treatment for this entity is prevention. A nasogastric tube permits location of the esophagus. If the esophagus is injured at the time of pneumonectomy, the esophageal tear should be repaired immediately in 2 layers—a mucosal repair first followed by esophageal muscle reapproximation. The repaired site should be covered with a pleural flap and methylene blue should be instilled into the esophagus to ensure it is secure in the repaired esophageal tear.

BRONCHOPLEURAL FISTULA AND POSTPNEUMONECTOMY EMPYEMA

The incidence of empyema after pneumonectomy should not exceed 3%.[1] In up to 10% of patients bronchopleural fistulae appear (disrupted healing of the main bronchus). The clinical signs of infection of the pleural space vary widely and may not appear for several months after the operation. Therefore, the possibility of empyema should be considered in any patient with signs of infection after pneumonectomy, no matter how far in the past they underwent the procedure. Unexplained fever, expectoration of serosanguineous fluid, drainage from the wound, or multiloculated air pockets or a decrease in the air–fluid level seen on a chest film should immediately arouse suspicion of an infected space and possibly a bronchopleural fistula.

The management of empyema has been radically changed by the contributions of Clagett and Geraci (1963).[13–17] It consisted of 1 or 2 segmental rib resections with intervening intercostal muscles and parietal pleura in the anterior portion of the thoracotomy incision and immediate pleurocutaneous fistula in the chest wall fenestration by suturing of the pleura to the skin with Vicryl sutures. Three times daily packing with sterile gauze and monitoring for sepsis is needed. Weekly monitoring of the bronchial stump by bronchoscopy is required and, when necessary, by esophagoscopy. The Clagett procedure has 3 components:

creating the chest wall window (fenestration), sterilizing the empyema cavity, and finally surgically closing the window. Stafford and Clagett (1972)[15–17] demonstrated obliteration of the empyema in 16 of 18 cases. Management consists of open drainage using a modification of the pleural flap operation of Eloesser (1969)[4] followed 4 to 8 weeks later by daily cleansing of the pleural space, bronchoscopy to monitor bronchial stump healing, filling the pleural space with dilute betadine solution, and tight closure of the incision.

Bronchopleural fistulas generally occur in the first operative week. Rarely do they occur months after a pneumonectomy. After a pulmonary resection and closed tube drainage, the persistence of a large air leak or the sudden appearance of a large leak of air followed by some fever and the development of purulent drainage may make one suspicious of a bronchopleural fistula. The presence of a fistula can be confirmed by bronchoscopy.

A bronchopleural fistula developing after a pneumonectomy is generally heralded by the sudden coughing up of a thin, bloody fluid. This fluid may be so copious as to flood the opposite lung and cause pneumonia and death. The patient should immediately reassume a position that will make the intrapleural fluid gravitate away from the opening in the bronchus, that is, sitting up or lying down with the side operated on dependent. All the pleural fluid that can be obtained should be aspirated promptly by thoracentesis. This treatment takes care of the immediate emergency. Closed tube drainage of the pleural space is then recommended. Intravenous broad-spectrum antibiotics after Gram stain and culture should be administered. When the mediastinum has stabilized, open drainage with chest wall fenestration, a pleural flap, and an immediate pleurocutaneous fistula should be performed. Pleural cavity packing is started 3 times daily and sepsis is monitored. If the patient is old and debilitated, open pleural drainage may be used indefinitely.[18] Subsequently, the fistula may close. If it closes, the infected pleural space can then be managed in the method described by Clagett.[13,15,17,18] If the fistula does not close spontaneously, a tailoring thoracoplasty[19] or closure of the fistula using an intercostal muscle flap, or pectoral muscular flap, or omentum should be performed.

FACTORS PREDISPOSING TO BRONCHOPLEURAL FISTULA

1. Common etiologic factors are believed to be endobronchial tuberculosis, drug-resistant organisms, and concomitant illness.
2. Preoperative radiation therapy interfering with bronchial microcirculation and endarteritis obliterans.
3. Improper surgical technique with stapled closure of the bronchus very close to the tracheal carina, creating tension in the bronchial stump closure.
4. Overzealous peribronchial dissection and consequent devascularization of the bronchus.
5. Presence of cancer at the bronchial resection margin.
6. Long bronchial stump resulting in the pooling of bronchial secretions and infection.
7. Disrupted bronchial blood circulation.
8. Faulty technique of bronchial stump closure.
9. Preexisting empyema.
10. Extended carinal resections.
11. Preoperative thoracic radiation.
12. Postoperative need for mechanical ventilation.
13. Right versus left pneumonectomy.
14. Poor nutritional status.
15. Diabetes.
16. Sepsis.
17. Age older than 70 years.
18. Underlying lung disease, including pulmonary tuberculosis, chronic infection, and chronic obstructive lung disease.
19. Preoperative immunosuppression and steroid therapy.
20. Postoperative sputum positive for acid-fast bacilli.

ESOPHAGOPLEURAL FISTULA AND EMPYEMA

This complication is an uncommon postoperative problem. It is the result of esophageal injury at the time of pneumonectomy. Extensive extrapleural dissection, especially on the right, and extensive lymph node dissection are probably the precipitating factors. Dumont and DeGraef[8] pointed out that the blood supply to the esophagus is segmental and that the part of the esophagus just below the carina has the poorest blood supply; this site of fistula formation is the commonest. The majority of fistulas after pneumonectomy occur on the right.

Takaro and colleagues[6] found 24 cases of esophagopleural fistula after pneumonectomy in 1960 occurring for tuberculosis or suppurative pulmonary disease with mortality rate of 49%. Erikson[7] in 1964 reported 3 cases of esophagopleural fistula occurring after right pneumonectomy for carcinoma of the lung. Benjamin and others[9] reported 3 cases of esophagopleural fistula after right pneumonectomy for carcinoma. Two cases occurred early in the postoperative period, and one occurred 8 months later.

Esophagoscopy and bronchoscopy were performed in each case to rule out the presence of tumor. Benjamin and colleagues[9] recommended empyema drainage followed by direct closure of the fistula with protection by a flap of pleura. After the fistula healed, the empyema was closed by the Clagett method. Engelman[10] and others reported a case of postpneumonectomy esophagopleural fistula successfully treated with a 1-stage procedure of intercostal pedicle flap closure of the fistula with an extensive thoracoplasty. The collapsed empyema space was then treated continuously irrigated with antibiotics.

The best treatment for this entity is prevention. A nasogastric tube will permit location of the esophagus. If the esophagus is injured at the time of pneumonectomy, the esophageal defect should be repaired and covered with a viable pleural flap and methylene blue should be instilled into the esophagus to determine leakage.

INVESTIGATIONS REQUIRED

The investigations that are required for diagnosis and management of postpneumonectomy sepsis are as follows.

Daily blood sampling for measuring white cell count and assessment of leukocytosis.

Daily serial chest radiographs to assess the postpneumonectomy space, air–fluid level, loculated air pockets in the pleural fluid, and contralateral lung for pneumonia.

Regular computerized chest computed tomography scan to assess the postpneumonectomy space and contralateral lung.

Regular fiberoptic bronchoscopy to assess the bronchial stump for impaired healing and defect.

Omnipaque bronchography and sinogram to assess for the bronchial stump leak.

Thoracentesis and chest tube drainage for bacteriologic examination of the pleural fluid in the postpneumonectomy space.

Omnipaque swallow and barium swallow to assess for postoperative esophagopleural fistula.

Esophagoscopy to assess esophagus for tear.

DEFINITION OF AND INTRODUCTION TO EMPYEMA THORACIS

The word empyema is used to denote the presence of pus in a natural body cavity. In thoracic medicine, that space is the empty pleural cavity created after a whole lung is removed by pneumonectomy. After pneumonectomy, the space is filled with serosanguinous fluid, which is a good

bacterial culture medium. The infecting bacteria causing empyema after pulmonary resection are often pneumococci (S pneumoniae), beta-hemolytic streptococci (S pyogenes), and S aureus. Anaerobic infections owing to peptostreptococci, Bacteroides, and fusobacteria are probably more common than is often reported. Mixed infections may occur, recording both anaerobic and aerobic organisms. It is clear that both anaerobic and aerobic cultures should be carried out routinely when infected fluid is obtained from the pleural cavity.

Gram-negative rods are found most commonly in empyema complicating esophagopleural fistula from esophageal trauma during pulmonary resection.

Clinical Manifestations

The clinical manifestation of postpneumonectomy empyema may be highly variable, depending both on the nature of the infecting organism and the competency of the patient's immune system. The spectrum ranges from an almost compete absence of symptoms to a severe illness with all the usual manifestations of systemic toxicity. The manner in which the empyema has arisen is also clearly relevant to the presenting findings, that is, whether it has followed pneumonia, surgical or other trauma or whether it is associated with mediastinitis or subdiaphragmatic sepsis.

Postpneumonectomy sepsis in the pleural space may develop for a variety of reasons. It may be related to intraoperative contamination from a lung abscess during surgical dissection. Bronchopleural fistula is another cause owing to unrecognized bronchial stump leak and bacterial contamination by infected bronchial secretions in the accumulating postpneumonectomy serosanguinous fluid, which is a good culture medium for the bacteria. Postoperative wound infection in the thoracotomy incision may extend into the pleural space and cause empyema. A subphrenic abscess may extend through the diaphragm and infect the postpneumonectomy pleural space. Poorly performed postoperative chest thoracentesis by needle or chest tube insertion has the potential to infect the pleural space.

Fever is common, although if the empyema cavity is well walled off or the patient is elderly, this symptom need not be present. General malaise and loss of weight are common features, as is pleuritic pain, which may take the form of dull chest wall discomfort. Dyspnea may result from compression of the contralateral lung from sympathetic pleural effusion, pulmonary embolism, atrial fibrillation, or cardiac tamponade owing to septic pericarditis and an associated pericardial effusion. A cough is frequently present, and, in the presence of a large bronchopleural fistula, large volumes of purulent sputum may be expectorated.

The suppurative process, if undrained and uncontrolled by appropriate antibiotics, may extend beyond the pleural cavity, with pointing occurring in an intercostal space often in the thoracotomy incision or often close to the sternum where the chest wall is thinnest. The term empyema necessitatis may be used to denote any such lesion that has ruptured through the skin surface to form a discharging sinus.

Diagnosis

The possibility of a complicating postpneumonectomy empyema should always be borne in mind in a patient who is running a febrile postoperative course. Whereas the clinical history and physical findings may be suggestive, the diagnosis can only be made with confidence when suspicious chest radiographic findings lead to thoracentesis.

The chest radiographic appearances of postpneumonectomy empyema may, in the early stages, be identical to those of an uncomplicated pleural effusion. The air–fluid level may have decreased, raising the possibility of bronchopleural fistula. The presence of loculated bubbles of air in the pleural fluid may raise suspicion for bronchopleural fistula.

A computed tomography scan of the thorax is similarly helpful. The pericardium should be assessed for pericardial effusion. The pneumonectomy space needs to be assessed for an air–fluid level and loculated air pockets. The contralateral lung should be assessed for aspirated fluid. A sample of pleural fluid must be obtained at thoracentesis to confirm the diagnosis.

Bronchoscopy and esophagogastroscopy are necessary. The bronchial stump needs to be examined for healing and fistula. The esophagus should be examined for injury.

A bronchogram is necessary by contrast study is using Omnipaque bronchography and sinogram to assess the bronchial stump.

Pathogenesis of Postpneumonectomy Empyema

Causes of nontraumatic pneumonectomy space sepsis include the following.[15]

Underlying thoracic disease

1. Pulmonary
   a. Lung abscess
   b. Bronchiectasis
   c. Tuberculosis
   d. Pneumonia
   e. Resection of lung cancer
   f. Iatrogenic esophageal tear during pulmonary resection
   g. Intraoperative errors
2. Osteomyelitis
   a. Sternum
   b. Ribs
   c. Vertebrae
3. Extrathoracic sepsis
   a. Subphrenic abscess extending through the diaphragm
   b. Transdiaphragmatic erosion of liver abscess
4. Preoperative chest injury from stabbings and gunshot wounds
5. Preoperative mediastinitis from complications during mediastinoscopy and esophageal tear

Investigation of empyema

1. Gross examination of the pleural fluid.
   a. Thin pus
   b. Thick pus
   c. Infected watery fluid
2. Pleural fluid aspiration for microscopic examination of the pleural fluid.
   a. White blood cells
   b. Bacteria
3. Microbiological examination.
   a. Type of bacteria
   b. Aerobic and anaerobic
   c. Bacterial culture
4. Complete blood sample measuring hemoglobin and white blood cell count every day.
5. Broad spectrum antibiotics selected from bacteriologic examination.
6. Bronchoscopy to assess healing of the bronchial stump.
7. Esophagoscopy to rule out esophageal iatrogenic injury during pulmonary resection.
8. Daily chest radiograph to assess the air–fluid level, a decrease in the fluid level, and the presence of multiloculated air pockets in the pneumonectomy fluid.
9. Assessment of the contralateral lung for aspiration pneumonitis from the infected postpneumonectomy space with a large bronchopleural fistula.
10. Chest computed tomography scan.
11. Two-dimensional echocardiogram to assess the pericardial space for pericarditis and pericardial effusion.

MANAGEMENT OF POSTPNEUMONECTOMY EMPYEMA

1. Preferred by most thoracic surgeons; the initial treatment is closed-tube thoracostomy with intent to cure.[16,17]
2. Bronchoscopy before discharge from the hospital.
3. The patient is fit for thoracotomy and bronchopleural fistula is evident without occurrence of pleural sepsis. The patient needs a bronchoscopy to assess the bronchus and to exclude persistent cancer in the bronchial margin. A thoracotomy should be undertaken to repair the bronchus and use vascularized pedicle to support bronchial repair. The choices are the intercostal muscle pedicle, pericardial fat pad, parietal pericardium pedicle, azygous vein flap by mobilization, ligation, and division of the proximal end at the azygous vein–superior vena cava junction, after which it is fileted open to cover the bronchus, and vascularized pedicle of omentum through upper laparotomy incision delivered into the chest through the retrosternal route.
4. Appropriate broad-spectrum antibiotic coverage must be continued for 4 weeks on the basis of bacteriologic examination.

Extent of Pneumonectomy and Postoperative Complications

Complications of pneumonectomy are classified as follows.

1. Standard pneumonectomy is a less demanding procedure, and the operative risk is less than 3%.
2. Carinal pneumonectomy is performed when the lung cancer has extended into the tracheal carina, requiring resection of the carina and the lung, and contralateral tracheobronchial anastomosis; the operative risk is increased to just higher than 5%.
3. Vocal cord dysfunction occurs when pneumectomy is on the left side and the left recurrent laryngeal nerve is vulnerable to injury.
4. Cardiac arrhythmias are frequent complication of thoracotomy and pneumonectomy.
5. Postpneumonectomy pulmonary edema and evolving hypoxia.
6. Chylothorax is recognized by the rapid accumulation of fluid in the pneumonectomy space and from fluid analysis for chylomicrons.
7. Pulmonary thromboembolism.
8. Bronchopleural fistula and empyema.
9. Esophagopleural fistula and empyema.
10. Postpneumonectomy syndrome is a rare complication after pneumonectomy. It

consists of an excessive mediastinal shift, resulting in the compression and stretching of the tracheobronchial tree and the esophagus. The aim of this study was to give a comprehensive overview of diagnosis, variety of symptoms and evaluation of surgical treatment of postpneumonectomy syndrome. Six women with a median age of 56.5 years (range, 49–65 years) developed postpneumonectomy syndrome after pneumonectomy for the treatment of lung cancer. Four presented with a right postpneumonectomy syndrome and 2 with a left postpneumonectomy syndrome. Symptoms consisted of shortness of breath in all patients and dysphagia as well as heartburn in 2 patients. Correction of postpneumonectomy syndrome required reexploration of the pneumonectomy space, reposition of the mediastinum followed by the insertion of single silicone prosthesis in 5 patients or fixation of the mediastinum with a xenopericardial graft in 1 patient.

Extent of Pneumonectomy, Clinical Manifestations, and Presentation of Postoperative Empyema

In Mearnskirk Hospital in Glasgow, 29 patients with postpneumonectomy empyema were treated by fenestration over a 12-year period.[20] This series was reported by Goldstraw.[20] Peter Goldstraw is Honorary Consultant Thoracic Surgeon to the Royal Brompton Hospital and Emeritus Professor of Thoracic Surgery at Imperial College London, UK. Seven of these patients were not considered fit enough for definitive closure and died of continuing disease or respiratory infection. Twenty-two patients went on to closure of their fenestra, and in 17 (77%) the pneumonectomy space was rendered permanently sterile. If the empyema recurred, treatment was repeated but proved less successful. Fenestration is an effective method of dealing with postpneumonectomy empyema, but also has several other advantages, particularly if the empyema is associated with a bronchopleural fistula (**Tables 1** and **2**).

Clinical Features of Empyema

Systemic features
  Pyrexia, usually high and remittent
  Rigors, sweating, malaise, and weight loss
  Polymorphonuclear leukocytosis
Local features
  Pleural pain, breathlessness, cough and infected sputum usually because of underlying lung disease, and copious purulent sputum owing to bronchopleural fistula

Clinical signs of fluid in the pleural space: dullness on percussion and absent breath sounds

EXTENT OF PNEUMONECTOMY AND POSTOPERATIVE COMPLICATIONS

Complications of pneumonectomy are classified as follows.

Standard pneumonectomy is a less demanding procedure, and the operative risk is less than 3%.

Carinal pneumonectomy is performed when the lung cancer has extended into the tracheal carina, requiring resection of the carina and the lung, and contralateral tracheobronchial anastomosis; the operative risk is increased to just higher than 5%.

Vocal cord dysfunction occurs when pneumectomy is on the left side and the left recurrent laryngeal nerve is vulnerable to injury.

Cardiac arrhythmias are frequent complication of thoracotomy and pneumonectomy.

Postpneumonectomy pulmonary edema and evolving hypoxia.

Chylothorax is recognized by the rapid accumulation of fluid in the pneumonectomy space and from fluid analysis for chylomicrons.

Pulmonary thromboembolism.

Bronchopleural fistula and empyema.

Esophagopleural fistula and empyema.

Postpneumonectomy Syndrome

Postpneumonectomy syndrome is a rare complication after pneumonectomy. It consists of an excessive mediastinal shift resulting in compression and stretching of the tracheobronchial tree and the esophagus. The aim of this study was to give a comprehensive overview of diagnosis, variety of symptoms and evaluation of surgical treatment of postpneumonectomy syndrome. Six women with a median age of 56.5 years (range, 49–65 years) developed postpneumonectomy syndrome after pneumonectomy for the treatment of lung cancer. Four presented with a right postpneumonectomy syndrome and 2 with a left postpneumonectomy syndrome. Symptoms consisted of shortness of breath in all patients and dysphagia as well as heartburn in 2 patients. Correction of postpneumonectomy syndrome required reexploration of the pneumonectomy space, reposition of the mediastinum followed by the insertion of single silicone prosthesis in 5 patients or fixation of the mediastinum with a xenopericardial graft in 1 patient.

SUMMARY
Natural History of Empyema Thoracis: Definition and Introduction of Empyema Thoracis

The word 'empyema' is used to denote the presence of pus in a natural body cavity. In thoracic medicine that space is the empty pleural cavity created after whole lung is removed by pneumonectomy. After pneumonectomy, the space becomes filled with serosanguinous fluid which is a good bacterial culture medium. The infecting bacteria causing empyema after pulmonary resection are often pneumococci (S pneumoniae), beta-hemolytic streptococci (S pyogenes), and S aureus. Anaerobic infections owing to

Table 1
Three phases of empyema pathogenesis – 3 phases

Phase of Empyema	Early Phase I – 1st Week	Intermediate Phase II – 2nd Week	Late Phase III – 3rd Week
Early acute exudative ⟶	Acute septic pleurisy; free serous infected fluid, thin and watery	–	–
Intermediate subacute "fibrinopurulent"	⟶	Subacute suppurative effusion gradually thickens, becomes more purulent; limiting adhesions develop with multiple loculations	–
Chronic "true purulent empyema" 4–6 weeks later	⟶		Localized abscess is formed with its walls lined by fibrinous deposit

Table 2
Symptoms and signs of empyema: clinical findings

Phase of Empyema		
Early - Phase I Acute Pleurisy, Exudative	Intermediate -Phase II Fibrinopurulent	Late - Phase III Empyema Pyopneumothorax
Sharp stabbing pain, aggravated by chest movements	General toxemia, dyspnea, fever, malaise, fatigue, and sweating episodes	General, toxemia, fever, malaise, loss of appetite, loss of weight
Pleural rub	Local – chest pain worsened by breathing	Local – chest pain
Chest movements and breath sounds are decreased by conscious efforts to decrease chest pain		
Moderate fever and dry cough usually accompany chest pain		

peptostreptococci, Bacteroides, and fusobacteria are probably more common than is often reported. Mixed infections may occur, recording both anaerobic and aerobic organisms. It is clear that both anaerobic and aerobic cultures should be carried out routinely when infected fluid is obtained from the pleural cavity.[21] Gram-negative rods are found most commonly in empyema complicating esophagopleural fistula from esophageal trauma during pulmonary resection.

Clinical Manifestations

The clinical manifestation of postpneumonectomy empyema may be highly variable, depending both on the nature of the infecting organism and the competency of the patient's immune system. The spectrum ranges from an almost compete absence of symptoms to a severe illness with all the usual manifestations of systemic toxicity. The manner in which the empyema has arisen is also clearly relevant to the presenting findings, whether it has followed pneumonia, surgical or other trauma, or whether it is associated with mediastinitis or subdiaphragmatic sepsis.

Postpneumonectomy sepsis in the pleural space may develop for a variety of reasons. It may be related to intraoperative contamination from a lung abscess during surgical dissection. Bronchopleural fistula is another cause owing to an unrecognized bronchial stump leak and bacterial contamination by infected bronchial secretions in the accumulating postpneumonectomy serosanguinous fluid, which is a good culture medium for the bacteria. Unrecognized postoperative wound infection in the thoracotomy incision may extend into the pleural space and cause empyema. Subphrenic abscess may extend through the diaphragm and infect the postpneumonectomy pleural space. A poorly performed postoperative

chest thoracentesis by needle or chest tube insertion has the potential to infect the pleural space.

Fever is common, although if the empyema cavity is well walled off or the patient is elderly this symptom need not be present. General malaise and loss of weight are common features, as is the pleuritic pain, which may take the form of dull chest wall discomfort. Dyspnea may result from compression of the contralateral lung from sympathetic pleural effusion, pulmonary embolism, atrial fibrillation, or cardiac tamponade owing to septic pericarditis and associated pericardial effusion. A cough is frequently present, and, in the presence of a large bronchopleural fistula, large volumes of serosanguinous fluid or frank purulent sputum may be expectorated (**Tables 1** and **2**).

The suppurative process, if undrained and uncontrolled by appropriate antibiotics, may extend beyond the pleural cavity, with pointing occurring in an intercostal space, often in the thoracotomy incision or often close to the sternum where the chest wall is thinnest. The term empyema necessitatis may be used to denote any such lesion that has ruptured through the skin surface to form a discharging sinus.

Diagnosis

The possibility of a complicating postpneumonectomy empyema should always be borne in mind in a patient who is running a febrile postoperative course. Whereas the clinical history and physical findings may be suggestive, the diagnosis can only be made with confidence when suspicious chest radiographic findings leads to thoracentesis and analysis of pleural fluid.

The chest radiographic appearances of postpneumonectomy empyema may, in the early stages, be identical to those of an uncomplicated pleural effusion. An air–fluid level may have decreased, raising the possibility of bronchopleural fistula. The presence of loculated bubbles of air in the pleural fluid may raise suspicion of bronchopleural fistula.

A computed tomography scan of the thorax is similarly helpful in establishing the diagnosis. The pericardium should be assessed for pericardial effusion. The pneumonectomy space needs to be assessed for the air–fluid level and loculated air pockets. The contralateral lung should be assessed for aspirated fluid. A sample of pleural fluid must be obtained at thoracentesis to confirm the diagnosis.

Bronchoscopy and esophagogastroscopy are necessary for establishing a diagnosis. The bronchial stump needs to be examined for leaks, healing, and formation and size of bronchial fistula. The esophagus should be examined for intraoperative transmural injury during pneumonectomy.

A bronchogram is necessary by contrast study is using Omnipaque bronchography and sinogram to assess the bronchial stump. Contrast thin liquid barium is helpful in assessing for esophageal–pleural fistula.

CLINICS CARE POINTS

- Bronchopleural fistula and empyema complicating pneumonectomy.

- Esophageal injury in the mediastinum during pulmonary resection and complicating postpneumonectomy empyema from esophagopleural fistula.

- Pathogenesis of sepsis in the postpneumonectomy space due to infecting bacteria.

- Factors predisposing to the formation of bronchopleural fistula.

- Clinical presentation of postpneumonectomy empyema.

- Management of postpneumonectomy empyema.

- Drainage procedures in the management of postpneumonectomy empyema.

REFERENCES

1. Boyd AD, Spencer FC. Bronchopleural fistulas. Ann Thorac Surg 1972;13:195.
2. James TW, Faber LP. Indications for pneumonectomy. Pneumonectomy for malignant disease. Chest Surg Clin 1999;9:291–309.
3. Clagett OT, Geraci JE. A procedure for the management of postpneumonectomy empyema. J Thorac Cardiovasc Surg 1963;45:141.
4. Eloesser L. An operation for tuberculous empyema. Ann Thorac Surg 1969;8:355.
5. Stafford ED, Clagett OT. Postpneumonectomy empyema. J Thorac Cardiovasc Surg 1972;63:771.
6. Takaro J, Walkup HE, Okano T. Esophagopleural fistula as a complication of thoracic surgery. A collective review. J Thorac Cardiovasc Surg 1960;40:179.
7. Eriksen KR. Esophagopleural fistula diagnosed by microscopic examination of pleural fluid. Acta Chir Scand 1964;128:771.
8. Dumont A, De Graef J. La fistule esophago-pleurale, complication tardive de la pneumonectomie. Lyon Chir 1961;57:481.
9. Benjamin I, Olsen AM, Ellis FH Jr. Esophagopleural fistula, a rare postpneumonectomy complication. Ann Thorac Surg 1969;7:139.
10. Engelman RM, Spencer FC, Berg P. Postpneumonectomy esophageal fistula successful one-stage repair. J Thorac Cardiovasc Surg 1970;59:871.
11. Zaheer S, Allen MS, Cassivi SD, et al. Postpneumonectomy empyema: results after Claggett procedure. Ann Thorac Surg 2006;82:279–86.
12. Shamji FM, Ginsberg RJ, Cooper JD. Open window thoracostomy in the management of post-pneumonectomy empyema with or without bronchopleural fistula. J Thorac Cardiovasc Surg 1983;86:818–22.
13. Darling GE, Abdurahman A, Yi QL, et al. Risk of a right pneumonectomy: role of bronchopleural fistula. Ann Thorac Surg 2005;79:433–7.
14. Deschamps C, Bernard A, Nichols FC 3rd, et al. Empyema and bronchopleural fistula after pneumonectomy: factors affecting incidence. Ann Thorac Surg 2001;72:243–7 [discussion: 248].
15. Wright CD, Wain JC, Mathisen DJ, et al. Postpneumonectomy bronchopleural fistula after sutured bronchial closure: incidence, risk factors, and management. J Thorac Cardiovasc Surg 1996;112:1367–71.
16. Conlan AA, Kopec SE. Indications for pneumonectomy. Pneumonectomy for benign disease. Chest Surg Clin N Am 1999;9:311.
17. Bribriesco A, Patterson GA. Management of postpneumonectomy bronchopleural fistula: from thoracoplasty to transsternal closure. Thorac Surg Clin 2018;28:323–35.
18. Le Roux BT, Mohlala ML, Odell JA, et al. Suppurative diseases of the lung and pleural space. Part 1, empyema thoracis and lung abscess. Curr Probl Surg 1986;23(1):1.
19. Naef AP, Discussion of Barker WL, Faber LP, et al. Management of persistent bronchopleural fistulas. J Thorac Cardiovasc Surg 1971;62:393.
20. Goldstraw P. Treatment of postpneumonectomy empyema: the case for fenestration. Thorax Dec 1979;34(6):740–5.
21. Dorman JP, Campbell D, Grover FL, et al. Open thoracostomy drainage of Postpneumonectomy empyema with bronchopleural fistula. J Thorac Cardiovasc Surg 1973;66(6):979–81.

Delays in Managing Lung Cancer
The Importance of Fast-Tracking in the Clinical Care

Farid M. Shamji, MBBS, FRCSC, FACS[a],*, Gilles Beauchamp, MD, FRCSC[b]

KEYWORDS

- Biology of lung cancer • Minimizing delays in treatment • Prognosis in lung cancer

KEY POINTS

- Investigations necessary in the diagnosis and staging of lung cancer.
- Factors of prognostic importance in lung cancer.
- Four intervals in the life history of lung cancer.
- Cell biology: cell proliferation and tumor growth.
- Tumor volume doubling time.
- Lymphatic spread of lung cancer: N1, N2, and N3.

INTRODUCTION

In no disease is early diagnosis more desirable, because surgical resection offers the only hope of cure. In the face of suggestive symptoms, a normal plain chest radiograph does not exclude the diagnosis, and investigation is essential. The various imaging changes seen on computerized tomography (CT scan) and PET scan provide strong suggestive evidence of lung cancer, but proof of diagnosis rests on histologic examination, material that may be obtained by one of the following diagnostic procedures.

Bronchoscopy

The centrally located neoplasms are within range of bronchoscopic vision and can be biopsied. Trap specimens of sputum aspirated by bronchial washing related to more peripherally situated tumors may show malignant cells.

Mediastinoscopy

Cervical mediastinoscopy for right and left lung cancer is important in the staging and planning surgical treatment of lung cancer. Equally important is the addition of left anterior mediastinotomy for lung cancer in the left upper lobe and left hilum when the lymphatic course is different.

Fine Needle Aspiration Biopsy

This is feasible for peripherally situated tumors with diminished risks of dissemination and local complications.

Thoracentesis and Pleural Biopsy

If there is a blood-stained pleural effusion or presence of pleural mass or thickening, a specimen should be obtained through a needle and examined for neoplastic cells.

a University of Ottawa, General Campus, Ottawa Hospital, 501 Smyth Road, Ottawa, Ontario K1H 8L6, Canada;
b Thoracic Surgery Unit, Department of Surgery, Maisonneuve-Rosemount, Hospital, University of Montreal, 5415 L'Assomption Boulevard, Montreal, Quebec H1T 2M4, Canada
* Corresponding author.
E-mail address: faridshamji@hotmail.com

Thorac Surg Clin 31 (2021) 417–427
https://doi.org/10.1016/j.thorsurg.2021.07.002

Lymph Node Biopsy

Biopsy by needle aspiration under ultrasound guidance of a palpable supraclavicular lymph node or by mediastinoscopy of enlarged mediastinal lymph node can provide adequate piece of tissue for reliable means of confirmation.

Exploratory Thoracotomy

In view of the grave prognosis, a diagnostic thoracotomy is justified if the preceding measures have failed or are inapplicable.

MANAGEMENT OF LUNG CANCER

The 3 important clinical pointers in the management of lung cancer are as follows:

1. Effect of delays in the diagnosis and surgical treatment of lung cancer
2. Effect of delays on prognosis in patients with non–small-cell lung cancer (NSCLC)
3. Effect of delays in the outcome of managing lung cancer

Can fast-tracking care for cancer lessen the delay and improve patient care? Efforts to reduce delays in managing lung cancer should not cease even though they may not affect the prognosis. It is universally acknowledged that the prognosis of lung cancer is very poor, with overall 5-year survival figures of approximately 10% to 15% worldwide.[1] What is less well recognized is that the picture has changed very little over the past 20 years, and that this is in sharp distinction to other solid tumors, in which not only are survival rates better, in the order of 60% to 90%, but they have been increasing (improving) fairly rapidly and continue to do so over a comparable time.

Comprehensive population-based registry data for 5-year survival of the 5000 patients in North America diagnosed with lung cancer in 1999 was 15% compared with 60%, 79%, 87%, and 92% for colorectal, cervical, prostate, and breast cancer, respectively.[2] There is merit therefore in considering what might influence and be responsible for this poor outcome in lung cancer.

"Lung cancer is a typically difficult cancer to treat, but even harder to cure when there is a late diagnosis. Those with lung cancer often take a long time to visit their doctor, sometimes because they feel there is a stigma around chest symptoms when you are a long-term smoker. We need more initiatives like this to find innovative new ways to facilitate early diagnosis."

FACTORS AFFECTING PROGNOSIS IN LUNG CANCER

The factors that affect prognosis in lung cancer are principally the stage and related performance status at presentation, histology (that is the biological activity of the tumor), and the changing histologic descriptors in adenocarcinoma spectrum disorder becoming most common cell type in NSCLC at 50% surpassing previously more common squamous cell type now reduced to 30%, comorbidity, age and sex of the patients, and the time interval between first symptom and treatment.

Some of these factors are not modified. In theory, however, reducing intervals between presentation and treatment might downstage patients and allow for an improvement in survival. There are excellent data to show the early-stage NSCLC, stage I and stage II, has better survival[3]; there is less good but nevertheless fairly convincing evidence that very early-stage disease (that is, small asymptomatic lesions measuring <10 mm size) have an even better prognosis. The size of the tumor, measured in millimeters, provides insight into the varying number of cancer cells in 1-mm, 5-mm, and 10-mm size tumors; tumor volume doubling time less than 30 days, 30 to 35 days, and 40 days and more.

There are, of course, other ways of reducing lung cancer mortality. In the very long term, over a period of decades, prevention is clearly key. In the longer term, over a 5-year to 10-year time span, the identification and treatment of very early asymptomatic disease offers good prospects of cure (by lung cancer screening).[4] Lung cancer screening program with low-dose CT was introduced 20 years ago for early identification of suspicious lung lesions and early treatment. At the present time, however, efforts to improve lung cancer mortality have to reside in reducing delays to treatment and ensuring better access to specialist appropriate care.[5] However, because the best appropriate care for cure is surgery and this modality has not changed appreciably, although now technically more adroit, for many years,[6] and because the cure rate will remain low unless a higher proportion of patients present and can be managed while at early stage I and stage II, the question of interval delays and their effect on prognosis is of great importance.

Professor Jon Emery, from the University of Melbourne Center for Cancer Research and Department of General Practice, will present initial results from the CHEST Trial at the Clinical Oncology Society of Australia Annual Scientific Meeting during Lung Cancer Awareness Month (November). He says that efforts to improve early detection of lung cancer are vital.

"Lung cancer remains Australia's biggest cancer killer and is expected to claim over 9000 lives this year. Survival rates for the cancer type remain low at less than 14% – mainly because over two-thirds of those with the disease are diagnosed too late to be successfully treated."

The CHEST Trial is the first of its kind to successfully encourage those at higher risk of lung cancer to seek medical attention when chest symptoms develop. The research involved more than 500 Australians who are long-term smokers, aged older than 55, with a history of heavy smoking, and who are therefore at higher risk of lung cancer.

Participants in the trial were given a one-on-one consultation with a research nurse as well as a self-help manual informed by psychological theory, to help them understand what symptoms to look for and promote them seeking help sooner. Researchers tracked which patients visited a general practitioner (GP) when they developed respiratory symptoms.

Professor Emery says the initiative is unique when compared with other trials, which have focused on CT scanning or symptom awareness in the general population.

"In the past, there have been campaigns to make all Australians aware of lung cancer symptoms, which include a chronic cough, wheezing, shortness of breath, fatigue, weight loss and coughing up blood. We wanted to trial an initiative specifically targeted at those who were at higher risk of developing lung cancer and empower them to act when respiratory symptoms appeared."

The study found that those who were given the intervention were significantly more likely to see their GP when symptoms developed, and researchers believe that the initiative could be a cost-effective way to help improve lung cancer survival rates.

STAGES IN THE DIAGNOSIS OF LUNG CANCER

The only prospect of cure for NSCLC is by surgical resection, which may entail a radical pneumonectomy for large centrally located tumor or, in most cases, lobectomy or segmental pulmonary resection for localized peripheral cancer. Sleeve carinal pneumonectomy or lung-sparing sleeve lobectomy may become necessary in special circumstances.

In considering the life history of a tumor and points at which medical intervention can take place, 4 intervals are pertinent:

1. Between first malignant change and first symptom
2. Between first symptom and presentation
3. Between first presentation and confirmation of diagnosis
4. Between diagnosis and staging/treatment

Interval Between First Malignant Change and First Symptom

This is the very long asymptomatic period between the first malignant change in the bronchial epithelium and the first symptom. It is a reasonable assumption that the change from Tx to T1 and then T2 or T3 or T4 is not only a local increase in size, but an increase in accompanying metastatic potential as well; that is, there is a greater chance that, as the tumor enlarges, the stage will increase in lymphatic metastases from N0 to N1, N2, N3, or distant metastases from M0 to M1a, M1b, and M1c.[7] There are reasonably good data, particularly from Japanese studies, that this is the case, certainly for tumors between 0.5 and 3 cm.[8,9] For example, in a study by Oda and colleagues,[9] the proportion of the 409 resected specimens that had nodal disease (N1, N2, N3) was 0% for primary tumors <10 mm in diameter, 21% for those of 11 to 20 mm, 23% for those of 21 to 30 mm, and 48% for tumors more than 30 mm in diameter. Unfortunately, most T1 lesions are asymptomatic. Tumors can enlarge markedly within lung tissue and remain silent clinically. Many of these have metastatic potential and do metastasize when they achieve a size of approximately 1 cm (10 mm). Thus, when the first symptoms begin there is, in practice, a high chance that the tumor will be at an advanced stage, either locally invasive T3 or T4 with nodal involvement N1-N2-N3, or it will present with metastatic symptoms, such as back pain.

Interval Between First Symptom and Presentation

The interval between the patient's first cancer-related symptom and presentation (within-patient delay) is currently under intense investigation as a possible target for health education action. The reasons why patients present when they do and with the symptoms they do is a highly complex phenomenon that is influenced by various factors such as age and health expectations, background symptoms, fear, and their impressions about health care.[10] However, it is likely that attempts to shorten this interval will increase the survival chances of only few patients with an eventual diagnosis of lung cancer.

Interval Between First Presentation and Confirmation of Diagnosis

The third interval is between first presentation to any doctor and a confirmed diagnosis in secondary care. A considerable amount of activity is presently taking place to encourage primary care physicians to recognize potential cancer symptoms and to expedite referral to specialists and for the specialists to rapidly diagnose and stage these patients. In the United Kingdom at present, and in parallel with European Health Care Systems, there are national recommendations for these pathways that are predicated on the assumption that reducing these intervals, as well as reducing patient distress, will improve survival.[11]

Interval Between Diagnosis and Staging/Treatment

The fourth interval is between a confirmed diagnosis, that is, when the patient is managed as a case of lung cancer, and staging/treatment. Once again, health care systems are investing considerable resources in reducing this and making it uniform. There is convincing evidence that, for some patients who are potentially curable, delays at this point can decrease their chances for survival.[12] Furthermore, the exponential growth pattern of tumors suggests that stage migration, that is, the change in a tumor staging from, for example, I to II, II to III, or III to IV, is likely to be a far more rapid event when the primary tumor is large or when there is early nodal disease than when the tumor is, for example, a small T1 lesion.[13] These points, based on considerations of tumor biology, suggest that survival should be improved if within-patient and within–health system delays are short.

STUDY BY MYRDAL AND COLLEAGUES

The article by Myrdal and colleagues[14] in this issue of *Thorax* from 2004, examined the impact of delay in diagnosis and treatment on the prognosis for lung cancer patients. It was based on retrospective analysis on patients diagnosed with NSCLC over a 5-year period.

Two types of delay were studied: (1) symptom to treatment delay, defined as the length of time from first onset of symptoms to the start of treatment, and (2) hospital delay, defined as the length of time from the hospital visit to the start of treatment. The impact of these separate delays on survival was then assessed.

The results showed that the mean first symptom to treatment delay was 5.8 months and was shortest in those patients with advanced disease (3.9 months). Only 9% of patients with stage I-II disease were treated within 3 months of first symptoms. Mean hospital delay was 2.5 months and appeared to be longer for those patients

with potentially curable lung cancer, but the difference was not statistically significant. On average, treatment was started 1.4 months earlier in patients with stage IV disease than in those with stage I-II disease. Survival was negatively influenced by a short delay time between first onset of symptoms and treatment: 3-year survival was 11% for patients within 3 months and 35% for delays of more than 6 months. Similarly, patients with the shortest hospital delay (<30 days) had a poorer prognosis.

The main conclusions of Myrdal and colleagues[14] were that delays in the investigation and treatment of lung cancer exceeded the recommended time scales advised by the Swedish Lung Cancer Study Group in most of their patients. They state that neither patient nor hospital delay appeared to negatively influence survival. Patients with advanced tumor stage who presented and received treatment within 30 days of the first hospital visit fared less well than those with a longer delay. They also suggested that, as NSCLC tumors have both varied cell doubling times and aggressiveness, further information is needed to allow identification of patients who have tumors that would benefit particularly from prompt treatment.

CELL BIOLOGY: CELL PROLIFERATION AND GROWTH OF HUMAN TUMORS

Tumor growth can be determined by estimating tumor volume as a function of time.[15] *Exponential growth of tumors* will occur if the rates of cell production and of cell loss or death are proportional to the number of cells present in the population. *Exponential growth* implies that the time taken for a tumor to double its volume is constant and often leads to the false impression that the rate of tumor growth is accelerating with time.

Increase in the diameter of a human tumor from 0.5 cm (5 mm) to 1.0 cm (10 mm) may escape clinical detection, whereas increase in the diameter of a tumor from 5 to 10 cm is more dramatic and is likely to cause new clinical symptoms. Both require 3 volume doublings; during exponential growth they will occur over the same period of time.

Estimates of the growth rates of untreated human tumors have been limited by the following constraints: (1) Only tumors that are unresponsive to therapy can ethically be followed without treatment; limited data are available from older studies, mostly for metastases, but almost all patients now receive treatment. There have been few measurements of the growth of primary tumors. (2) Accurate measurements can be made only on tumors from selected sites. Most studies have examined lung metastases using serial radiographs, although CT and MRI scans (Robert Cusimano and Farid M. Shamji's article, "Superior Vena Cava Resection and Reconstruction with Resection of Primary Lung Cancer and Mediastinal Tumor," in this issue) now allow accurate estimates of tumor volumes in most organs of the body. (3) The limited observation period between the time of tumor detection and either death of the host or the initiation of some form of therapy represents only a small fraction of the history of the tumor's growth.

Despite these limitations, there are many published estimates of the growth rate of human tumors. Steel[16] reviewed published measurements of the rate of growth of 780 human tumors, and estimates of volume doubling time for several types of tumors are summarized in **Table 1**. A few general conclusions may be stated:

1. There is a wide variation in growth rate, even among tumors of the same histologic type and site of origin.
2. Representative mean doubling times for lung metastases of common tumors in humans are in the same range of 2 to 3 months.
3. There is a tendency for childhood tumors and adult tumors that are known to be responsive

to chemotherapy (eg, lymphoma, cancer of the testis) to grow more rapidly than less responsive tumors (eg, cancer of the colon).
4. Metastases tend to grow more rapidly than the primary tumor in the same patient.

Tumors are unlikely to be detected until they grow to approximately 1 g, and tumors of this size will contain approximately 1 billion (10^9) cells. There is indirect evidence that many tumors arise from a single cell, and a tumor containing approximately 10^9 cells will have undergone approximately 30 doublings in volume before clinical detection (because of cell loss, this will involve more than 30 consecutive divisions of the initial cells). After 10 further doublings in volume, the tumor would weigh approximately 1 kilogram (10^{12} cells), a size that may be lethal to the host. Thus, the range of size over which the growth of a tumor may be studied represents a rather short and late part of its total growth history (**Figs. 1** and **2**). There is evidence (eg, for breast cancer) that the probability of metastatic spread increases with the size of the primary tumor, but the long preclinical history of the tumor may allow cancer cells to metastasize before detection. Thus, early clinical detection may be expected to reduce but not to prevent the subsequent appearance of metastases.

Table 1
Volume doubling time (Td) for representative human tumors

Tumor Type	Number of Tumors	Volume Doubling Time,[a] Weeks
Primary lung cancer		
Adenocarcinoma	64	21
Squamous cell carcinoma	85	12
Anaplastic carcinoma	55	11
Breast cancer		
Primary	17	14
Lung metastases	44	11
Soft tissues metastases	66	3
Colon/rectum		
Primary	19	90
Lung metastases	56	14
Lymphoma		
Lymph node lesions	27	4
Lung metastases of		
Carcinoma of testis	80	4
Childhood tumors	47	4
Adult sarcomas	58	7

[a] Geometric mean values.
Data from Steel GG. Growth Kinetics of Tumors: Cell Population Kinetics in Relation to the Growth and Treatment of Cancer. Clarendon Press; 1977.

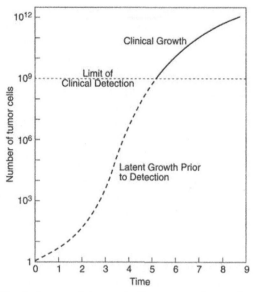

Fig. 1. Exponential growth. (*From* Tannock IF, Hill R, Bristow R, Harrington L. Chapter 9: Cell Proliferation and Tumor Growth. The Basic Science of Oncology. 4th ed. McGraw-Hill Professional: 2004.)

The growth rate of a tumor in its preclinical phase can only be estimated indirectly. In patients, one may study the time to appearance of recurrent tumors after treatment that is curative in only some of the patients, so that growth in others may be assumed to derive from a small number of residual cells. These studies support the concept that growth is more rapid in the preclinical phase of a disease, such as breast cancer, but there is little evidence for deceleration of growth during the clinical phase of rapidly progressive malignancies such as Wilms' tumor or Burkitt lymphoma.

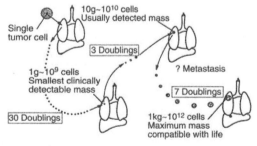

Fig. 2. A human solid tumor must undergo approximately 30 to 33 doublings in volume from a single cell before it achieves a detectable size at a weight of 1 to 10 g. Metastases may have been established before detection of the primary tumor. Only a few further doublings of volume lead to a tumor whose size ($\geq$5 cm) is incompatible with life. (*From* Tannock IF, Hill R, Bristow R, Harrington L. Chapter 9: Cell Proliferation and Tumor Growth. The Basic Science of Oncology. 4th ed. McGraw-Hill Professional: 2004.)

Deceleration of growth of large tumors is probably due to increasing cell death and decreasing cell proliferation as tumor nutrition deteriorates. Also, tumors often contain a high proportion of nonmalignant cells such as macrophages, lymphocytes, and fibroblasts, and the proliferation and migration of these cells will influence changes in tumor volume. Tumor growth may also be slow at very early stages of development (see **Table 1**). Tumor cells may have to overcome immunologic and other host defense mechanisms, and they cannot expand to a large size until they have induced proliferation of new blood vessels (*angiogenesis*) to support them.

FACTORS AFFECTING PROGNOSIS IN LUNG CANCER

The factors that affect prognosis in lung cancer are principally the stage and related performance status at presentation, histology (that is the biological activity of the tumor), and the changing histologic descriptors with adenocarcinoma spectrum disorder becoming the most common cell type in NSCLC at 50% after once more common squamous cell type now reduced to 30%, comorbidity, age and sex of the patients, and the time interval between first symptom and treatment.

Some of these factors are not modified. In theory, however, reducing intervals between clinical presentation and treatment might downstage patients and allow for an improvement in survival. Asking the first question about clinical presentation with emphasis on the nature of symptoms and how this determines the prognosis is the beginning in the first step. Staging of the cancer is the second step. There must be clear understanding of the clinical presentation, analysis of pertinent symptoms, and relating this to prognosis. The importance of all the presenting symptoms is relevant before conducting a focused physical examination, and the investigations will be the third step in the process. Staging of lung cancer cannot be a hurried process and there are excellent data to show that early-stage disease (stage I, stage II, stage IIIA) has better survival,[3] and there is less good but nevertheless fairly convincing evidence that very early-stage disease (that is, small <10 mm diameter asymptomatic lesions) have an even better prognosis. Staging of lung cancer needs more understanding than simply labeling the cancer in different stages of development, as stage I, stage II, and stage III. The size of the tumor, measured in millimeters, provides insight into the number of cancer cells in 1 mm, 5 mm, and 10 mm sized tumors; tumor volume doubling time less than 30 days, 30 to 35 days, and 40 days and more. A deeper understanding of the clinical presentation and analysis of the clinical history is essential, requiring focused understanding of each symptom.

The nonspecific clinical presentation about causation of lung cancer that needs special attention is as follows: occupation in mining iron ore, asbestos, uranium, beryllium, and nickel; heavy cigarette smoking and the precise relationship between cigarette smoking and bronchial carcinoma and the carcinogen exposure; and the amount of cigarette smoking. Cigarette smoking is not the only cause of bronchial carcinoma; other causative factors include passive smoking, exposure to exhaust fumes, and cooking oil fumes.

The clinical presentation of symptom is in 1 of 5 ways: (1) with one, some or all of the cardinal symptoms of respiratory disease and none are specific for lung cancer: cough, hemoptysis, chest pain, dyspnea, and wheeze; (2) without symptoms and because of an abnormality detected on chest radiograph made for routine purpose: lung nodule or mass that could be due to tuberculosis, pneumonia, granuloma due to fungal infection, amyloid deposit, or lung cancer, lymphoma; (3) hoarseness due to laryngitis or tumor, recurrent laryngeal nerve palsy, superior vena cava obstruction for which there are many causes, seizures, pathologic fracture due to weakness in the long bones or spine; (4) with nonspecific symptoms such as cachexia with loss of appetite and weight, insomnia, dyspepsia, and so on; (5) with what may be called infrequently humoral or neural concomitants of the disease: pulmonary paraneoplastic syndromes that include pulmonary osteoarthropathy, hypercalcemia, syndrome of inappropriate antidiuretic hormone secretion, carcinoid syndrome and carcinoid crisis, gynecomastia, galactorrhea, clubbing, myopathy, and autonomic neuropathy, sensory and motor neuropathy, Lambert-Eaton Syndrome, limbic encephalopathy, dermatomyositis, and neuropathy; (6) exposure to carcinogens in prolonged cigarette smoking, exposure to cooking oil fumes in poor ventilated areas, exposure to diesel fumes, exposure to radon gas, exposure in mining of iron ore, uranium, asbestos, beryllium, and nickel, and carcinogenic viruses HPV 16 and 18.

CELL BIOLOGY TO ANALYZE CELL PROLIFERATION AND TUMOR GROWTH

Tumor growth can be determined by estimating tumor volume as a function of time. *Exponential growth of tumors* will occur if the rates of cell production and of cell loss or death are proportional to the number of cells present in the population. *Exponential growth* implies that the time taken for a tumor to double its volume is constant and often leads to the false impression that the rate of tumor growth is accelerating with time.[17]

Exponential Growth

Hypothetical growth curve for a human tumor, showing the long latent period in months before detection. Tumors may show an early lag phase and progressive slowing of growth at large size. The Time factor in the graph is in months (see **Fig. 1**).

A human solid tumor must undergo approximately 30 to 33 doublings in volume from a single cell before it achieves a detectable size at a weight of 1 to 10 g. Metastases may have been established before detection of the primary tumor. Only a few further doublings of volume lead to a tumor whose size (≥5 cm) is incompatible with life (see **Fig. 2**).

Increase in the diameter of a human tumor from 0.5 cm (5 mm) to 1.0 cm (10 mm) may escape clinical detection, whereas increase in the diameter of a tumor from 1.0 cm to 3.0 cm permits clinical and radiological detection, and from 5 to 10 cm is more dramatic and is likely to cause new clinical symptoms. Both require 3 volume doublings; during exponential growth they will occur over the same period of time.

Estimates of the growth rates of untreated human tumors have been limited by the following constraints: (1) Only tumors that are unresponsive to therapy can ethically be followed without treatment; limited data are available from older studies, mostly for metastases, but almost all patients now receive treatment. There have been few measurements of the growth of primary tumors. (2) Accurate measurements can be made only on tumors from selected sites. Most studies have examined lung metastases using serial radiographs, although CT and MRI scans now allow accurate estimates of tumor volumes in most organs of the body. (3) The limited observation period between the time of tumor detection and either death of the host or the initiation of some form of therapy represents only a small fraction of the history of the tumor's growth.

Despite these limitations, there are many published estimates of the growth rate of human tumors. Steel (1977)[18] reviewed published measurements of the rate of growth of 780 human tumors and estimates of volume doubling time for several types of tumors are summarized in **Table 1** and a few general conclusions may be stated:

5. There is a wide variation in growth rate, even among tumors of the same histologic type and site of origin.

6. Representative mean doubling times for lung metastases of common tumors in humans are in the same range of 2 to 3 months.
7. There is a tendency for childhood tumors and adult tumors that are known to be responsive to chemotherapy (eg, lymphoma, cancer of the testis) to grow more rapidly than less responsive tumors (eg, cancer of the colon).
8. Metastases tend to grow more rapidly than the primary tumor in the same patient.

Tumors are unlikely to be detected until they grow to approximately 1 g (10 mm), and tumors of this size will contain approximately 100 million (10^8) cells. There is indirect evidence that many tumors arise from a single cell, and a tumor containing about 10^8 cells will have undergone approximately 30 doublings in volume before clinical detection (because of cell loss, this will involve more than 30 consecutive divisions of the initial cells).[13,14] After 10 further doublings in volume, the tumor would weigh approximately 1 kg (10^{12} cells), a size that may be lethal to the host. Thus, the range of size over which the growth of a tumor may be studied represents a rather short and late part of its total growth history (see **Fig. 1**). There is evidence (eg, for breast cancer) that the probability of metastatic spread increases with the size of the primary tumor, but the long preclinical history of the tumor may allow cancer cells to metastasize before detection. Thus, early clinical detection may be expected to reduce but not to prevent the subsequent appearance of metastases.

The growth rate of a tumor in its preclinical phase can only be estimated indirectly. In patients, one may study the time to appearance of recurrent tumors after treatment that is curative in only some of the patients, so that growth in others may be assumed to derive from a small number of residual cells. These studies support the concept that growth is more rapid in the preclinical phase of a disease, such as breast cancer, but there is little evidence for deceleration of growth during the clinical phase of rapidly progressive malignancies such as Wilms' tumor or Burkitt lymphoma.

Deceleration of growth of large tumors is probably due to increasing cell death and decreasing cell proliferation as tumor nutrition deteriorates. Also, tumors often contain a high proportion of nonmalignant cells, such as macrophages, lymphocytes, and fibroblasts, and the proliferation and migration of these cells will influence changes in tumor volume. Tumor growth may also be slow at very early stages of development (see **Figs. 1** and **2**). Tumor cells may have to overcome immunologic and other host defense mechanisms, and they cannot expand to a large size until they have induced proliferation of new blood vessels (*angiogenesis*) to support them.

The following was noted in the retrospective analysis:

42% of patients had adenocarcinoma, a figure probably 3 times higher than in comparable UK populations, which may influence the overall natural history of this group of patients with NSCLC.

Recall of first symptoms is likely to be difficult for patients, given this serious diagnosis and will probably add bias to the analysis: 34% of patients could not recall their first symptom.

Those patients who presented with an incidental finding on a chest radiograph were more likely to be operable (small peripheral tumor not causing any symptoms).

A review of the literature by Jensen and colleagues[17] showed that the time intervals between intervals between first symptom and contacting a doctor varied widely from a median of 7 days to 6 months.

The effect of delay on prognosis has been examined before. According to Bozcuk and Martin,[19] the prognostic consequences of delays in diagnosing and treating lung cancer was studied and, like Myrdal and colleagues, found that treatment (hospital delay) did not affect survival, regardless of disease stage. Billing and Wells found that the length of delay did not correlate with tumor stage for potentially resectable patients.[19,20]

Setting up a quick access 2-stop clinic in one center led to a substantial increase in the number of patients who had successful surgical resection.[21] Delay for radical radiotherapy resulted in progressive disease, making patients unsuitable for treatment implying that even a modest delay decreased their chance of cure. For asymptomatic patients with stage III/IV lung cancer, delaying palliative radiotherapy treatment did not negatively affect quality of life, symptom control, or survival.[22] In one study, staging for potentially operable patients required a mean of 5.1 diagnostic tests per patient (mainly to exclude metastasis), necessitating on average an extra 20 days in the diagnostic workup.[23] Patients suitable for surgery also need more detailed workup, which may include cardiopulmonary exercise testing, mediastinoscopy, and so forth.

The study by Myrdal and colleagues[14] suggests that increased delay (patient or hospital)has no negative influence on survival, and this is probably true for most patients because of the high proportion of patients who present with stage III/IV disease. However, for those with a large but potentially radically treatable tumor, delay may be crucial. It is these patients perhaps who need to be identified and "fast tracked" through the diagnostic pathway.

The effect of delays on prognosis in patients with NSCLC was investigated by Myrdal and colleagues[14] in the journal Thorax in 2004. In the background it was mentioned that the effect of delay on survival in lung cancer remained uncertain. It was suggested that prompt management of NSCLC can influence prognosis. The study was undertaken by Myrdal and colleagues[14] to examine the relation between delay and prognosis in patients with NSCLC and to investigate the delay from first symptom and from first hospital visit to start of treatment.

METHODS

Two types of delay (symptom to treatment delay and hospital delay) were investigated in 466 patients treated for NSCLC at 2 institutions in central Sweden. Delays in relation to clinical characteristics were compared and the effects of delay times and other relevant factors on survival were assessed in multivariate analyses.

RESULTS

Thirty (5%) patients received treatment within 4 weeks of the first hospital visit and 52% within 6 weeks. Median symptom to treatment delay was 4.6 months and median hospital delay 1.6 months. Older age, advanced tumor stage, and nonsurgical treatment were independently related to poor survival. Both prolonged hospital delay and symptom to treatment delay provided additional information when considered separately. In a final multivariate model, only increased symptom to treatment delay gave significant information of a better prognosis. There was an association between a short delay and a poor prognosis, which was most pronounced in patients with advanced disease.

CONCLUSION

When considering the whole population and all stages of tumor together, shorter delay was associated with a poorer prognosis. This is likely to reflect the fact that patients with severe signs and symptoms receive prompt treatment. These findings indicate that the waiting time for treatment in patients with NSCLC is longer than recommended.

Waiting times for health care services are a constant problem. In cancer care, recommendations about maximum waiting times are sometimes made without knowledge of the possible influence of delay on survival. It is known that surgery in early-stage lung cancer can result in 5-year survival rates of 75% to 80%,[1] whereas there is no evidence that immediate treatment of patients with unresectable locally advanced NSCLC influences the prognosis.[2] However, the overall influence of the delay time in the diagnosis of NSCLC on survival remains poorly understood.[3–5] It appears that delay in the management of NSCLC is often longer than recommended in clinical practice.[6] Some studies have indicated that delay negatively affects the prognosis,[4,8] whereas others have not shown such an association.[3,5] In a recent Swedish study, no association was found between prolonged delay time (by the patient or the doctor) and advanced tumor stage.[9]

The objective of this study was twofold: (1) to examine the relation between delay and survival in patients receiving treatment for NSCLC, and (2) to investigate the delay time from the first symptom and from the first hospital visit to the initial treatment.

These points, based on considerations of tumor biology, suggest that survival should be improved if, within-patient and within–health system, clinical care delays are short. The factors that are important in prognosis include the following descriptors:

1. Cell type
2. Size of the primary tumor
3. Lymphatic spread to N1, N2, and N3 lymph nodes
4. Angiolymphatic invasion
5. Distant metastasis: brain, bone, adrenal, liver, and lung and the importance of disease-free interval

SUMMARY AND FUTURE CONSIDERATIONS

Efforts should be modified to reduce delays in patients with lung cancer. The delay between appearance of the first symptom and treatment is dependent on many factors. Presentation of the patient to the family doctor, decision by the family doctor to refer for radiography, and waiting time to see a chest specialist make up the steps in the delay to a first hospital visit. The symptoms of lung cancer may be vague and nonspecific. A history of hemoptysis without obvious lung infection will generally alert both patient and clinician. Cough is a less robust symptom but significant new persistent cough (that is more than 3 weeks) should arouse suspicion. Many patients with lung cancer have chronic obstructive pulmonary disease, so increasing breathlessness is a part of their overall clinical progression and may not be a reliable specific symptom for lung cancer. Half of all patients do not have symptoms in primary care, which suggest a diagnosis of lung cancer. It is therefore difficult to see how earlier referral to a chest physician can be achieved. In secondary care, some centers use direct referrals from a radiologist to a chest physician. A chest physician reads chest radiographs every day, and relevant urgent appointments and investigations are implemented directly by the physician.[15,18,24–27]

To reduce hospital delay time further will require an increase in resources and reengineering of clinical services (for example, "one-stop" clinics). However, in some patients it will still necessarily take longer time to obtain the diagnosis as they may need several investigations before a positive diagnosis is made.

We should not cease our efforts to reduce delays. Efforts should be made to reduce delays in patients with lung cancer. There are 3 reasons for this. First, the psychological stress on patients and their families who have a possible diagnosis of lung cancer is enormous. Delays only serve to worsen this. Second, there is a small group of patients with potentially radically treatable disease (especially those in whom this may be a borderline decision) who may have a different outcome if delays occur. Third, there should be large rewards from being able to identify patients at an early (asymptomatic) stage when radical treatment is possible.

The results of this study by Myrdal and colleagues[14] indicate that neither longer symptom to treatment delay time nor longer hospital delay time are associated with a poorer prognosis, corroborating findings in earlier studies.[3,5] On the contrary, the prognosis was poorer in patients with a shorter delay. A similar pattern has been observed in studies of the influence of referral delay on breast cancer.[11] Moreover, the results showed that patients with limited disease had to wait significant longer for treatment than those with advanced disease.

There was an interaction between tumor stage and delay; that is, the association between short delay and poor outcome was most pronounced in patients with advanced disease. This probably indicates that the severity of signs and symptoms at presentation influences the speed of the medical decision process and also correlates with prognosis.[28] The effect of delay on prognosis was less pronounced in patients with stage I-II disease.

CLINICS CARE POINTS

- Investigations necessary are bronchoscopy, mediastinoscopy, fine needle aspiration, thoracentesis and pleural biopsy, lymph node biopsy.
- Factors affecting prognosis in lung cancer.
- Stages in the diagnosis of lung cancer expressed in four points.
- Cell biology about cell proliferation and cancer growth.
- Tumor volume doubling time.

REFERENCES

1. Janssen-Heijnen MLG, Gatta G, Forman D, et al. Variation in survival of patients with lung cancer in Europe. Eur J Cancer 1998;34:2191–6.
2. Northern and Yorkshire Cancer Registry and Information Aervice (NYCRIS). A report on incidence and management for the main sites of cancer 1999. Leeds: NYCRIS; 2002. p. 1–56.
3. Mountain CF. Revisions in the international system for staging lung cancer. Chest 1997;111:1710–7.
4. van Klaveren RJ, Habbena JDF, Pedersen JH, et al. Lung cancer screening by low-dose spiral computed tomography. Eur Respir J 2001;18:857–66.
5. Muers MF, Howard RA. Management of lung cancer. Thorax 1996;51:557–60.
6. British Thoracic Society and Society of Cardiothoracic Surgeons of Great Britain and Ireland Working Party. Guidelines on the selection of patients with lung cancer for surgery. Thorax 2001;56:89–108.
7. International Association for the Study of Lung Cancer. Stage Grouping for the 8th Edition of the TNM Classification for Lung Cancer.
8. Konaka C, Ikeda N, Hiyoshi T, et al. Peripheral non-small cell lung cancers 2.0cm in diameter: proposed criteria for limited pulmonary resection based upon clinicopathological presentation. Lung Cancer 1998;21:185–91.
9. Oda M, Watamabe Y, Shimizu J, et al. Extent of mediastinal node metastasis in clinical stage 1 non-small cell cancer: the role of systematic nodal dissection. Lung Cancer 1998;22:23–30.
10. Muers MF, Holmes WF, Littlewood C. The challenge of improving the delivery of lung cancer care. Thorax 1999;54:540–3.
11. NHS Executive. The National Cancer Plan. A plan for investment, a plan for reform. London: Department of Health; 2000.

12. O'Rourke N, Edwards R. Lung cancer treatment waiting times and tumor growth. Clin Oncol 2000; 12:141–4.

13. Geddes DM. The natural history of lung cancer: a review based on rates of tumor growth. Br J Dis Chest 1979;73:1–17.

14. Myrdal G, Lambe M, Hillerdal G, et al. Effect of delays on prognosis in patients with non-small cell lung cancer. Thorax 2004;59:45–9.

15. Tannock IF, Hill RP, Bristow RG, et al. The basic science of oncology. In: Harrington LA, Tannock IF, Hill RP, et al, editors. Cell proliferation and tumor growth. 4th edition. New York: McGraw-Hill Medical Publishing Division; 2005. p. 167–93. Chapter 9.

16. Bozcuk H, Martin C. Does treatment delay affect survival in non-small cell lung cancer? A retrospective analysis from a single UK center. Lung Cancer 2001;34:243–52.

17. Jensen AR, Mainz J, Overgaard J. Impact of delay on diagnosis and treatment of primary lung cancer. Acta Ontol 2002;24:147–52.

18. Steel GG. Growth kinetics of tumors: cell population kinetics in relation to the growth and treatment of cancer. Oxford, UK: Clarendon Press; 1977.

19. Billing JS, Wells FC. Delays in the diagnosis and surgical treatment of lung cancer. Thorax 1996;51: 903–6.

20. Koyi H, Hilllerdal G, Branden E. Patient's, and doctor's delays in the diagnosis of chest tumors. Lung Cancer 2002;35:53–7.

21. Laroche C, Wells F, et al. mproving surgical resection rate in lung cancer. Thorax 1998;53:445–9.

22. Falk SJ, Girling DJ, et al. Immediate versus delayed palliative thoracic radiotherapy in patients with unresectable locally advanced non-small cell lung cancer and minimal thoracic symptoms: randomized control trial. BMJ 2002;325:465–8.

23. Herder GJM, Verboom P, Smit EF, et al. Practice, efficacy, and cost of staging suspected non-small lung cancer: a retrospective study in two Dutch hospitals. Thorax 2002;57:11–4.

24. Melamed MR, Flehinger BJ, Zaman MB, et al. Detection of true pathologic stage I lung cancer in a screening program and the effect on survival. Cancer 1981;47:1182–7.

25. Pearson FG. Current status of surgical resection for lung cancer. Chest 1994;106:337–339S.

26. Lederle FA, Niewoehner DE. Lung cancer surgery. A critical review of the evidence. Arch Intern Med 1994;154:2397–400.

27. Melamed MR, Flehinger BJ. Screening for lung cancer. Chest 1984;86:2–3.

28. Shamji FM, Deslauriers J. Thoracic surgery clinics: lung cancer, Part I screening, diagnosis, and staging; fast-tracking investigation and staging of patients with lung cancer, Elsevier; 2013. p. 187–91.

The Lymphatic Spread of Lung Cancer
An Investigation of the Anatomy of the Lymphatic Drainage of the Lungs and Preoperative Mediastinal Staging

Farid M. Shamji, MBBS, FRCSC, FACS[a],*, Gilles Beauchamp, MD, FRCSC[b], Harman Jatinder S. Sekhon, MD, MSc, PhD[c]

KEYWORDS

- Pulmonary lymphatic system • Lymphatic drainage • Lymph flow • Lymph nodes
- Lymphatic metastases • Mediastinal lymph node metastases

KEY POINTS

- Staging of lung cancer, seed and soil theory by S Paget, aerogenous metastases, history of pulmonary lymphatic drainage, physiologic function of the lymphatic system.

INTRODUCTION

The knowledge of lymphatic spread of lung cancer permitted the study of anatomy of lymphatic drainage of the lungs. The history of anatomy of lymphatic drainage of the lungs began in the 15th century.

The anatomy of the lymphatic system is important in both health and disease. The lymphatic system is complex, and the normal system will become abnormal in the disease state. One of the functions of the lymphatic system is to return excess tissue fluid filtering out of blood capillaries back to the bloodstream to maintain homeostasis. The flow of lymph from any region, therefore, usually reflects the extent of blood capillary filtration in that area. *What is now known is that in the lungs, the flow of pulmonary lymph is normally very little*—less than from most body tissues when considered in relation to the large volume of blood flowing in the pulmonary circulation per minute. The output of blood from the right ventricle into the pulmonary circulation at rest in the healthy adult subject is about 5500 mL/min and it matches the output from the left ventricle into the systemic circulation. Under normal circumstances, about *20 L of interstitial fluid* escape every day from the systemic circulation near the arteriolar end of the blood capillaries into the tissue spaces. Of this amount of interstitial fluid, 16 L to 18 L are reabsorbed into the blood flowing in the capillaries near the venular end, and the remaining 2 L to 4 L are returned to the venous circulation in the neck via the lymph.[1,2]

The pulmonary circulation differs from the systemic circulation in being the low-pressure system at 25/8 mm Hg and in the amount of fluid that filters out of the pulmonary capillaries, which is normally very little and, as such, of physiologic importance so as not to interfere with gas exchange in the alveoli.

In the human, pulmonary lymph flows to the lymph nodes around the lobar bronchi and thence to extrapulmonary lymph nodes located around

[a] University of Ottawa, General Campus, Ottawa Hospital, 501 Smyth Road, Ottawa, Ontario K1H 8L6, Canada; [b] Thoracic Surgery Unit, Department of Surgery, Maisonneuve-Rosemount Hospital, University of Montreal, 5415 L'Assomption Boulevard, Montreal, Quebec H1T 2M4, Canada; [c] Department of Pathology and Laboratory Medicine, The Ottawa Hospital, CCW, Room 4240, Box 117, 501 Smyth Road, Ottawa, Ontario K1H8L6, Canada
* Corresponding author.
E-mail address: faridshamji@hotmail.com

Thorac Surg Clin 31 (2021) 429–440
https://doi.org/10.1016/j.thorsurg.2021.07.005
1547-4127/21/© 2021 Elsevier Inc. All rights reserved.

the main bronchi and trachea and its bifurcation (tracheobronchial lymph nodes). These send their efferents to a right and left mediastinal lymph trunks, which may join the thoracic duct, but usually drain opening directly into the brachiocephalic vein of their own side. Ultimately, lymph from the lungs goes either to the right lymphatic duct (right bronchomediastinal duct) or to the thoracic duct which empties into the venous confluence of the subclavian and internal jugular vein in the neck on the right and left sides.

THE LYMPHATIC SYSTEM

The anatomy of the lymphatic system is important in both health and disease to understand in relation to lymphatic spread of cancer. Three main components of lymphatic system are:

1. Lymphatic capillaries
2. Collecting lymphatic vessels
3. Lymph nodes

Lymph consists of lymph cells and fluid that has filtered out of the blood capillaries according to Starling forces. The lymph cells are mainly T lymphocytes. The lymphatic system collects interstitial tissue fluid and coveys it to the bloodstream through the thoracic duct and right thoracic lymphatic trunk; these are the larger collecting vessels (thoracic duct and right thoracic lymphatic trunk) opening into the venous system in the low neck near the confluence of 2 major veins (internal jugular vein from the head-neck region and subclavian vein from the upper limb) forming the 2 brachiocephalic veins.[1,2]

The lymphatic system comprises the lymphatic capillaries and vessels, the lymph nodes, and aggregates of lymphatic tissue in the spleen, thymus, and around the alimentary tract. The lymphatic capillaries are larger than those of the vascular system; they are composed of a single layer of endothelial cells. The lymph vessels resemble veins and possess many paired valves and regularly traverse lymph nodes along their course. The ultrastructure of the small lymph vessels differs from that of the capillaries in several details: there are no visible fenestrations in the lymphatic endothelium; there is very little if any basal lamina under the endothelium; and the junctions between endothelial cells are open with no tight intercellular junctions.

A lymph node is an aggregation of lymphoid tissue along the course of a lymph vessel. It is bean-shaped with several afferent lymphatic vessels (conveying lymph to the node) entering its convex surface, and an efferent vessel (carrying lymph away from the node) leaving at its hilum. The efferent vessel then becomes afferent for the next lymph node.

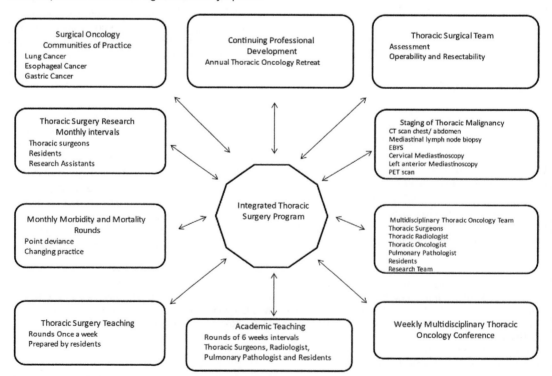

Fig. 1. Picture of a lymph node. (*Courtesy of* Farid Shamji, Ontario, CA.)

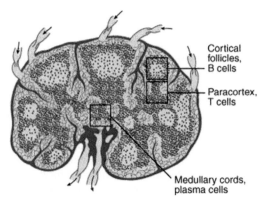

Cortical follicles, B cells

Paracortex, T cells

Medullary cords, plasma cells

Fig. 2. Anatomy of a normal lymph node. (*Courtesy of Edita Delic, Ontario, CA.*)

The lymph node is surrounded by a fibrous capsule from which fibrous trabeculae pass inwards. It is filled with a reticular network of fine collagen fibers, and the cells are primitive lymphocyte precursors, mature B and T lymphocytes, and macrophages. The 3 regions of the lymph node are cortex with cortical follicles containing B cells, paracortex with T cells, and medulla with medullary cords of plasma cells (**Fig. 1**).

In a human, there are about 500 lymph nodes that range in size from very small size of a pin's head 1 mm to almost as big as an olive almost 25 mm. They are distributed throughout the body, with clusters found in the axillae, groins, neck, chest, and abdomen (**Fig. 2**).

Numerous lymphocytes and a few monocytes lie freely within the meshwork, but they are absent peripherally, leaving a subcapsular sinus lymph space. The cells of the outer part of the node (cortex) are densely packed with lymphocytes and form oval masses called follicles. The center of the follicle and the hilar (medullary) regions of the node contain loosely packed lymphocytes. Lymphocytes are key elements in the production of immunity.

HISTORY OF PULMONARY LYMPHATIC DRAINAGE

See Ref.[3] and **Table 1**.

PHYSIOLOGIC FUNCTION OF THE LYMPHATIC SYSTEM

1. Filtering mechanism—restricts propagating cancer cells and resists the spread of infection.

Table 1
History of lymphatic drainage

Year	History
1563	Eustachius observed thoracic duct in horse and called it "Vena Alba Thoracis."
1627	Asellius discovered lymph vessels in dog's mesentery and termed them "Venae Lactae."
1653	Thomas Bartholinus wrote his "Vasa Lymphatica."
1758	John Hunter researched into absorbent vessels in the dog's mesentery at the Great Piazza, supposed to be the continuation of the extreme ends of the arteries, which were not large enough to carry red cells, only carrying the serum or lymph demonstrating lymph nodes and vessels by injection of mercury.
1955	Kinmouth introduced lymphangiography for investigating lymphatic routes of most regions in man
1954–1958, 1960	Nohl-Oser investigated pulmonary lymphatics by studying lymphatic spread of lung cancer. Lymph nodes draining the lungs were divided into 2 main groups: (a) the pulmonary lymph nodes which are invariably removed by a simple pneumonectomy and (b) the mediastinal lymph nodes. The *intrapulmonary spread* and the lymphatic drainage of each pulmonary lobe by dissections of lung specimens resected for bronchial carcinoma. The study of the *mediastinal spread* was undertaken by analysis of the results of mediastinoscopy or scalene node biopsy in patients suffering from lung cancer.

2. Transport excess tissue fluid from interstitial space to the bloodstream. The flow of lymph from any region, therefore, usually reflects the extent of capillary filtration in that area. In the lungs, the lymph flow is normally very little — less than from most tissues, especially when considered in relation to the blood flow (equal to the cardiac output).

The very small lymph flow from the lungs, reflecting a low filtration rate through the pulmonary capillary wall, is brought about partly by the low pulmonary capillary pressure of only 5 to 10 mm. Hg in the pulmonary circulation and partly by the fine structure of the capillary wall. The oncotic pressure from plasma protein inside the capillaries stays at 25 mm Hg compared to the low oncotic pressure in the interstitial fluid due to lower protein content compared to that in the capillary blood.

It is of particular importance in the lung that any accumulation of interstitial fluid, especially protein-rich fluid, be prevented, so that gaseous exchange between alveoli and capillaries shall not be hindered. To this end, lungs are supplied with an abundant lymphatic network, especially in the visceral pleura and deeper in the lung tissue accompanying the bronchi, the pulmonary artery, and the pulmonary veins.[3]

One of the characteristic features of the anatomic distribution of pulmonary lymphatics is their absence from the walls of the alveoli. Any excess interstitial fluid in the region between the alveolar epithelial layer and the capillary

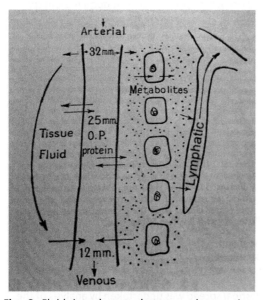

Fig. 3. Fluid interchanges between plasma, tissue spaces, and lymphatics. (*Data from* Refs.[4–8]; and *Courtesy of* Edita Delic, Ontario, CA.)

endothelium or in the alveoli themselves must be taken up by the terminal lymph vessels in the region of the alveolar ducts. Most of the lymph formed in the lung is directed by centrally pointing valves inwards toward the hilum (*centripetal lymph flow*). The flow of lymph toward the hilar nodes depends on a gradient of pulmonary pressure as well on these valves. Some of the lymph, however, that forms in the periphery of the lung, may pass by communicating vessels into the subpleural vessel which drains into the hilar nodes after traversing the surface of the lung (*centrifugal lymph flow*). Most of the lymph from all parts of the lungs usually drain into the right lymphatic duct through a lymph node on the right side of the trachea except the upper section of the left lung which drains into the thoracic duct.

The anatomy of the lymphatic system and the formation of lymph fluid and lymph flow is important to understand in relation to lymphatic spread of cancer (**Fig. 3**). A malignant tumor always directly invades the surrounding tissues. The cancer cells eventually enter channels like the lymphatics and blood vessels, and groups of cells are then carried to other parts as tumor emboli to distant sites where they become lodge, and if able to survive, proliferate to form secondary growths or metastases. Local invasion and embolic spread are the 2 main characteristics of malignant tumors. Most of the embolized cancer cells in the bloodstream and lymph die. Only the selected few cancer cells are able to take root to grow into secondary deposits. The "seed" (cancer cells) may be widespread, but only where the "soil" (selected organ – favored programmed sites) is suitable does growth occurs. What factors govern this are not known, but it appears that certain sites are particularly favored and biochemically programmed by the primary tumor to receive cancer cells.

Interstitial tissue fluid in the tissue spaces, on entering into the lymph capillaries, becomes lymph. The formation of interstitial fluid depends on the relationship between the hydrostatic pressures in the blood capillaries and the osmotic pressure of the plasma proteins (colloid oncotic pressure) as defined in the Starling hypothesis in 1896.

Von Hayek in 1960[4] described the lymphatic system from each lung, as follows:

1. Abundant lymphatic vessels within the lung parenchyma
   - Beneath visceral pleura
   - Interlobular septum
   - Submucosa of bronchial walls
   - Perivascular connective tissue
   - Peribronchial connective tissue
2. Pulmonary lymph nodes (N1)

- Intrapulmonary nodes
- Interlobar nodes (lymphatic sump of Borrie on the right side)
- Tracheobronchial node
- Bronchopulmonary lymph nodes
  - Hilar
  - Interlobar
3. Mediastinal lymph nodes (ipsilateral N2 and contralateral N3)
   Superior mediastinum:
   - Anterior mediastinal (subaortic window station 5 LN, preaortic arch station 6 LN)
   - Right and left paratracheal (station 2, 4, 3 LNs)
   - Anterior and posterior subcarinal (station 7 LNs)
   Inferior mediastinum:
   - Inferior pulmonary ligament (station 9 LN)
   - Paraesophageal (station 8 LN)

INVESTIGATION OF INTRAPULMONARY SPREAD OF LUNG CANCER

By correlating the location of the cancer in the lung in a specific pulmonary lobe with the site of lymph node metastases, it is possible to determine the intrapulmonary pathways of spread from each lobe. This gave rise to the concept of identifying sentinel lymph node and lymph node dissection pertaining to the lobe in question.

Intrapulmonary lymph nodes: lie at the points of division of segmental bronchi or bifurcations of the pulmonary artery will be the first station to encounter cancer cells in the lymph vessels: *N0 or N1 descriptor*.

Bronchopulmonary lymph nodes subdivided into "hilar" and "interlobar" lymph nodes: the second station to "see" cancer cells: *N1 Descriptor*.

Interlobar lymph nodes: lymphatic sump of Borrie is in the depths of interlobar fissures, situated in the angles formed by the bifurcation of main bronchus into lobar bronchi: the third station to encounter cancer cells: *N1 Descriptor*.

Hilar nodes: located along the main stem bronchi: the fourth station to receive cancer cells: *N1 Descriptor*.

It has been found that cancer cells may travel through the encountering stations of lymph nodes and not establish metastases. In all the lymph nodes, the subcapsular sinuses receive the incoming cancer cells. To establish metastases from free-floating cancer cells, it is required that a collection of cancer cells first form a group and the supply of nutrition to the cancer cells is by diffusion. Until the group of cancer cells survives and reaches a minimum size of between 1 and 3 mm then neoangiogenesis is initiated by vascular

endothelial growth factor (VEGF) and other growth factors to provide nutritive elements and the micrometastases then grow to become recognizable macrometastases to between 7 and 10 mm when PET scan will become positive.

RIGHT LYMPHATIC SUMP OF BORRIE: *N1 DESCRIPTOR*

- Collection of lymph nodes grouped around the bronchus intermedius—between the upper lobe bronchus above and the middle lobe and lower lobe apical segmental bronchi below.
- All 3 lobes of the right lung drain into this sump
  - RUL drains into the sump lymph nodes lying on the lateral aspect of the bronchus intermedius.
  - RLL drains into the sump lymph nodes on the lateral and medial aspect of the bronchus intermedius. Medially situated lymph nodes are contiguous with the posterior subcarinal lymph nodes, which then drain into the right paratracheal lymph nodes.

Clinical application: N1 descriptor

1. Right upper lobectomy is adequate for early growths of the right upper lobe as they rarely metastasize to lymph nodes below the level of the sump.
2. For right lower lobe growth, right lower and middle lobectomy or pneumonectomy will accomplish complete resection of cancer with ablation of all the nodes in the sump.
3. Right upper lobe growths rarely metastasize to subcarinal lymph nodes.
4. Right lower lobe growths frequently metastasize to subcarinal lymph nodes.

LEFT LYMPHATIC SUMP: *N1 DESCRIPTOR*

- Collection of nodes found in the left major interlobar fissure
- The following nodes are invariably found:
  - Large constant node found in the bifurcation between the upper lobe and lower lobe bronchi.
  - Large constant node found above and posterior to the left main pulmonary artery before it enters the major fissure.
  - Nodes in the angles of branches of left main pulmonary artery.

Clinical application: N1 descriptor

1. Left lymphatic sump node clearance by lobectomy is difficult as there is no intermediate stem bronchus on the left side. For this reason, there is a worse prognosis following resection of the left lower lobe for lung cancer. For this reason, pneumonectomy rather than lobectomy has a greater chance of competing curative resection
2. Upper lobe growths rarely metastasize below the level of the sump and lobectomy alone for competing curative resection is feasible.

Investigation of Mediastinal Lymphatic Spread

In 1959, Dr Eric Carlens[7] of the Karolinska Institute in Stockholm introduced *cervical mediastinoscopy* and biopsy of the superior mediastinal lymph nodes for sarcoidosis. Four years later, late Dr FG Pearson during a visit to the Karolinska Institute as a postgraduate student from Toronto, met Dr Eric Carlens for the first time. It was Dr Eric Carlens who showed him the procedure and the required instruments. After this historical visit, it was from surgical intuition that, late Dr FG Pearson recognized the benefit of the procedure in the management of lung cancer, and he initiated *cervical mediastinoscopy*[8–11] for the first time in lymphatic staging of lung cancer.

Left anterior mediastinotomy for lymphatic staging of lung cancer was introduced later in 1966 by Dr Thomas McNeill and Dr J Maxwell Chamberlain[12] at the Roosevelt Hospital in New York for cancer in the left upper lobe and left hilum after recognition of the different lymphatic drainage pathway from these locations compared to the rest of the lungs. The lymphatic drainage was into the anterior chain of lymph nodes in the subaortic window and along the course of left phrenic nerve in front of the transverse aortic arch; both lymph node stations were NOT accessible by cervical mediastinoscopy. Left anterior mediastinotomy (Pic 2) provided the necessary surgical access to the mentioned lymph nodes. This pattern of lymphatic drainage from the lungs was recognized 6 years later from the 1972 publication by Dr HC Nohl-Oser, Consultant Thoracic Surgeon to Harefield, Hillingdon, and West Middlesex Hospitals in London on "AN INVESTIGATION OF THE ANATOMY OF THE LYMPHATIC DRAINAGE OF THE LUNGS AS SHOWN BY THE LYMPHATIC SPREAD OF BRONCHIAL CARCINOMA and Anatomic Disposition of the Mediastinal Lymph Nodes."[13]

The importance of the procedure in the objective management of lung cancer was universally accepted. With the introduction of the staging technique, it was now possible to be *selective* in the surgical exploration of those patients with operable and resectable lung cancer in up to 95% of cases; instead of 50% which was the common occurrence previously when all the patients with lung cancer underwent surgical exploration. Thus, began the process of being *selectivity* as the basis of the surgical management of lung cancer. *Left anterior mediastinotomy* was introduced later by Dr T McNeil and J Maxwell Chamberlain for cancer in the left upper lobe and left hilum because of the recognition of the different lymphatic pathway compared to the rest of the lungs. The lymphatic drainage was into the *anterior chain of lymph nodes* in the subaortic window and along the course of the left phrenic nerve in front of the transverse aortic arch, not accessible by cervical mediastinoscopy. Left anterior mediastinotomy provided the necessary surgical access to the mentioned lymph nodes. The completeness of mediastinal staging of lung cancer required the addition of left anterior mediastinotomy to cervical mediastinoscopy to access the mentioned lymph nodes on the left side.

The mediastinal lymph nodes accessible for biopsy included: *N2 descriptor*.

- Right and left paratracheal nodes
- Anterior subcarinal node
- Tracheobronchial node
- Pretracheal node

The lymph nodes which are not accessible for biopsy include: *N2 descriptor*.

- Anterior mediastinal nodes: which lie in front of the great vessels of the aortic arch along the course of the phrenic nerve and in the subaortic window.
- Posterior subcarinal lymph node
- Inferior mediastinal nodes in the pulmonary ligament and in front of the esophagus.

Anatomic disposition of mediastinal lymph nodes: which are not accessible for biopsy at cervical mediastinoscopy include:
Anterior mediastinal nodes: *N2 descriptor*.

- Overlie upper portions of pericardium
- Right side—parallel and anterior to the phrenic nerve
- Left side—near the origin of pulmonary artery and ligamentum arteriosum
- Along the inferior border of the left innominate vein
- Along the course of phrenic nerve on the aortic arch

Posterior mediastinal nodes: *N2 descriptor*.

- Posterior subcarinal lymph node
- Lymph node found in the inferior mediastinum—situated in the pulmonary ligament usually 2 or 3 nodes lie below the inferior pulmonary vein
- Mainly paraesophageal nodes
- Left sided predominance with connections with paraaortic nodes in the abdomen and left adrenal gland
- On the right side—paraesophageal node lies retrotracheal near the arch of the azygous vein

Tracheobronchial lymph nodes: *N1 descriptor*.

Lie in 3 groups about the bifurcation of trachea
1. Inferior tracheobronchial nodes (subcarinal): *N2 descriptor*
   - Bifurcation or subcarinal nodes
   - Within pretracheal fascial envelope
   Reached during cervical mediastinoscopy
2. Superior tracheobronchial nodes: *N1 descriptor*
   Located in the obtuse angle between trachea and main bronchus on both sides
   Outside the pretracheal fascia
   Right side—situated medial to the arch of the azygous vein and above the right main pulmonary artery
   Left side—lie in concavity of aortic arch, closely related to the recurrent laryngeal nerve and form a continuous link with anterior mediastinal nodes
3. Anterior tracheal group of nodes: *N2 descriptor*
   Lie in front of the lower trachea and right main bronchus
   Link inferior tracheobronchial (subcarinal) nodes to right superior tracheobronchial nodes
4. Paratracheal nodes: *N2 descriptor*
   In the superior mediastinum
   Right side—anterolateral to trachea, overlapped laterally by superior vena cava
   Larger and more numerous nodes
   It is important to recognize that these form a link between superior tracheobronchial nodes below and inferior deep cervical nodes above (scalene nodes)

LYMPHATIC DRAINAGE OF LUNGS TO THE MEDIASTINUM (NARUKE MEDIASTINAL LYMPH NODE MAP)

1. Lymphatic drainage from right lung to the superior mediastinum is ipsilateral 96% and occasionally contralateral 4% right superior tracheobronchial node drains into right

Table 2 Stage grouping of TNM classification for lung cancer			
Stage	**T**	**N**	**M**
Occult carcinoma	TX	N0	M0
0	T1s	N0	M0
IA1	T1mi	N0	M0
	T1a	N0	M0
IA2	T1b	N0	M0
IA3	T1c	N0	M0
IB	T2a	N0	M0
IIA	T2b	N0	M0
IIB	T1a	N1	M0
	T1b	N1	M0
	T1c	N1	M0
	T2a	N1	M0
	T2b	N1	M0
	T3	N0	M0
IIIA	T1a	N2	M0
	T1b	N2	M0
	T1c	N2	M0
	T2a	N2	M0
	T2b	N1	M0
	T3	N0	M0
	T4	N1	M0
IIIB	T1a	N3	M0
	Tib	N3	M0
	Tic	N3	M0
	T2a	N3	M0
	T2b	N3	M0
	T3	N2	M0
	T4	N2	M0
IIIC	T3	N3	M0
	T4	N3	M0
IVA	Any T	Any N	M1a
	Any T	Any N	M1b
IVB	Any T	Any N	M1c

paratracheal nodes and finally into the right scalene node (*M1 descriptor*)
2. Lymphatic drainage from the left lung to the superior tracheobronchial lymph node is contralateral 25% from the left lower lobe and about 12% from the left upper lobe. The contralateral spread occurs through subcarinal and anterior tracheal lymph nodes
3. Both right and left lower lobes drain into paraesophageal and posterior subcarinal lymph nodes (*N2 descriptor*)
4. Anterior chain of lymph nodes on the left side drains into the left scalene lymph node (*M1 descriptor*)

Classification of Mediastinal Lymph Nodes: NARUKE MEDISTINAL and BRONCHOPULMONARY

LYMPH NODES[14–17] recommended by the Japan Lung Cancer Society Journal of Oncology Vol 4, Issue 5, pp 568-577 (**Table 2**)

1. Superior mediastinal or highest lymph node—N2
2. Paratracheal lymph node—N2
3. Pretracheal lymph node—N2
   3a Anterior mediastinal lymph node—N2
   3b Retrotracheal mediastinal or posterior mediastinal lymph node—N2
4. Tracheobronchial lymph node—N1
5. Subaortic lymph node—N2
6. Paraaortic (ascending aorta) lymph node—N2
7. Subcarinal lymph node (anterior and posterior)—N2
8. Paraesophageal lymph node (below carina)—N2
9. Pulmonary ligament node (inferior)—N2
10. Hilar lymph node—N1
11. Interlobar lymph node—N1
12. Lobar lymph node—upper lobar, middle lobar, and lower lobar—N1
13. Segmental lymph node—N1
14. Subsegmental lymph node—N1

TNM CLASSIFICATION FOR LUNG CANCER

- PRIMARY TUMOR
    TX: primary tumor cannot be assessed
    T0: no evidence of primary tumor
    Tis: carcinoma-in-situ
    T1: primary tumor ≤3 cm; not visualized by bronchoscopy
      T1mi: minimally invasive adenocarcinoma
      Tia: tumor ≤1 cm
      Tib: ≥1 cm but ≤2 cm
      Tic: tumor ≥2 cm but ≤3 cm
    T2: primary tumor 3 cm but ≤5 cm
      involves main bronchus
      invades visceral pleura
      associated atelectasis with pneumonitis
        T2a ≥3 cm but ≤4 cm
        T2b ≥4 cm but ≤5 cm
    T3: tumor ≥5 cm but ≤7 cm, with direct invasion of the chest wall or in the mediastinal structures: chest wall, phrenic nerve, parietal pericardium
    T4: tumor ≥7 cm with invasion of mediastinal structures: muscular diaphragm, heart, great vessels, trachea, esophagus, recurrent laryngeal nerve, vertebral body
- Regional lymph node
    NX: regional lymph nodes inaccessible
    M0: no lymphatic metastases
    N1: metastatic spread to ipsilateral intrapulmonary hilar, segmental or subsegmental lymph nodes
    N2: metastatic spread to ipsilateral mediastinal lymph nodes
    N3: metastatic spread to contralateral mediastinal or contralateral hilar lymph nodes, ipsilateral or contralateral supraclavicular or scalene lymph nodes
- Distant metastasis
    M0: no distant metastasis
    M1: distant metastasis present
      M1a: separate tumor deposit in contralateral lobe, malignant pleural or pericardial effusion, pleural or pericardial tumor deposits
      M1b: solitary single extrathoracic metastasis
      M1c: multiple extrathoracic metastases.

PRINCIPLES OF METASTASIS

As long as cancer occurs, metastasis remains a major clinical problem; paradoxically, the more effective local treatment is in prolonging life, the greater the risk of metastasis.[18] The primary tumor is seldom the cause of death and the risk of dying is related to the widespread formation of metastases. The metastases cause local destruction of tissues and interfere with the physiologic function of the affected organ, a pathophysiological deterioration which is not cancer-specific.

The likelihood of developing metastasis is related to the growth rate of the cancer, the faster the growth rate, the greater the risk of developing metastases. This behavior is exemplified by the fastest-growing small cell cancer of the lung in comparison to squamous cell cancer and adenocarcinoma. This is evident from the tumor volume doubling time (Fig). Cancer cells become detached from the primary tumor early in the course of its development and spread through the lymphatic vessels and venules to distant sites. Only the innate tumor immunity against the foreign antigen of cancer cells slows down the growth of metastatic deposits and prolong survival.

The mode of spread of cancer cells has given rise to much speculation, and fortunately, there is now a better understanding of the process. It is necessary to understand the mechanism behind the formation of metastases in the metastatic cascade. It begins with a *reduction in cell adhesiveness* and *detachment of cancer cells* from the primary cancer. The detached cancer cells begin the process of *intravasation and facilitated local invasion* in the surrounding tissues by *motility* resembling the white blood cells. This is aided by the secretion of enzymes and toxins by the tumor cells and host stroma. *The local infiltration into the surrounding tissues is the salient feature of all malignant tumors.* The invading cancer cells penetrate various natural passages, moving in the line of least resistance, which affords an easy route for further spread. The most important of these are the *local* lymphatics and blood vessels and in both the malignant cells may become detached as emboli and spread by permeation along the vascular endothelium to reach distant sites. If the cells survive and supported by nutrition through diffusion multiply producing a secondary isolated mass of tumor. *This is a metastasis.* Under 3 mm size, it is invisible, and nutrition is provided by diffusion to keep cancer cells alive. After reaching more than 3 mm size, growth is now facilitated by angiogenesis and transform from micrometastasis to become visible by PET scan macrometastases at 7 mm to 10 mm size.

LYMPHATIC SPREAD

The detachment of groups of tumor cells in an invaded lymphatic leads to the production of emboli, which become lodged in the *subcapsular sinus* of the regional draining lymph node. The embolized cancer cells may travel unchecked through the first draining lymph node station to the next one where they may get *arrested by adhesions*. If the cells survive and grow, the node soon becomes replaced by the tumor, and further spread occurs to the next group of glands by way of efferent channel. Another method of lymphatic spread is by clumps of cancer cells growing on the endothelium and spreading on endothelial cells by *permeation* to reach the next group of lymph nodes.

The process of *angiogenesis* and *neovascularization* occurs in the metastases initiated by angiogenic VEGF and other growth factors released by the tumor cells once a size of 3 mm is reached. Under 3 mm size, the cancer cells receive nourishment to keep them alive by diffusion. The new blood vessels during angiogenesis provide nutrition to the tumor cells, which now begin to multiply quickly and grow from *micrometastases* to become recognizable *macrometastases* on PET scan once a size of 7 mm to 10 mm is reached. The normal architecture of the lymph node is gradually replaced by continued cancer cell growth and in time cancer cells invade into the perinodal tissues through the capsule of the lymph node. This extranodal invasion is a poor prognostic indicator shortening survival and not favorably affected by surgery. The affected lymph node has in turn potential ability to promote further spread of cancer cells by the *cascade mechanism.* Eventually, all the lymph drains into the venous

circulation, and the first capillary network the tumor cells met is in the lung.

BLOOD-BORNE SPREAD

Vascular invasion into the *local* blood vessels is in the *thin-walled venules* requiring enzyme-related breakdown of the subendothelial basement membrane. Malignant cells invading small vessels or veins become detached and are then carried by the bloodstream to some distant site where they reach a capillary network. There the emboli become impacted, proliferate, and develop into secondary tumors. The same process of embolization and permeation along the endothelium will occur in venules carrying malignant cells to distant sites to produce distant metastasis through the arterial and venous circulation. The invasion of large veins is seen most frequently in lung cancer because of the large number of vessels available. The tumor becomes covered by thrombus and fibrin provides a network on which the tumor cells grow.

DISTANT METASTASES

The distribution of secondary tumors might be expected to be related to the blood supply, but this is not the case. Cardiac and skeletal muscle have an abundant blood supply, and yet are rarely the site of metastasis. The spleen likewise is not usually involved.

It has been found that tumor cells are present in the bloodstream in cases of malignant disease, but the frequency of this is undecided. The cells are not plentiful, and the reported incidence is perhaps 10%. There is no general agreement as to the significance of finding tumor cells in the blood, for it does not seem to be related to prognosis. It is probable that many of the cells die. Only the selected few are able to take root to grow into secondary deposits. What factors govern this are not known, but it appears likely that certain sites are particularly favored. The "seed" may be widespread, but only where the "soil" is suitable does growth occur. The *seed-and-soil hypothesis* is essentially due to *Dr E. Fuchs in 1882*[19] and was so acknowledged by *Dr S Paget*[20] in his much-quoted paper in *1889* in English. Paget remarked that "When a plant goes to seed, its seeds are carried in all directions, but they can only live and grow if they fall on congenial soil...then regards as metastasis."

This is termed *selective metastasis* and the favored sites in lung cancer are:

- *Liver*, a common site of blood-borne metastases because the liver affords an excellent nutritive medium for tumor cells having dual blood supply from portal vein bring nutrients absorbed from the small intestine and hepatic arterial circulation.
- *Ipsilateral or contralateral lung*, the frequent site of metastases supported by oxygen and rich dual blood supply: pulmonary circulation for gas exchange and nutritive bronchial arterial circulation.

AEROGENOUS SPREAD IN LUNGS

This is the *S*pread of primary lung cancer cells *T*hrough alveolar *Air Spaces (STAS)*.[21] This is a new concept of spread through air spaces (STAS), which was introduced for pulmonary *adenocarcinomas* (ADC) in the 2015 World Health Organization (WHO) classification for lung cancer. The available data demonstrates that STAS is of high prognostic impact and associated with specific clinic-pathological characteristics following validation in 2 large independent cohorts from the United States and Germany.

According to the 2015 WHO classification, STAS is defined as "micropapillary clusters, solid nests, or single cells spreading within air spaces beyond the edge of the main tumor." Besides the existing criteria for invasion (a histologic subtype other than a lepidic pattern; myofibroblastic stroma associated with invasive tumor cells; vascular or pleural invasion), STAS was thereby established as a fourth category that defines invasion for ADC.

Before the definition of STAS, early reports indicated that aerogenous tumor spread and free-floating cell clusters from ADC but also metastases from colorectal cancer are unfavorable prognostic features. Furthermore, Onozato and colleagues[22] described so-called tumor islands and their adverse prognostic impact, a morphologic feature closely related to STAS in 2013. In principle, tumor islands can be separated from STAS by specific criteria. Of note, using 3D reconstruction approaches, it was demonstrated that the tumor islands are connected to the main tumor at different levels. Subsequent clinicopathological correlations revealed a significant association of tumor islands with smoking, high-grade (solid or micropapillary) predominant pattern, *KRAS* mutations, and higher nuclear grade. Furthermore, tumor islands were significantly associated with a worse recurrence-free survival.

Papillary or micropapillary patterns of ADC or cell clusters floating within pools of mucin in mucinous or specifically colloid adenocarcinomas are internationally accepted features of an invasive tumor although a stromal invasion or infiltration through the basal membrane is not necessarily present in these cases.

DISTANT METASTASES

The distribution of secondary tumors might be expected to be related to the blood supply, but this is not the case. Cardiac and skeletal muscle have an abundant blood supply, and yet are rarely the site of metastasis. The spleen likewise is not usually involved.

It has been found that tumor cells are present in the bloodstream in cases of malignant disease, but the frequency of this is undecided. The cells are not plentiful, and the reported incidence is perhaps 10%. There is no general agreement as to the significance of finding tumor cells in the blood, for it does not seem to be related to prognosis. It is probable that many of the cancer cells die and release cancer DNA into the blood. This is detected by liquid biopsy and provides information about the status of the cancer metastases: eliminated and cured by treatment, still persistent and active invisible on imaging studies (PET is the best for detection of metastases), or recurrent after initial treatment considered curative.

Only the selected few cancer cells are able to take root (*seed-and-soil*)[23] to grow into secondary deposits. What factors govern this are not known, but it appears likely that certain sites are particularly favored. The "seed" may be widespread, but only where the "soil" is suitable does growth occur.

This is termed *"selective metastasis"* and the favored sites from primary lung cancer are:

- *Liver* is a common site of blood-borne metastases because the liver affords an excellent nutritive medium for tumor cells by having a dual blood supply from the portal vein rich in nutrients absorbed from the small intestine and oxygenated hepatic arterial circulation.
- *Ipsilateral or contralateral lung*, the frequent site of metastases supported by oxygen and rich dual blood supply: from pulmonary circulation for gas exchange and from nutritive bronchial arterial circulation.
- *Skeletal metastases*, the bones are frequent sites of secondary deposits from lung cancer. Of all the lung cancer cell types, it is the small-cell carcinoma that is particularly liable to metastasize quickly to the skeleton and other organs such as the liver, adrenal glands, and brain on account of its inherent biological aggressiveness. The most common distant sites are long bones and spine, brain, adrenal

glands, and liver. Bone metastases cause osteolysis and this is seen radiologically as an area of radiolucency and may lead to pathologic fracture.

- *Brain* is not an infrequent site of secondary tumor deposits, solitary or multiple. Surrounding vasogenic edema is a frequent occurrence seen on imaging studies and MRI is the best for detection of the tumor deposit and the accompanying edema. The tumor deposit way be silent or manifest with neurologic (seizures or motor deficit) or psychiatric symptoms.
- Of the endocrine glands, the *adrenal* is the one which most frequently contains metastases, usually in the medulla. Lung cancer, especially the small cell variety, frequently metastasizes to this site, and the route of spread may be lymphatic from the inferior posterior mediastinal lymph node (left one is preferred for lymphatic spread) or blood-borne causing unilateral or bilateral deposits.
- The *skin* is occasionally the site of metastases, which tend to erupt as discrete nodules.

SUMMARY

A thorough knowledge of pulmonary lymphatic drainage is essential in the clinical staging of mediastinal lymph nodes in the planning of best selection of treatment for lung cancer. There are 4 choices of treatment, which are as follows: surgical, definitive chemoradiotherapy, induction chemoradiotherapy, and immunotherapy. This requires a safe and standard method of performing mediastinal lymph node biopsy according to the lymph node map (Naruke map and IASLC map) by minimally invasive cervical mediastinoscopy and left anterior mediastinotomy. This depends on sound knowledge of the mediastinal anatomy with utmost care for the vital mediastinal structures: airway (trachea and main bronchi), left recurrent laryngeal nerve and ascending aorta in the left paratracheal space, azygous vein and superior vena cava in the right paratracheal space, esophagus and its relationship in the subcarinal space, the right recurrent laryngeal nerve as it loops around the proximal right subclavian artery, right main pulmonary artery in its relationship to the tracheal carina, left main pulmonary artery and left recurrent laryngeal nerve in the subaortic window and the transverse aortic arch and the overlying left phrenic nerve in the left chest, and the origin of left innominate vein in the superior left paratracheal space. All these structures are physiologically vital and have to be protected from inadvertent injury during the staging

operations; the potential for surgical complications from inadvertent injury is real and due diligence and proper care have to be exercised.

CLINICS CARE POINTS

- Knowledge of lymphatic spread of lung cancer is reflected in the study of anatomy of lymphatic drainage.
- In the normal state, in the lungs, the flow of pulmonary lymph is normally very little in relation to the large volume of blood flowing in the pulmonary circulation per minute.
- The anatomy of the lymphatic system is important in both health and disease to understand in relation to lymphatic spread of lung cancer.
- Anatomy of normal lymph node is important in surgical discipline.
- Fluid interchanges between plasma, tissue spaces, and lymphatics is important to understand.
- Investigation of mediastinal lymphatic spread is relevant in lung cancer.
- Staging of lung cancer.
- Seed and soil theory of Dr. S Paget.
- Aerogenous metastases.

REFERENCES

1. Albertine KH, Staub NC. Blood vessels and lymphatics in organ system. In: Abramson DL, Dobrin PB, editors. Chapter 11: organization of pulmonary lymphatic system. Academic Press, Inc; 1984. p. 397–401.
2. Parent RA, Peake JL, Pinkerton KE. Comparative biology of the normal lung. In: Chapter 3. The Human Lung. Gross and sub gross anatomy of the lungs, pleura, connective tissue septa, distal airways, and structural units. 1960.
3. Leeson CR, Leeson TS, Paparo AA. Lymphoid organs. In: Textbook of histology. 5th edition. W.B. Saunders Company; 1985. p. 263–90. Chapter 9.
4. Von Hayek H. Lymph vessels, lymph nodes and lymphoid tissue. In: The human lung, vol. 1. New York: Hafner Publishing Company; 1960. p. 298–314.
5. Ganong WF. Review of medical physiology. In: Dynamics of blood and lymph flow. Chapter 30. 21st edition. Los Altos, California: LANGE Medical Publications; 2003. p. 579–98.

6. Wright S. Applied physiology. In: Keele CA, Neil E, editors. 12th edition. London: Oxford University Press; 1971. p. 77–87. Part II, Section 4.

7. Carlens E. Mediastinoscopy: a method for inspection and tissue biopsy in the superior mediastinum. Dis Chest 1959;4:343–52.

8. Pearson FG. Mediastinoscopy: a method of biopsy in the superior mediastinum. Can J Surg 1963;6:423.

9. Pearson FG. Mediastinoscopy: a method of biopsy in the superior mediastinum. J Thorac Cardiovasc Surg 1965;49:11–21.

10. Pearson FG. An evaluation of mediastinoscopy in the management of presumably operable bronchial carcinoma. J Thorac Cardiovasc Surg 1968;55: 617–25.

11. Pearson FG, Nelems JM, Henderson RD, et al. The role of mediastinoscopy in the selection of treatment for bronchial carcinoma with involvement of superior mediastinal lymph nodes. J Thorac Cardiovasc Surg 1972;64:382–90.

12. McNeil TM, Maxwell Chamberlain J. Anterior mediastinotomy in 1966. Ann Thorac Surg 1981;32(2):109.

13. Nohl-Oser HC. An investigation of the anatomy of the lymphatic drainage of the lungs. Ann Roy Coll Surg Engl 1972;51:157–76.

14. Naruke T, Suemasu K, Ishikawa S. Lymph node mapping and curability at various levels of metastasis in resected lung cancer. J Thorac Cardiovasc Surg 1978;76:832–9.

15. Naruke T, Tsuchiya R, Kondo H, et al. Lymph node sampling in lung cancer: how should it be done? Eur J Cardiothorac Surg 1999;16(Supp 1):S17–24.

16. Naruke T, Goya T, Tsuchiya R, et al. The importance of surgery in non-small cell cancer of lung with mediastinal lymph node metastasis. Ann Thorac Surg 1988;1988(46):603.

17. Goldstraw P, Chansky K, Crowley J, et al. The IASLC lung cancer staging project: proposals for revision of the TNM stage groupings in the forthcoming (Eighth) Edition of the TNM classification for lung cancer. J Thorac Oncol 2015;11(1):39–51.

18. Weiss L. Principles of metastasis. In: Mechanisms of metastatic patterns. Academic Press; 1985. p. 200–56.

19. Fuchs E. Das Sarkom des Uvealtractus. In: Graefe's Archiv für opthalmologie, XII, 2. Wien; 1882. p. 233.

20. Paget S. "The distribution of secondary growths in cancer of the breast". Lancet 1889;1:571–3.

21. Gaikwad A, Souza C, Inacio JR, et al. Aerogenous metastases: a potential game changer in the diagnosis and management of primary lung adenocarcinoma. AJR Am J Roentgenol 2014;203(6):1–22.

22. Onozato ML, Kovach AE, Yeap BY, et al. Tumor Islands in resected early-stage adenocarcinomas are associated with unique clinicopathological and molecular characteristics and worse prognosis. Am J Surg Pathol 2013;37(2):287–94.

23. Akhtar M, Haider A, Rashid S, et al. Paget's 1889 "Seed and Soil" theory of cancer metastasis: an idea whose time has come. Adv Anat Pathol 2019; 26(1):69–74.

Standardized Postoperative Adverse Event Data Collection to Document, Inform, and Improve Patient Care

Farid M. Shamji, MBBS, FRCSC, FACS[a],*, Molly Gingrich, H BSc, MSc[b],
Caitlin Anstee, BA[c], Andrew J.E. Seely, MD, PhD, FRCSC[d]

KEYWORDS

- Historical context, standardized data collection • Audit and feedback in Thoracic Surgery
- National integration • Surgeon self-assessment • Positive deviance rounds
- Morbidity and Mortality Rounds • The Clavien-Dindo Classification System

KEY POINTS

- Thoracic surgery is associated with substantial risk for postoperative adverse events.
- Standardized postoperative data collection.
- Requirement for high quality in data collection.
- Postsurgical audit and feedback practices.
- National integration of both standardized data collection and audit feed back.

INTRODUCTION

There is great potential for standardized postoperative adverse events data collection to document, inform, audit, and feedback, all to optimize patient care. Adverse events, defined as any deviation from expected recovery from surgery, have harmful implications for patients, their families, and clinicians. Postoperative adverse events occur frequently in thoracic surgery, predominately due to the high-stakes (ie, high potential for cure) and high-risk (ie, vital physiology and anatomy and pre-existing disease) nature of the surgery. Many surgical complications begin in the operating room and are preventable, highlighting the importance of surgeon education, practice standardization, and continuing review. As we discuss, engaging surgeons in audit and feedback practices informed by standardized data collection would generate consensus recommendations to reduce adverse events and improve patient outcomes.

HISTORICAL CONTEXT

Throughout history, prominent surgeons have recognized the detrimental impact that postsurgical complications have on patient outcomes. As early as 1363, the French physician and surgeon Guy de Chauliac[1] stated in his *Chirurgia Magna,* "let the surgeon be bold in all *sure* things, and fearful in *dangerous* things; let him avoid all *faulty* treatments and practices." The British surgeon and anatomist

a University of Ottawa, General Campus, Ottawa Hospital, 501 Smyth Road, Ottawa, Ontario K1H 8L6, Canada; b 501 Smyth Road Box 708, Ottawa, Ontario K1H 8L6, Canada; c Division of Thoracic Surgery, Department of Surgery, The Ottawa Hospital, 501 Smyth Road, Ottawa, Ontario K1H 8L6, Canada; d Department of Surgery, Division of Thoracic Surgery, Thoracic Surgery & Critical Care Medicine, The Ottawa Hospital, University of Ottawa, Ottawa Hospital Research Institute, Assistant Kelly White, 501 Smyth Road - Box 708, Ottawa, Ontario K1H 8L6, Canada
* Corresponding author.
E-mail address: faridmashamji@gmail.com

Thorac Surg Clin 31 (2021) 441–448
https://doi.org/10.1016/j.thorsurg.2021.07.003
1547-4127/21/© 2021 Elsevier Inc. All rights reserved.

Sir Astley Cooper[2] highlighted the importance of surgical education in his nineteenth century *Introductory Lecture*, stressing that "operations cannot be *safely* undertaken by any man, unless he possesses a thorough knowledge of anatomy" and that "physiologic knowledge is of the utmost importance to the profession of surgery." To prevent complications, he stated that "it is the duty of the surgeon never to advise an operation unless there is a probability that it will be attended with success."[2]

As health care availability expanded through the twentieth century, surgeons, hospitals, and entire health care systems continued to acknowledge the value of surgical quality improvement and reductions to postsurgical adverse events. In the 1970s, Experimental Medical Care Review Organizations were established in the United States to combine review with quality improvement strategies.[3] The realization in the 1980s that data-informed clinical practice guidelines improved quality of care led to the generation of the Agency for Health Care Policy and Research, tasked with addressing practice variation and developing clinical recommendations.[3] Similarly, the National Quality Forum and its Strategic Framework Board were established to set health care quality standards.[4] Although variations of these initiatives have continued through the early 2000s, yet practice-specific standardized, continuous systems of data-informed quality improvement aimed at addressing serious and preventable postsurgical adverse events are still lacking.

THE NATURE OF THE PROBLEM

Postoperative adverse events are common in thoracic surgery, occurring in 30% to 60% of patients.[5–7] Among the most common adverse events are prolonged air leak and atrial fibrillation, with patients older than 70 years at particularly high risk.[5] The harmful effects of adverse events on both patients and health care providers are far reaching with consequences including physical and psychological harm. Patients may suffer an increased risk of mortality,[7,8] impaired postoperative recovery,[9] increased length of hospital stay,[9–11] greater readmissions,[12,13] and in cases of cancer treatment, worsened oncological outcomes associated with septic complications (Harrison et al, unpublished data, 2015). Poor patient experiences are often subsequently reported, and patients may lose trust in the health care system.[14] Physicians suffer reduced staff morale and the possible legal consequences of making errors, including ensuing litigations against the responsible medical professional and the hospital.[15]

In Canada, an estimated 37% to 51% of adverse events are potentially preventable and strain an already burdened health care system by an additional $400 million per year.[16] Although some adverse events may occur because of the high-risk nature of thoracic surgery, unacceptably high rates of practice variation have been identified and contribute to poor patient outcomes.[17–21] This shortcoming should be addressed through a program of systemwide standardized data collection coupled to audit and feedback-based quality improvement initiatives that generate consensus recommendations to inform practice standardization and better surgical practice.

Adverse events in health care: learning from mistakes

Large national reviews of patient charts estimate that approximately 10% of hospital admissions are associated with an adverse event. An adverse event is defined as an injury that the patient suffers after an operation resulting in prolonged hospitalization, medication errors, hospital-acquired pressure sores and infections, falls and fractures, disability, complications and morbidity, or death, which are caused by health care management. Apart from having a significant impact on patient morbidity and mortality, adverse events also result in increased health care costs due to longer hospital stays. Furthermore, a substantial proportion of adverse events are preventable. By identifying the nature and rate of adverse events initiatives to improve care can be developed. In most adverse events, a surgical service was providing the care at the time the adverse event occurred; the median proportion across the studies was 58% for surgical compared with 24% for medical services.

STANDARDIZED DATA COLLECTION

The collection of standardized data is required to evaluate and inform improvements to patient care and should be based on (1) clear data definitions, (2) a system for data collection, (3) a means to transfer data safely, and (4) methods to ensure that data is of high quality.

Clear Data Definitions

Identical data must be collected on all patients across institutions to allow for valid comparison and effective knowledge transfer. The process of data collection can be applied to a multiplicity of procedures related to patient care, and thus the definition of a minimum set of data elements is essential. Definitions should be standardized, yet adaptable, to maintain relevance with evolving

Table 1 The Clavien-Dindo classification system	
Grades	**Definition**
I	Any deviation from the normal postoperative course without the need for pharmacologic treatment or surgical, endoscopic, and radiological interventions
II	Requiring pharmacologic treatment with drugs, blood transfusion, and total parenteral nutrition
III	Requiring surgical, endoscopic, or radiological intervention
IIIa	Interventions not under general anesthesia
IIIb	Interventions under general anesthesia
IV	Life-threatening complication including CNS complications requiring ICU
IVa	Single-organ dysfunction (including dialysis)
IVb	Multiorgan dysfunction
V	Death of a patient

Adapted from Dindo D, Demartines N, Clavien PA. Classification of surgical complications: a new proposal with evaluation in a cohort of 6336 patients and results of a survey. Ann Surg. 2004;240(2):205-213.

surgical practice and harmonization with other international databases. Regular revision overseen by a steering committee may be required to remove irrelevant variables, clarify existing variables, or add new variables of interest.

Acquisition of data must take into consideration (1) patient-related factors, (2) disease-related factors, and (3) treatment-related factors, with knowledge of all 3 essentials for a well-conducted clinical audit. At minimum, collected data should include (1) clinical information and surgical risk factors, (2) the operation performed, (3) hospital length of stay, and (4) intraoperative or postoperative adverse events including both incidence and severity (eg, graded according to the Clavien-Dindo classification system based on the degree of therapy required to treat the adverse event; **Table 1**). Collection of both incidence and severity allows the impact of adverse events to be better monitored, and the use of such a standardized grading system further supports objective and reproducible adverse event reporting.

The current gold standard of data elements is the American College of Surgeons National Surgical Quality Improvement Program (NSQIP), composed of definitions designed to measure and improve the quality of surgical care.[22] Although an excellent surgical initiative, NSQIP is not thoracic surgery specific, and therefore many adverse events are not included. The Thoracic M&M (TM&M) Classification System of data elements was developed to obtain the same major adverse events identified through NSQIP, as well as the large number of minor thoracic surgery-specific adverse events that would otherwise not be captured.[6] The Society of Thoracic Surgeons has likewise designed its own widely used database to address the same inconsistencies.[23] Harmonization between databases should be a future goal to ensure that interinstitutional data between centers is comparable regardless of the data definition system implemented.

A System for Data Collection

Data collection should be prospective and integrated into care, documented on a daily basis from surgical residents' and patients' clinical notes. A collegial effort is fundamental to this process and new responsibilities are likely to be imposed on some surgical team members, although input from all care providers is necessary for the collection of accurate and complete data. To facilitate data collection, storage, and feedback, a Web-based software tool is ideal to allow clinicians access from any device connected to the hospital network. For example, the Thoracic Surgery Quality Monitoring, Information Management, and Clinical Documentation software (TSQIC, www.tsqic.org/) can be used to collect information on surgical volume, priority of surgery, disease diagnoses, procedure class, and surgical approach/incision. The software is dynamically modifiable and can be updated at all participating sites to ensure harmonization. Although TSQIC has been successful at The Ottawa Hospital and other Canadian thoracic surgery centers, any system that allows for simple, thorough, and accurate data reporting may achieve similar results.

A Means to Transfer Data Safely

Data collected locally should initially be stored within the local hospital server, protected behind the hospital firewall. Communication between individual data collection devices and the hospital server should be encrypted with Secure Socket Layer to maintain data security. Demographic, diagnostic, operative, and adverse event data from multiple centers should be consolidated within a large, protected database, with data transferred by local data managers through a secure submission portal at scheduled intervals. Centralization of data serves to both increase security and improve the capacity for interinstitutional data comparison.

Methods to Ensure that Data Are of High Quality

Multiple levels of data quality monitoring should be introduced to ensure that data are complete, valid, and consistent. When the original, local file is created, an algorithm should be applied to detect missing or incorrect data fields that are then fed back to the data manager. Upon upload to the central server, the algorithm should again be applied to ensure that corrections were made. A central research coordinator should review all files before final acceptance and communicate any inconsistencies with the local data manager for review. A final delayed review 3 to 6 months following data submission can highlight any missing data fields that may now be known, such as the discharge date of a patient who was still hospitalized at the time of data transfer.

The integration of these elements of standardized data collection ensures that information collected is reproducible, reliable, and comparable at both the individual and institutional level. At academic centers, engagement of a thoracic surgery research personnel further supports the success of any data collection initiative. Subsequently and most importantly, integration with audit and feedback practices facilitates using the data to improve care.

AUDIT AND FEEDBACK IN THORACIC SURGERY

Standardized data on their own will not necessarily indicate whether clinical care has been of high quality, because the occurrence of adverse events may be influenced by patient factors, disease factors, treatment factors, and other elements of the health care system. Audit and feedback involve the regular review of surgical results to identify both achievements and shortcomings in the surgical unit and individual performance and provide a complementary approach that is undertaken with the objective of assessing quality of care and enhancing surgical practice.

Informed by this data, audit and feedback may occur through several means. Most commonly, the Morbidity and Mortality (M&M) rounds enable exceptional surgical cases to be presented for teaching and discussion (see section Morbidity and Mortality (M&M) Rounds). However, a favourable method involves the addition of systematic data summary and presentation that includes surgeon self-assessment and positive deviance rounds (sections Surgeon Self-Assessment and Positive Deviance Rounds). Collegial discussion leads to the generation of consensus recommendations that surgeons implement into practice (section Actionable Recommendations). Thus, audit and feedback have the capacity to alter individual surgeon behavior and performance when applied collectively and continuously, reducing adverse event incidence, and optimizing patient care.

Morbidity and Mortality Rounds

Best practice M&M rounds are an established quality improvement practice in surgery and essential for successful audit and feedback. Allowing for regular clinical case review, M&M rounds provide ongoing education to health care professionals.[24] M&M rounds are most effective when based on the following principles: (1) incorporation of data review, (2) case selection based on severity and preventability, (3) analysis and discussion of systemic and cognitive errors, (4) identification of actionable consensus recommendations, and (5) recognition of remediable action to be undertaken.[25] M&M rounds should be implemented at least monthly and begin with a review of the surgical volume and adverse event rates from the previous month and previous quarter to inform participants of the current status of their division. It is essential that accurate and reliable adverse event data be routinely collected to facilitate this process. Next, cases presented during M&M rounds should include a severe and/or preventable adverse event, generally grade IV or V (see **Table 1**), that may have resulted from a systemic or cognitive issue. This issue could apply to the preoperative, intraoperative, or postoperative phases of care and include a range of elements such as improper evaluation of fitness for surgery, incorrect use of surgical equipment, or poor communication among the surgical team. Following the case presentation, collegial discussion should be focused on identifying how the systemic and/or cognitive issue led to the adverse event presented and result in the generation of actionable consensus recommendations. Interprofessional involvement should be encouraged so that a range of perspectives are incorporated, with nurses, physiotherapists, pharmacists, social workers, and other allied health care professionals invited to attend and participate in discussions. Following the rounds, the discussion and recommendations generated should be summarized by a facilitator and distributed to both attendees and those who were unable to attend. Importantly, consensus recommendations should be tabled and discussed at divisional meetings to determine the appropriate actions to be taken to address the identified issues.

Surgeon Self-Assessment

The ability for surgeons to objectively compare their operative data with that of their peers is essential for performance assessment. Software can be used to summarize and feedback surgical data, allowing surgeons to compare their current outcomes for individual thoracic surgery procedures to past performance, the performance of anonymized peer colleagues, division averages, or the full census of patients undergoing thoracic surgery. Software can allow for the subdivision of data based on disease type, priority of surgery, surgical approach, procedure class, disease system, and complication, with integration of risk adjustment tools further increasing the validity and benefit of such software and its analyses. Importantly, surgeon self-assessment can be integrated into other quality improvement processes including positive deviance rounds (see Section Positive Deviance Rounds).

Positive Deviance Rounds

Self-assessment is limited if surgeons who perform poorly lack the knowledge of what or how to change. Positive deviance rounds provide complementary value by combining best evidence with best experience to generate actionable consensus recommendations that all agree upon. Based on the global health observation that in every community there are individuals whose uncommon practice leads to improved health outcomes,[26] positive deviance seminars draw on standardized data collected from individual surgical centers to anonymously identify best performing surgeons (ie, those displaying positive deviance). Four components are essential to the implementation of effective and positivistic rounds: (1) selection of procedure and adverse event/outcome, (2) presentation of literature

review (ie, best evidence), (3) identification of surgeons displaying positive deviance (ie, best experience), and (4) collegial discussion and generation of actionable consensus recommendations. Before the positive deviance rounds, a thoracic surgical procedure and corresponding adverse event or outcome is chosen, such as air leak after lobectomy or length of stay after pneumonectomy. The positive deviance rounds begin with the presentation of a literature review by a surgical fellow or member of surgical staff regarding the chosen procedure and outcome, summarizing relevant key trials, recent reviews, and existing recommendations. Next, the group is shown individual-level surgeon data, anonymized to protect surgeons' identities. The group identifies the surgeons with the best outcomes (ie, those demonstrating positive deviance) and may agree to disclose the identity of the surgeons, who will then be asked to describe their clinical techniques and why they believe their practice leads to superior outcomes. A collegial discussion of the findings of the literature review and the strategies used by the surgeons displaying positive deviance collectively results in the generation of actionable consensus recommendations that all commit to practicing. This process should be repeated for multiple procedures and outcomes, with 2 or 3 topics typically discussed at each positive deviance round and implemented at both the local (ie, intrainstitutional) and national (ie, interinstitutional) levels.

Actionable Recommendations

To have impact, standardized data collection and associated audit and feedback processes must lead to action. Clear, actionable, consensus recommendations for change are thus a critical component of both M&M rounds and positive deviance seminars. The culmination of successful quality improvement processes, actionable recommendations provide clinicians with clear guidelines for practice change. At a single hospital, recommendations generated through data-informed audit and feedback led to the reduction of 3 major adverse events, highlighting the capacity for consensus recommendations to impact patient care.[27]

Recommendations generated during M&M rounds and positive deviance seminars can be tabled at divisional meetings, reviewed by best practice committees, distributed through institutional or national surgical networks, and monitored over time to assess impact. Continuous recommendation generation and review is thus essential for the broad distribution of best practice guidelines to reduce adverse events and improve patient care.

NATIONAL INTEGRATION

The impact of standardized data collection and audit and feedback is greatest when implemented in multiple centers working as a quality collective, if possible at a national level. Collection of identical data elements across centers establishes a national data set that supports intercenter comparisons. Nationally coordinated audit and feedback provides greater benefits than single-center based initiatives, particularly in specialized surgical domains where a limited number of specialist surgeons are spread across the country (eg, there are ~125 Canadian thoracic surgeons in ~30 centers). A national network of standardized data collection and audit and feedback not only links large urban centers but also allows for the participation of small centers that would otherwise be unable to implement collegial audit and feedback practices and improves the ability to distribute recommendations across the country. National integration allows for greatest surgeon participation, extends impact to the greatest number of patients, and achieves the greatest improvement in patient outcomes.

FUTURE DIRECTIONS

A standardized system of postoperative data collection provides an effective means to document adverse events, inform audit and feedback practices, and improve patient care. The recommendations generated during quality improvement processes can influence clinical guidelines and health system planning. Postoperative adverse event databases serve as an inexpensive randomized controlled trial-ready platform that enables future clinical trials and provides an opportunity to complete prospective and retrospective studies and comparative-effectiveness research. Increasing the collection of postoperative data allows for the standardized documentation and study of rare pathologies, procedures, and complications that may otherwise be overlooked. The applications of standardized data collectively reduce adverse events and improve surgical outcomes, optimizing patient care.

The purpose and conduct of medical audit, from educational perspective, is a means of quality control for medical practice by which the profession shall regulate its activities with the intention of improving overall patient care. The quality assurance depends on patients' satisfaction as well as that of the doctors. The medical profession needs to be educated about the structure, the process, and the outcome. The structure equates to resources found within the hospital; this means not only beds but also operating rooms, equipment, technology, staffing, investigations, and administration of these resources. The process equates to efficiency and function of the staff, both by assessment of diagnosis and the treatment of patients and the use of resources for such a function. The outcome concerns the patient, not only the patient's outcome from surgery but also the surgeon's expectation, the patient's expectation, and the community's expectation through community health councils and any legal means. Outcome is when quality of care becomes preeminent. However, outcome does vitally involve the patient's motivation, personality, determination, education, and beliefs; how they express outcome; and how they see it. These attributes although very important, are equally difficult to assess and to be given appropriate weight.

In the future, the audit systems will have to be based on an integrated hospital information system with a central database with all hospital staff and facilities involved. It will be based on interface schemes, rather than isolated medical audit systems, and probably will only be found in those hospitals with adequate computer resource management and hospital information systems.

Medical audit developments will involve individual requirements, statistical analysis, word processing, a database, a standard coding classification, the ability to recode outpatient/inpatient data and adverse events, and an adequate and sensible classification of diseases and disorders.

Audit of all aspects of medical practice has been around and undertaken for many years. The medical journals have reported the review of clinical practice from the time of their initial publication, and groups of clinicians have met and discussed clinical problems and their management for centuries. The main change now is in accountability. Clinicians are expected to account for all decisions appertaining to each clinical case and give reasons if problems arise. This, of course, has both medical and resource implications so that clinical colleagues and hospital management expect to audit these decisions. The justification for this is that resources are limited and so must be used most efficiently. The role of audit has become polarized into 2 linked areas:

1. Review of clinical decision making and management
2. Making the most efficient use of resources for the patients.

Audit has achieved a great deal, but further effort is required to ensure that audit continues to contribute to the improvement in quality of care for patients. The value of audit will improve as data collection becomes adequate with data validation. Resources are needed if medical audit is to be successful and worthwhile. The critical resource is an attitude of mind. *Surgical education* is important just as the *application of knowledge*. Proper documentation and collection of clinical data is essential. Regular meetings to analyze the outcome of the audit is required. It is all about *"Working for the Patient,"* and this must be the premise for embarking on every audit. The desire for improvement and change must be in the forefront of mind and thinking.

CLINICS CARE POINTS

- Although vital for treatment of chest cancers, thoracic surgery is associated with substantial risk of postoperative adverse events, as chest operations impair respiration and circulation and are often performed on patients with preexisting cardiopulmonary disease.

- Standardized postoperative data collection based on clear data definitions, a system for data collection, a means to transfer data safely, and methods to ensure that data are of high quality should all be implemented to effectively document adverse events.

- Postsurgical audit and feedback practices informed by standardized postoperative adverse events documentation and data collection allow for collegial discussion and the generation of actionable consensus best practice recommendations to reduce practice variation and adverse event incidence.

- National integration of both standardized data collection and audit and feedback ensures that data can be compared across centers, allows for the broad surgeon participation and learning, and extends impact to the greatest number of patients.

REFERENCES

1. de Chauliac, G. Chirurgia magna. (1363).
2. Cooper, A. The Principles and Practice of Surgery: founded on the Most Extensive Hospital and Private Practice, During a Period of Nearly Fifty Years. (1836).
3. Chassin MR, Loeb JM. The Ongoing Quality Improvement Journey: Next Stop, High Reliability. Health Aff 2011;30:559–68.
4. Burstin H, Leatherman S, Goldmann D. The evolution of healthcare quality measurement in the United States. J Intern Med 2016;279:154–9.
5. Seely AJE, Ivanovic J, Threader J, et al. Systematic classification of morbidity and mortality after thoracic surgery. Ann Thorac Surg 2010;90:936–42 [discussion: 942].
6. Ivanovic J, Seely AJE, Anstee C, et al. Measuring surgical quality: comparison of postoperative adverse events with the american college of surgeons NSQIP and the Thoracic Morbidity and Mortality classification system. J Am Coll Surg 2014;218:1024–31.
7. Andalib A, Ramana-Kumar AV, Bartlett G, et al. Influence of postoperative infectious complications on long-term survival of lung cancer patients: a population-based cohort study. J Thorac Oncol 2013;8:554–61.
8. Khuri SF, Henderson WG, De Palma RG, et al. Determinants of long-term survival after major surgery and the adverse effect of postoperative complications. Ann Surg 2005;242:326–41 [discussion: 341–3].
9. Irshad K, Feldman LS, Chu VF, et al. Causes of increased length of hospitalization on a general thoracic surgery service: a prospective observational study. Can J Surg 2002;45:264–8.
10. Khan NA, Quan H, Bugar JM, et al. Association of postoperative complications with hospital costs and length of stay in a tertiary care center. J Gen Intern Med 2006;21:177–80.
11. Baker GR, Norton PG, Flintoft V, et al. The Canadian Adverse Events Study: the incidence of adverse events among hospital patients in Canada. CMAJ 2004;170:1678–86.
12. Brown LM, Thibault DP, Kosinski AS, et al. Readmission after Lobectomy for Lung Cancer: Not All Complications Contribute Equally. Ann Surg 2019. https://doi.org/10.1097/SLA.0000000000003561.
13. Dickinson KJ, Taswell JB, Allen MS, et al. Unplanned Readmission After Lung Resection: Complete Follow-Up in a 1-Year Cohort With Identification of Associated Risk Factors. Ann Thorac Surg 2017;103:1084–91.
14. Harrison R, Walton M, Manias E, et al. The missing evidence: a systematic review of patients' experiences of adverse events in health care. Int J Qual Health Care 2015;27:424–42.
15. Lipira LE, Gallagher TH. Disclosure of Adverse Events and Errors in Surgical Care: Challenges and Strategies for Improvement. World J Surg 2014;38:1614–21.
16. Etchells E, Koo M, Daneman N, et al. Comparative economic analyses of patient safety improvement strategies in acute care: a systemic review. BMJ Quality Safety 2012;21:448–56.
17. Finley, C. J., Schneider, L. & Shakeel, S. Approaches to high-risk, resource intensive cancer surgical care in Canada. (2019).
18. Iyer AKV, Yadav, S. Postoperative care and complications after thoracic surgery. In: Firstenberg MS,

editor. Principles and Practice of Cardiothoracic Surgery. INTECH OPEN, 2013.

19. Finley CJ, Jacks L, Keshavjee S, et al. The effect of regionalization on outcome in esophagectomy: a Canadian national study. Ann Thorac Surg 2011; 92:485–90 [discussion: 490].

20. Finley CJ, Bendzsak, Tomlinson G, et al. The effect of regionalization on outcome in pulmonary lobectomy: A Canadian national study. J Thorac Cardiovasc Surg 2010;140:757–63.

21. Miller JD, Jain MK, de Gara CJ, et al. Effect of surgical experience on results of esophagectomy for esophageal carcinoma. J Surg Oncol 1997;65:20–1.

22. Khuri SF, Daley J, Henderson W, et al. The Department of Veterans Affairs' NSQIP: the first national, validated, outcome-based, risk-adjusted, and peer-controlled program for the measurement and enhancement of the quality of surgical care. National VA Surgical Quality Improvement Program. Ann Surg 1998;228:491–507.

23. Shahian DM, Jacobs, Edwards FH, et al. The society of thoracic surgeons national database. Heart 2013; 99:1494–501.

24. Benassi P, MacGillivray L, Silver I, et al. The role of morbidity and mortality rounds in medical education: a scoping review. Med Education 2017;51:469–79.

25. Shahian DM, Jacobs, Edwards FH, et al. Enhancing the Quality of Morbidity and Mortality Rounds: The Ottawa M&M Model. Acad Emerg Med 2014;21: 314–21.

26. Marsh DR, Schroeder DG, Dearden KA, et al. The power of positive deviance. BMJ 2004;329:1177–9.

27. Ivanovic J, Mostofian F, Anstee C, et al. Impact of Surgeon Self-evaluation and Positive Deviance on Postoperative Adverse Events After Non-cardiac Thoracic Surgery. J Healthc Qual 2018;40:e62–70.

The History and Evolution of Surgical Instruments in Thoracic Surgery

Farid M. Shamji, MBBS, FRCSC[a],*, Kristin Waddell, BScN[b],
Gilles Beauchamp, MD, FRCSC[c]

KEYWORDS

- Thoracic surgery • Thoracic surgical instruments

KEY POINTS

- Thoracic surgical instruments were designed by surgeons in different surgical disciplines and there has been no major changes introduced ever since.
- The names of different surgeons, now deceased, were mentioned in the chapter in order to bring familiarity.
- The essential requirements in the operating theatre for medicolegal reasons and safety were described, including the necessary steps observed during the conduct of operation, and familiarity and knowledge of surgical instruments, and surgical dissection.

INTRODUCTION

Surgery is as old as man, and its evolution has been moulded in every age by current technical and scientific advances, not forgetting the demands made upon it by social circumstances and religion. It is both an art and a science, while its practice largely depends on the human relations between doctor and patient. It is extremely difficult to define where surgery begins or ends, and its separation from medicine is largely based on the very different paths which the two disciplines took in ancient times.[1]

Appreciation and knowledge of the normal human physiology, anatomy, biochemistry, chemical pathology, microbiology, surgical pathology, and pathogenesis of diseases forms the essential basis of modern surgical care and treatment. Nevertheless, the culminating event in the management of the surgical patient is the operation itself, and familiarity with the surgical instruments to be used specifically for the particular operation and the skills useful in the operating theater—technical surgical precision and attention to operative details—remain the determining factors in limiting intraoperative adverse events and postoperative morbidity (illness) and mortality (death).[2]

The operation should be carried out carefully and expeditiously without breaks in the surgical technique. Adequate exposure is accomplished by combination of adequately monitored anesthetic relaxation, carefully planned surgical approach and incision, selection of surgical instruments specific for the operation, knowledgeable and thoughtful surgical assistants, and focus on maintaining adequate surgical exposure with proper retraction. The illumination of the surgical field should be bright, and instruments and ancillary monitoring equipment should be checked

K. Waddell: Nursing responsibilities are to act as a liaison between the hospital and the surgeons; organizing equipment for cases and bringing in equipment for cases when a special request is made; and training nurses in thoracic surgery.

a University of Ottawa, General Campus, Ottawa Hospital, 501 Smyth Road, Ottawa, Ontario K1H 8L6, Canada; b General Campus, Ottawa Hospital, 501 Smyth Road, Ottawa, Ontario K1H 8L6, Canada; c Thoracic Surgery Unit, Department of Surgery, Maisonneuve-Rosemount Hospital, University of Montreal, 5415 L'Assomption Boulevard, Montreal, Quebec H1T 2M4, Canada
* Corresponding author.
E-mail address: faridshamji@hotmail.com

Thorac Surg Clin 31 (2021) 449–461
https://doi.org/10.1016/j.thorsurg.2021.06.002

and in good working order. Cooperation and communication in the operating room should remain the high priority. The operating team must be acquainted with the surgeon's preference and methods and be able to anticipate his/her needs. Competent surgical skills and anesthetist skills are necessary. Tissues must be handled gently and approximated accurately, and hemostasis carefully secured, protecting from injury those structures outside the operative field, all of which necessitates availability of appropriate surgical instruments and assistance.

The smooth coordination of these factors depends to a large part on the assistants' intelligence, surgical knowledge, forethought, and familiarity with the complexity of the modern operating theater. Every day in the operating room around the world, there is regular use of surgical instruments by the cardiothoracic surgeons. These instruments were designed by some of the most talented and famous surgeons of the time in this specialty. The driving force in designing these instruments was their ingenuity, observations, clinical needs, surgical talents, and surgical skills. The knowledge of these instruments and those who designed them is most essential in this branch of surgery.[3–5]

The specialized surgical instruments have been designed for the performance of various thoracic technical operations.[6] Not all of these are necessary or even useful in the hands of a competent thoracic surgeon. In general, it is best to use those instruments which have good applicability and to avoid using unusual or complicated devices. The instruments that have been found particularly helpful are being mentioned and used to develop familiarity with their application before operation is essential.

TYPES OF CARDIOTHORACIC SURGICAL INSTRUMENTS AND RESPECT IN HANDLING

Group 1: Most frequently used *bone instruments* are mentioned:[6]

These include the costotomes, rongeurs, periosteal elevators, special bone-cutting instruments, sternal saw and knife, and rib approximators:

1. Tudor Edwards Guillotine for cutting ribs at any point except the neck, where the double action large bone-cutting rib shears is more useful.
2. First Rib Roos Costotome
3. Large Bone-cutting Shears
4. Tudor Edwards Rib Shears
5. Bailey Rib Approximator
6. Ronguer used are duck-billed and broad tipped for smoothing the ragged sharp ends of rib after excision

7. Powered Sternal Saw
8. Lebsche Sternum-cutting Knife and Mallet
9. Semb Bone-holding Forceps during rib resection
10. Lambotte Bone-holding forceps used in thoracic surgery as rib approximator to facilitate closure of incision
11. Lewis Rib Periosteal Elevator
12. Alexander Periosteal Elevator
13. Cameron-Haight Periosteal Elevator
14. Slim Jim Periosteal Elevator
15. Doyen Rib Strippers—right and left
16. Doyen Periosteal Elevator
17. Awl with Wrench for Sternal Closure

Group 2: Most used *retractors* are,

- For spreading ribs after making thoracotomy incision,
  1. Tudor Edwards Rib Retractors in three sizes; small (intended for children), medium, and large (intended for patients with unusually large chest)
  2. Finochietto Rib Retractor in three sizes; small, medium, and large
  3. Henley Rib Retractor
  4. Tuffier Retractor
  5. Morse-Favaloro Rib Spreader
  6. Baby Reinhoff Rib Retractor (modification of Tuffier Rib Retractor for use in infants and small children)
- For retraction lung during pulmonary resection
  1. Deaver Retractors—two widths
  2. Allison Lung Retractor
- For retracting chest wall muscle and tissues
  1. Large Blunt Rake Retractor for use on the muscle of the chest wall
  2. Small Richardson-Type Retractor used in each end of the thoracotomy incision to retract muscles when the rib is being cut across
  3. Small Rake Retractors has many uses
  4. Langenbeck Retractor
  5. Davidson Scapular Retractors in two widths for retraction of scapula during making of thoracotomy incision and during thoracoplasty. It is usually a comfortable instrument for an assistant to hold during the operation.

Group 3: *Special Instruments* for general use in thoracic surgical procedures:

1. Curved hemostatic forceps having long handles and short pointed Jaws. It is invaluable in many thoracic operations
2. Full-length hemostatic forceps is useful because of its length and slender jaws

3. Thump forceps with atraumatic teeth, for grasping mucosa, and available in long and short sizes
4. Wangensteen needle holder is invaluable in the performance of a high intrathoracic esophagogastric anastomosis
5. Adson needle holder for anastomotic work
6. Sweet bent (angled) scissors for division of esophagus during esophagectomy
7. Angled scissors for division of bronchus
8. Allison lung curved blunt-tipped dissecting long heavy scissors used in pulmonary resection during dissection on major blood vessels
9. Long Mayo–type lung-dissecting scissors
10. Metzenbaum scissors, long and short
11. Long flexible right-angle clamp, modified Mixter-type forceps used to grasp the esophagus distal to the level of transection during esophagectomy and to grasp the bronchus in the same manner during lobectomy or pneumonectomy
12. Bulldog clamps for temporary occlusion of blood vessels, long and short, straight and curved
13. Vascular Clamps: Satinsky Clamp, Curved and Angled DeBakey Clamp, Derra Clamp, Lambert-Kay Clamp, Potts Clamp
14. Judd Allis forceps
15. Potts Angled Scissors
16. Duval lung grasping forceps
17. Turner Babcock grasping forceps
18. Babcock Lung grasping forceps
19. DeBakey Atraumatic dissecting forceps
20. Lees Bronchial Clamp
21. Kochers clamp straight and curved
22. Swedish DeBakey forceps

Group 4: *Mediastinoscopy* setup:

1. Light source
2. Light Carrier
3. Carlens Traditional Mediastinoscope Long and Short
4. Current Videoscope Mediastinoscope
5. Biopsy Forceps Straight and Upbiting, Small and Large, Laryngeal Biopsy Forceps
6. Sponge prepared to be ready for immediate use from 4 by 8 gauze or vaginal pack for packing in the mediastinum for hemostasis
7. Inflatable Bag for Neck Extension
8. Arterial Line Right Wrist—anesthetize preference if necessary
9. Surgical Prep from Neck to Upper Abdomen and draping to maintain access for immediate median sternotomy, if necessary, for control of mediastinal bleeding

10. Endotracheal tube exiting from the left corner of mouth
11. Use traditional mediastinoscope or videomediastinoscope according to the surgeon's preference

Group 5: Flexible Video-Gastroscopy setup:

1. Small-diameter endotracheal tube exiting from the left corner of the mouth
2. Biopsy forceps
3. Boston Scientific Balloon for esophageal stricture dilation
4. Savary or Maloney Bougies for dilation under fluoroscopy following the rule of three: 9 mm, 11 mm, and 12.8 mm on first attempt and the next time 4 weeks later to use 11 mm, 12.8 mm, and 14 mm. Gradually progress to 20 mm guided by measurements 3F = 1 mm

Minimum diameter necessary to permit adequate swallowing is 13.0 mm according to Schatzki's rule.

Group 6: Rigid Esophagoscope:

1. Negus Rigid Scope
2. Pilling Rigid Scope
3. Berciward Laryngo-Pharyngoscope

Group 7: Esophageal Dilatation setup:

1. Fluoroscopy C-Arm in position
2. Bougies Required: Maloney 28F, 32F, 36F, 40F, 44F, 48F, 50F, 52F (3F = 1 mm)
   Savary 6 mm to 20 mm
   Gum-Tipped 8F to 36F

Group 8: Bronchoscopy:

1. Rigid Pilling and Storz Bronchoscopes: 7 by 40 and 8 by 40 for female; 8 by 40 and 9 by 40 for male
2. Balloon for Tracheal Stricture Dilatation with MLA mask
3. Sanders Injector for oxygenation
4. Video-Fiberoptic Bronchoscopes

Group 9: Transcervical Thymectomy setup:

1. Gomez Retractor
2. Thymectomy Retractor
3. Penrose drain
4. Inflatable Bag for Neck Extension and Widening of Anterior Superior Mediastinum; the bag is deflated after the sternal retractor is in position in the mediastinum and the sternum lifted up avoiding hyperextension of the neck
5. Head Light
6. Sternotomy setup to be ready

THORACIC SURGICAL INSTRUMENTS—HISTORICAL EVOLUTION AND THE DESIGNERS

1. *Arthur Tudor Edwards* (1890–1946) was a *Welsh Thoracic Surgeon*, who worked at the Westminster Hospital, the Royal Brompton Hospital and Queen Mary's Hospital, Roehampton and *pioneered lung surgery* in particularly pulmonary tuberculosis and lung tumors.[6] He designed the chest retractor which was named after him. He was also responsible for the training of notable surgeons including Dwight Harken, Sir Clement Price Thomas, and Sir Russell Brock.

2. A *Pennington clamp*, also known as a *Duval clamp*, is a surgical clamp with a triangular head for use in some OB/GYN procedures, particularly caesarian section. Under the name "Duval clamp", they are frequently used much like a Foerster clamp to atraumatically grasp lung tissue. The clamp is named after *David Geoffrey Pennington*, an *Australian Surgeon* who is a pioneer of microsurgeries.

   Duval Lung Grasping Forceps lightweight, ratcheted, finger ring forceps used for grasping large tissue and organs, such as the stomach and lungs. The triangular, fenestrated tips are horizontally serrated providing a large, secure grasping surface. This feature makes this instrument versatile for handling slippery or weak tissue as well.

3. *Allison Lung Retractor*, designed by Philip Rowland Allison (1907–1974), is a hand-held surgical instrument used in cardiothoracic procedures in which it is necessary to retract the lung. Its open design and thin flat wires are gentle on the delicate lung tissue. This lung retractor is crafted with a solid hooked handle and a flat, spatula-shaped blade. The lightweight design and wide, flat blade ensure the least amount of excessive pressure on lung tissue to maintain the maximum amount of ventilation through the procedure. This instrument is available in two blade sizes to accommodate a wide range of patients and surgical scenarios.
   ○ Allison Lung Retractor

4. The two American Mayo brothers opened the *Mayo Clinic* in Rochester in 1919 seeing patients on 1 day and operating on the next day. They concentrated their efforts on treating foregut disorders and thyroid disease. Their pioneering spirit led to their designing of the *Mayo Scissors*, still widely used in the operating theaters. These are relatively large and heavy to be used in purposeful surgical approach. *Straight Mayo Scissors* are used for cutting sutures. *Curved Mayo Scissors* are used for cutting fibrous tissue.
   1. Mayo straight scissors
   2. Mayo curved scissors

Myron Metzenbaum (1876–1944)

Having small hands, wearing size 6 gloves, and difficulty in manipulating the standard surgical instruments led him to develop *Metzenbaum Scissors* for use during tonsillectomies. Their wide use in many different types of operation ever since is related to being thin and sleek surgical instrument and used for delicate tissue dissection. *Metzenbaum scissors* are surgical scissors designed for cutting delicate tissue and blunt dissection. The scissors come in variable lengths and have a relatively long shank-to-blade ratio. They are constructed of stainless steel and may have tungsten carbide cutting surface inserts. The blades can be curved or straight, and the tips are usually blunt. This is the most common type of scissors used in organ-related operations.

- Metzenbaum Scissors

Davidson Scapular Retractor is hand-held and used in shoulder and posterolateral thoracic procedures to retract scapula.

5. *Enrique Finochietto* was born in Argentina and was Italian by birth. He was just 16 years old when he joined the Faculty of Medicine at the University of Buenos Aires in Argentina. He spent his early career in Europe learning new surgical techniques. He was skillful in technical drawing and designed many surgical instruments, including the specifically designed and still in use thoracic rib spreader, affectionately known as the *Finochietto Retractor*, specifically designed to separate the ribs in thoracotomy incisions. The Burford-Finochietto rib spreader has replaceable blades.
   - Finochietto Rib Spreaders Rib Retractors
6. *Theodore Tuffier* (1857–1929):

   Theodore Tuffier was a French pioneering innovator surgeon who designed in 1914 and introduced the *Rack-and-pinion–type stainless steel rib spreaders* (with a *thumbscrew* to lock it in place) and widely used and affectionately known as the *Tuffier Retractor*. This was modified in 1936 by Argentinian surgeon *Enrique Finochietto* to have fenestrated blades (blades with "windows") and a hand-cranked lever to both separate the arms in a staged fashion and lock them in place at each stop.

The Tuffier retractor and especially the Burford-Finochietto retractor (and its variants) are ubiquitous in open thoracic surgery. Recently, a new intelligent, automated rib spreader in development demonstrated results superior to the Finochietto-style retractors.

Tuffier Rib Spreader

7. *Carl Boye Semb* (1895–1971):

    Carl Semb was an internationally renowned Norwegian surgeon and professor at the *University of Oslo* (1951–1965). He grew up in Oslo, Norway, and designed the *Semb Bone Holding Forceps* angled on one side and has serrated jaws. Carl Semb was President of the Nordic Surgical Society (1955–56).

    • Carl Boye Semb

8. Robert Masters Kerrison (1776–1847)

Robert Masters Kerrison was an English physician who designed the *Kerrison rongeur*. It took more than 100 years before the Kerrison rongeur was modified and took its current form.

A rongeur is heavy-duty surgical instrument with a sharp-edged, scoop-shaped tip, used for gouging out bone. *Rongeur is a French word meaning rodent or "gnawer".* A rongeur can be used to open a window in bone, often in the skull, to access tissue underneath. They are used in neurosurgery, pediatric surgery, maxillofacial surgery, and orthopedic surgery to expose areas for operation.

A rongeur is used in oral maxillofacial surgery to remove bony fragments or soft tissue. It is also used in hand surgery to cut traumatic amputated bone to allow skin to be closed over the defect. A rongeur can also be used in cadaver dissection laboratory to break through ribs when removing the anterior chest wall.

    • Kerrison Rongeur

9. Jules-Émile Péan (1830–1898):

Jules-Émile Péan was one of the greatest French surgeons of the 19th century, born in France.

A *Haemostat* (also called a Haemostatic clamp, Arterial forceps, or Péan after *Jules-Émile Péan*) is a *surgical* tool used in many surgical procedures to control bleeding. For this reason, it is common in the initial phases of surgery for initial incision to be lined with hemostats which close blood vessels awaiting *ligation*. Hemostats belong to a group of instruments that *pivot* (similar to scissors, and including needle holders, tissue holders, and various clamps) where the structure of the tip determines the function.

The hemostat has handles that can be held in place by their locking mechanism. The locking mechanism is typically a series of interlocking teeth, a few on each handle, that allow the user to adjust the clamping force of the pliers. When locked together, the force between the tips is approximately 40 *N* (9 *lbf*).

    • Pean Mosquito Forceps, Hemostat Artery Forceps

10. *Osteotome*: An osteotome is an instrument used for cutting or preparing bone. Osteotomes are similar to a *chisel* but bevelled on both sides. They are used today in *plastic surgery*, *orthopedic surgery*, and *dental implantation*.

    • Osteotomes

11. Oscar Huntington Allis (1836–1921)

Oscar Allis introduced the Allis clamp in 1883. It remains part of the modern surgeon's armamentarium. This is also called the *Allis Forceps*, commonly used surgical instrument worldwide. Allis forceps is a straight grasping pair of forceps.

The Allis clamp is a surgical instrument with sharp teeth, used to hold or grasp heavy tissue. It is also used to grasp fascia and soft tissues such as *breast* or *bowel* tissue. Allis clamps can cause damage, so they are often used in tissue about to be removed. When used to grasp the *cervix* to stabilize the uterus, such as when an *intra*-uterine device is being inserted, an Allis clamp has the advantage of causing less bleeding than the more commonly used tenaculum.

An *Allis clamp* (also called the *Allis forceps*) is a commonly used surgical instrument.

Allis hemostats.

Allis intestinal forceps.

Allis Micro-Line pediatric forceps.

Allis sign: In fracture of the neck of the femur, the trochanter rides up, relaxing the fascia lata, so that the finger can be sunk deeply between the great trochanter and the iliac crest.

    • Allis Tissue Forceps

Sidney Yankauer (1872–1932)

Sidney Yankauer was an American otolaryngologist who developed the suction tip that bears his name in 1907. The *Yankauer suction tip* (pronounced yang'kow-er) is an *oral suctioning* tool used in medical procedures. The Yankauer suction instrument has become the most common medical suction instrument in the world.

It is typically a firm plastic suction tip with a large opening surrounded by a bulbous head and is designed to allow effective suction without damaging surrounding tissue. This tool is used to suction oropharyngeal secretions to prevent aspiration. A Yankauer can also be used to clear operative sites during surgical procedures, and its suctioned volume counted as blood loss during surgery.

12. Emil Theodor Kocher (1841–1917):

Emil Theodor Kocher was a *Swiss surgeon* and medical researcher who received the 1909 *Nobel Prize in Physiology or Medicine* for his work in the physiology, pathology, and surgery of the *thyroid* gland. Among his many accomplishments are the introduction and promotion of aseptic surgery and scientific methods in surgery, specifically reducing the mortality of *thyroidectomies* below 1% in his operations.

The *Kocher's Forceps* is named after *Emil Theodor Kocher*. The forceps is designed the same way as Spencer Wells Artery Forceps; however, the blades are a bit longer than Spencer's Forceps, and it has a tooth at the terminal end of one blade and groove in the other. The blades have transverse serrations. The ratchet mechanism locks the instrument securing the structure picked up by the forceps. The forceps may be straight or curved.

• *The Kocher's is hemostatic forceps.* It is specifically designed to catch the bleeders that are deep within tissue; hence, it is ideally used on tough structures such as palms, soles, or scalp. The forceps catches the structure that is bleeding and crushes the bleeder that results in clogging. The tooth gripped the structure firmly, so that the tissue does not slip.

Aseptic Surgery

It is unclear whether Kocher directly knew *Joseph Lister*, who pioneered the antiseptic (using chemical means to kill bacteria) method, but Kocher was in correspondence with him. Kocher had recognized the importance of aseptic techniques early on, introducing them to his peers at a time when this was considered revolutionary. In a hospital report from 1868, he attributed the lower mortality directly to the "antiseptic Lister's wound bandaging method," and he could later as the director of the clinic order strict adherence to the antiseptic method.

Contributions to Neurosurgery

Kocher also contributed significantly to neurology and *neurosurgery*. In this area, his research was pioneering and covered the areas of *concussion*, neurosurgery, and intracranial pressure (ICP). Furthermore, he investigated the surgical treatment of *epilepsy* and spinal and cranial trauma. He found that in some cases, the epilepsy patients had a brain tumor which could be surgically removed. He hypothesized that epilepsy was caused by an increase in ICP and believed that drainage of cerebrospinal fluid could cure epilepsy.

Surgical Successes

Three main factors contributed to Kocher's success as a surgeon, according to Bonjour (1981). The *first* factor was his consequent implementation of *antiseptic wound treatment* which prevented infection and later death of the patients. The *second* factor, according to *Erich Hintzsche*, was *monitoring of the anesthesia* where he used special masks and later used *local anesthesia* for *goiter* surgery which decreased or removed the dangers of anesthesia. As a *third* factor, Hintzsche mentions the minimal blood loss which Kocher achieved. Even the *smallest source of blood during surgery was precisely controlled and inhibited by Kocher*, initially because he thought that decomposing blood would constitute an infection risk for the patient.

Named in his honor:
• The *Kocher lunar crater* was named in his memory.
• An asteroid (2087) Kocher also commemorates his name.
Eponymous attributes:
• *Kocher's forceps*, a surgical instrument with serrated blades and interlocking teeth at the tips used to control bleeding
• *Kocher's point*, common entry point for an intraventricular catheter to drain cerebral spinal fluid from the cerebral ventricles
• Kocher maneuver, a surgical maneuver to expose structures in the retroperitoneum
• *Kocher-Debre-Semelaigne syndrome*, hypothyroidism in infancy or childhood characterized by lower extremity or generalized muscular hypertrophy, myxoedema, short stature, and cretinism
• *Kocher's collar incision* is used in thyroid surgery
• *Kocher's subcostal incision*, cholecystectomy
• *Kocher's sign*, eyelid phenomenon in hyperthyroidism and Basedow's disease
  ○ Kocher Clamp

13. William Wayne Babcock (1872–1963):

He was an American Surgeon, graduated in Baltimore, who invented this popular Tissue-Holding

Forceps. *What are Babcock's Forceps?* The forceps is a tissue clamp and has a ratchet mechanism, ring handles, and blades with a *triangular orifice*, along with a horizontal groove at the terminal end in one blade and a ridge in the other blade. When the instrument is closed, the ridge fits into the groove securing the held structure from slipping. The instrument is nontraumatic.

What is its function? The Babcock's is invented to hold tubular organs; the orifices in the blades accommodate some part of the tissue and reduce the intraluminal pressure, which protects the organs from getting damaged. The surgical procedure is as follows: There are numerous surgical procedures where Babcock's is used. It is most commonly used during appendicectomy (removal of appendix) to hold either appendix or caecum. Moreover, it is used to hold small bowel during exploratory laparotomy and sometimes during resection anastomosis. To this day, the Babcock clamp is widely used in many surgical specialities, including thoracic surgery.

Turner-Babcock Forceps: Turner-Babcock Forceps are similar to standard Babcock forceps but have solid tips versus fenestrated tips. They are finger rings, ratcheted forceps often used to hold portions of the intestines or other delicate tissue. The tips are circumferential and triangular with horizontal serrations. This product is straight, and the overall length is 9 to 1/2 inches.

- Babcock Tissue Forceps
14. *Lee Bronchus Clamp* is ideally suited for use in some cardiothoracic surgical procedures. This clamp features a long slightly curved shank and a jaw that is set at an obtuse angle making it ideal in clamping the bronchus. The slender design of this instrument allows it to pass with minimum damage and trauma to the surrounding structure. Additionally, the clamp is narrow enough to only be clamping a minimum amount of bronchus to reduce the likelihood of damage to the bronchus.

This figure of the right-angled Lees Atraumatic Bronchus Clamps provides secure closures of the bronchial lumen during cardiothoracic procedures. The clamp has two ratcheted finger ring handles, a long shaft and neck, and two right-angled blades. The jaws have 2 × 3 DeBakey-style serrations to enable stronger grasps on smooth tissues and round structures. The overall length of the clamp is 25.5 cm, and the terminal jaw is 42-mm long.

- *Lees Atrauma Bronchus Clamp Angled 90*: The LEES Bronchus Clamp has a jaw length of 1 to $\frac{1}{2}$ in (4 cm) and an overall length of 9 to $\frac{1}{4}$ in (23.5 cm).

15. Howard A. Kelly (1858–1943):

After only 1 year as a Professor of Obstetrics at the University of Pennsylvania (1888–1889), he was recruited to become the first Professor of Obstetrics and Gynecology at John Hopkins (1889–1899) by Dr William Osler. During his tenure, Kelly assisted in fostering the development of many surgical techniques and procedures of the female reproductive and genitourinary tract. Kelly remained a surgeon innovator into his old age, advocating the use of electrosurgery in 1932. He designed the tissue *Kelly Clamp* which is one of the most widely used and known surgical instruments.

- Kelly Box Lock Forceps
- Kelly Artery Forceps

16. Eugene L. Doyen (1859–1916):

Eugene Doyen was a French surgeon remarkable in being both excellent and expeditious. Additionally, he was a noted bacteriologist. He was one of the first to introduce electrocoagulation and use blood aspiration by suction in the operative field. He designed many surgical instruments which allowed rapid and precise movements during the operations when brevity of time was essential in the face of dangerous anesthesia and absence of artificial ventilation. The right and left rib strippers and periosteal elevator bear his name.

Doyen Rib Raspatories

17. John Alexander (1891–1954)

John Alexander was a Philadelphia native who graduated in medicine from the University of Pennsylvania. After graduating in 1916, he traveled to France to serve his country in World War I. After the war, he began his career at the University of Michigan. He was able to maintain his academic position and continued with his career and developed the first formal thoracic surgery program at the University of Michigan. He was a surgeon innovator, and with *Cameron Haight*, he designed a periosteal elevator called the *Cameron Haight Periosteal Elevators*.

- Cameron Haight Periosteal Elevators

18. Cameron Haight (1901–1970):

Cameron Haight was an American physician who graduated from Harvard Medical School and began his surgical training at the University of Michigan. He came under the influence of *John Alexander*, and under his guidance, he excelled in the field of congenital tracheoesophageal fistula repair. He had success in pneumonectomies. He designed a periosteal elevator and developed nasotracheal suctioning. His surgical innovation was displayed in the designing of the periosteal elevator. *Cameron Haight Periosteal Elevator* is double-ended with a round blade 12-mm wide and straight edge 15-mm wide, and its overall length is 13in (33 cm). Cameron-Haight Periosteal Elevator is commonly used to elevate layers of soft tissue from the underlying thoracic outlet syndrome (TOC) surgery to protect the vasculature near the first rib. This elevator is double-headed with one end featuring a chiseled sharp tip for scraping away tissues near to bone while the opposing end is more rounded and less sharp for more delicate manipulation of soft tissue.

Cameron Haight Elevator is used for stripping periosteum from both surfaces of the ribs.

- Cameron Haight Periosteal Elevators

19. Victor P. Satinsky (1912–1997):

Victor Satinsky was born in Philadelphia, and by birth, he was Russian. His sharp intellectual capacity and creativity developed quickly. He attended the Jefferson Medical College graduating in 1938. Soon after, while in residency at Mount Sinai in New York, he joined the United States Army in World War II. While looking after wounded solders, he needed to treat those with chest injuries. As a result of the wartime experience, his interest in cardiothoracic surgery excelled resulting in becoming the research director of the Hahnemann Cardiovascular Institute (1961–1977). He developed at least *30 major medical innovations and designed a vascular clamp for optimal vascular control during cardiac operation, which is still in use today.*

1. Satinsky Vascular Clamps
2. Cooley-Satinsky Vascular Clamp
3. Satinsky-DeBakey Vascular Clamp

20. Alfred Washington Adson (1887–1951)

Alfred Washington Adson was an American physician, military officer, and surgeon. He was born at Terril, Iowa, and was Norwegian by birth. He was in medical practice with the Mayo Clinic and the Mayo Graduate School of Medicine of the University of Minnesota at Rochester, Minnesota. He was associated with the development of the Section of Neurologic Surgery which was first established at Mayo in 1919. He functioned as its chair until 1946. He undertook pioneering neurosurgery and gave his name to a medical condition, a medical sign, a medical diagnostic maneuver, and medical instruments.

He described thoracic surgical sympathectomy for treating Raynaud's disease. He was a founding member of the American Board of Surgery. His skill as a surgeon innovator extended to designing instruments for proper handling of tissues, laminectomy retractors, and fine-toothed tissue forceps that bears his name. Adson needle holder is used for anastomotic work.

Adson undertook *innovative neurosurgery* for the treatment of *glossopharyngeal neuralgia, Raynaud's Disease, Hirschsprung's disease*, and *essential hypertension*. He was a colonel in the US Army Medical Reserve Corps.

Eponymous Attributes to Alfred Adson

- *Adson-Coffey syndrome*: named by Adson and Jay R Coffey, also called TOS, a condition which involves pressure on the nerve bundle that leaves the *thoracic cavity* in the region of the armpit.
- *Adson maneuver*: used to elicit *Adson's sign*. A loss of the radial pulse on the side affected by *TOS* when the patient fills their lungs and turns their head with stretched neck, to the affected side.
- *Adson-Graeff forceps*: 125-mm-long tissue forceps.
- *Beckman-Adson retractor*: used for holding open surgical incisions.
- *Adson dissecting forceps*: used for holding fine tissue.

21. Popular Different Types of Drains and Purpose:

The purpose of a drain is to prevent fluid (blood or other) buildup in a closed ("dead") space, which may cause either disruption of the wound and the healing process or become an infected abscess, with either scenario possibly requiring a formal drainage/repair procedure (and possibly another trip to the operating room). The drain is also used to evacuate an *internal abscess* before surgery when an *infection* already exists. Clots and other solid matter in the drainage fluid may occlude the tubing, preventing the device from draining properly.

- Adson Forceps

Surgical drains can be broadly classified into 4 categories:

1. *Jackson-Pratt drain* (also called a JP drain) is a *closed-suction* medical device that is commonly used as a *postoperative drain* for collecting bodily fluids from surgical sites. The device consists of an internal drain connected to a grenade-shaped bulb via plastic tubing. *Jackson-Pratt drain* consists of a perforated round or flat tube connected to a negative pressure collection device. The collection device is typically a bulb with a drainage port which can be opened to remove fluid or air. After compressing the bulb to remove fluid or air, negative pressure is created as the bulb returns to its normal shape.
   • Jackson Pratt Drain
2. *Penrose drain* is a soft, flexible rubber tube used as a surgical drain, to prevent the buildup of fluid in a surgical site. The Penrose drain is named after the American gynecologist *Charles Bingham Penrose (1862–1925)*. A Penrose drain removes fluid from a wound area. Frequently it is put in place by a surgeon after a procedure is complete to prevent the area from accumulating fluid, such as blood, which could serve as a medium for bacteria to grow in. In podiatry, a Penrose drain is often used as a tourniquet during a hallux nail avulsion procedure or ingrown toenail extraction. It can also be used to drain cerebrospinal fluid to treat a *hydrocephalus patient*.
3. *Blake drain* is a round silicone tube with channels that carry fluid to a negative pressure collection device. Drainage is thought to be achieved by capillary action, allowing fluid to travel through the open grooves into a closed cross-section, which contains the fluid and allows it to be suctioned through the tube.
4. *Negative pressure wound therapy* (*NPWT*) involves the use of enclosed foam and a suction device attached; this is one of the newer types of wound healing/drain devices which promotes *faster tissue* granulation, often used for large surgical/trauma/nonhealing wounds.

NPWT, also known as a vacuum-assisted closure, is a therapeutic technique using a suction pump, tubing, and dressing to remove excess exudate and promote healing in acute or chronic wounds and second- and third-degree burns. The therapy involves the controlled application of sub-atmospheric pressure to the local wound environment, using a sealed wound dressing connected to a vacuum pump. The use of this technique in wound management increased dramatically over the 1990s and 2000s,[5] and a large number of studies have been published examining NPWT.[6] NPWT has many indications for use:

i. Dehisced surgical wounds
ii. Closed surgical wounds
iii. Pressure injuries or pressure ulcers
iv. Diabetic foot ulcers
v. Management of the open abdomen (laparotomy)
vi. Venous insufficiency ulcers
vii. Skin flaps and grafts

Overview

NPWT promotes wound healing by applying a vacuum through a special sealed dressing. The continued vacuum draws out fluid from the wound and increases blood flow to the area.[3] The vacuum may be applied continuously or intermittently, depending on the type of wound being treated and the clinical objectives. Typically, the dressing is changed two to three times per week.[4] The dressings used for the technique include foam dressings and gauze, sealed with an occlusive dressing intended to contain the vacuum at the wound site. Where NPWT devices allow delivery of fluids, such as saline or antibiotics to irrigate the wound, intermittent removal of used fluid supports the cleaning and drainage of the wound bed.[7,8]

In 1995, Kinetic Concepts was the first company to have an NPWT product cleared by the US Food and Drug Administration. After increased use of the technique by hospitals in the US, the procedure was approved for reimbursement by the Centers for Medicare and Medicaid Services in 2001.

   • NPWT
5. *Redivac drain*, a high negative pressure drain in which suction is applied through the drain to generate a vacuum and draw fluids into a bottle.
6. *Pigtail drain*, has an exterior screw to release the internal "pigtail" before it can be removed.
7. *Argyle Chest tube*, is a flexible plastic tube that is inserted through the chest wall and into the pleural space or mediastinum.

OPERATING THEATER SUITE

The *three zones* to be respected in the theater suite and the appropriate surgical and nursing staff behavior required are as follows:

To minimize bacterial contamination, the operating theater is traditionally divided into three zones:

1. *The outer perimeter outside the theater* encompasses those areas outside the operating

theater itself, used for sterilization of materials, scrubbing, stretcher, storing nonessential equipment, and in some hospitals, induction of anesthesia.

2. *The middle zone inside the theater* is the domain of the circulating nurse, the anesthetist and his equipment, and nonsterile equipment such as collection bottles, tubing, monitoring equipment, and the diathermy chassis. The circulating nurse delivers necessary supplies to the sterile field from storage areas, handles nonsterile equipment needed in the operation, keeps track of sponges, instruments, and specimens as they move to and from the operating table.

3. *The inner zone inside the theater* is completely sterile and consists of the operative field, that portion of the patient draped by sterile sheets, the surgeon, and his/her assistants, the instrument nurse, and under her/his control the instrument table. Everything entering this area must be sterile as it comes into contact with the operative field.

OPERATING THEATRE RULES AND GUIDANCE

The *essential requirements* during the operation in the operating theater for medicolegal reasons and safety are as follows:

1. The team must be on time to start the case, and delay is to be avoided.
2. All imaging studies related to the case must be available, be on display, and reviewed by the surgical team.
3. Unnecessary conversations inside the operating theater must be discouraged and avoided.
4. Noise level inside the operating theater must be kept at minimum.
5. Operative plan and conduct of the operation must be reviewed and discussed with the anesthetist and the responsible operating room nurses by the attending surgeon. There is a need for intraoperative monitoring, sharing of the airway for tracheal operation, cross-table ventilation, urinary bladder catheter, proper placement of arterial and intravenous lines, intraoperative radiography, electrical equipment, and positioning of the patient to facilitate exposure of the operative field.
6. Respectful behavior toward everyone involved in the case is essential.
7. Properly conducted surgical pause is mandatory.
8. Seriousness during the operation should be observed.

9. Checking the patient, the chart, the operative consent form, and preoperative investigation is the responsibility of the operating room nurses, the surgeon, and his/her assistant before the patient enters the operating room.
10. Strict adherence to the surgical scrub for skin preparation and draping of the operative field.
11. Administration of prophylactic intravenous broad-spectrum antibiotic 1 hour before making the surgical incision.
12. Administration of one dose of prophylactic subcutaneous heparin.
13. The pathologist for frozen section should be notified beforehand.
14. Mislabeling of the specimens taken for analysis must not occur.
15. Conversation should be kept to a minimum as it is distracting and significantly contributes to droplet contamination of the operative field.
16. By and large, traffic through the inner two zones of the operating theater should be restricted to essential personnel. Observers crowding around the operating team in an attempt to see the field must be discouraged to avoid bacterial contamination.

THE OPERATION

The necessary steps to be diligently observed during the conduct of operation are as follows:

1. *Proper surgical exposure* of the deeply placed operative field is essential, and this depends upon proper use of the correct retractors; knowledge and familiarity with the different types of retractors is absolutely essential. Improperly used retractors can cause serious injury to essential structures in the field. The tissues under a retractor should be carefully padded. The proper placement of the retractors is the sole responsibility of the operating surgeon. The most effective exposure can be achieved if the surgeon permits the retractor holder to see what he/she is doing. Good retraction must be maintained right to the end of the operation.
2. *Maintaining clear operative field* with sponges and suctioning are essential functions of the assistant to keep the field clear of blood. This action must be taught to the assistant to remain vigilant and avoid unnecessary motions.
3. *Securing surgical hemostasis* by ligation and electrocoagulation for control of bleeding vessels in an essential requirement during the operation. This requires a team effort and not a lesson to be taught to the assistant during

the operation unless the assistant is learned and surgically competent when the first and foremost safety for the patient's welfare prevails.

4. *Adequate surgical knowledge* about the different gauge needles, round tapered or cutting shanks, and the appropriately selected gauge is essential, as well as the type of sutures to be used for control of major bleeding blood vessel, repair of connective tissues, vascular anastomosis, and bowel anastomosis or repair of defect. The difference between varying fine and heavy sutures and appropriate recorded labeling must be known by the surgical team at all times.

FAMILIARITY AND KNOWLEDGE OF SURGICAL INSTRUMENTS

Familiarity with the types and names of surgical instruments available at a particular hospital greatly facilitates the operation. This is when preparedness becomes the essence in conduct of safe operation and outcome.

The basic surgical instruments include,

1. *Surgical knife (scalpel):* This is the razor-like cutting instrument used for incision and dissection. It is available as a separate handle to which is coupled a disposable blade. Both the handles and blades come in a variety of sizes and shapes. To ensure optimal control and safety, only a very sharp-edged fresh blade should be used. Contact with dense tissues and metallic materials will quickly dull the razor edge and calls for replacement with a fresh blade.

2. *Scissors:* Different types of scissors are available for dissection, division of tissues, and cutting of sutures. The character of the tissue being dissected dictates the size and sturdiness of the scissors selected. Those with curved blades lend themselves to dissection while those used for cutting sutures are generally straight with blunt tips.

3. *Tissue forceps (Thump Forceps):* These tweezer-like instruments are available with a variety of grasping tips, ranging from gently serrated ones to those with interlocking (mousetooth) teeth. These are used for grasping tissues, sponges, sutures, needles, and so forth. Those forceps with fine teeth are atraumatic for secure handling of delicate tissues.

4. *Hemostatic forceps (Spencer Wells):* These are hinged clamps with a ratchet lock device in the handle. They are available in carious sizes, both straight and curved. The interlocking serrated blades are used to hold and compress blood vessels for control of bleeding. They are often used for dissection or grasping of tissues.

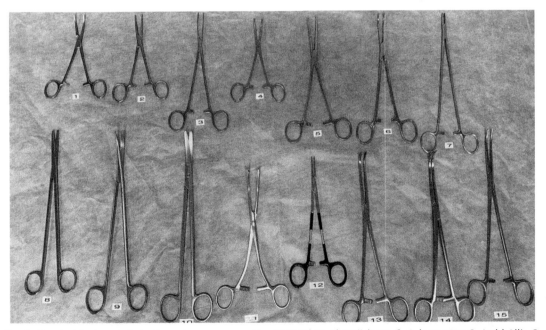

Fig. 1. Surgical instruments in thoracic surgery used by Dr Farid M. Shamji (Part 1). 1. hemostat, 2. Judd Allis, 3. Kelly Clamp, 4. Curved Kocher, 5. Straight Kocher, 6. Lower, 7. Crile wood Needle Driver, 8. Metzenbaum scissors, 9. Bronchial Scissor, 10. Alison Scissors, 11. Duval, 12. Fraser, 13. Finochietto forceps, 14. Semb forceps, 15. Swedish DeBakey. (*Courtesy of* Kristen Waddell, BScN, RN, Ontario, CA.)

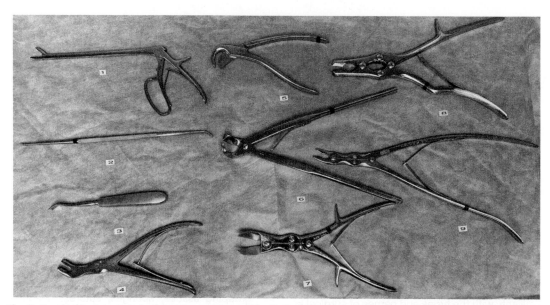

Fig. 2. Surgical instruments in thoracic surgery used by Dr Farid M. Shamji (Part 2). 1. First Rib Urschel Rongeur, 2. Slim Jim Elevator, 3. Bifurcated Rasparatory 12 mm, 4. Leksell Rongeur, 5. Collins rib shear, 6. Roos Rib Shear, 7. Stille-Horsley (Liston Key) Rib Cutter, 8. Sauerbruch Rongeur, 9. Dale Roos Rongeur. (*Courtesy of* Kristen Waddell, BScN, RN, Ontario, CA.)

Most varieties crush the tissue within their jaws; however, atraumatic vascular clamps occlude a vessel lumen without injuring its wall.

5. *Retractors:* These are instruments used to provide exposure by distracting wound ages and adjacent structures from the operative field. The two basic types include the hand retractor and the self-retaining retractor. Each type consists of a handle and retracting blade. The form and size of the blades vary considerably,

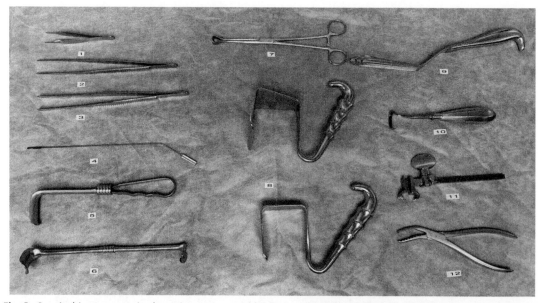

Fig. 3. Surgical instruments in thoracic surgery used by Dr Farid M. Shamji (Part 3). 1. Adson Tissue Forceps with teeth, 2. DeBakey Tissue forceps, 3. Russian Tissue Forceps, 4. Obturator Rummel, 5. Richardson appendectomy retractor, 6. Double ended Richardson, 7. Turner Babcock, 8. David Scapula retractor wide and narrow, 9. Allison Lung Retractor, 10. Doyen, 11. Bailey Rib Approximator, 12. Semb Bone Holding Forceps. (*Courtesy of* Kristen Waddell, BScN, RN, Ontario, CA.)

allowing for application in a wide range of anatomic situations. They vary from self-retaining retractors with bidirectional pull of opposing blades to effect retraction and to maintain their fixed position in locations as the thoracic wall (*Finochietto retractor*); lung retractor is designed to retract the lung with its open design and thin flat wires which are gentle on the delicate lung tissue (*Allison Lung Retractor*), right angle short blade on long handle retractor for soft tissues, and small rake-like retractors for drawing back subcutaneous tissues.

6. *Needle holder*: This instrument is similar to hemostatic forceps, with the jaws modified to securely hold and guide the curved surgical needles.

7. *Other specialized surgical instruments:* This group includes blunt dissectors, sponge-holders, tenacula, suction tips, stapling devices, hemostatic clips and clip holders, intestinal clamps, ligature carriers, and so forth and should be familiar to the surgical assistant.

SURGICAL DISSECTION DURING THE OPERATION

Dissection by the surgeon is facilitated by the maneuvers of the assistant. Dissection is performed sharply with a knife or scissors, or bluntly with finger, gauze dental or peanut pledget, forceps and blunt dissecting instruments.

Application of the various techniques to varying situations can only be learned by practical experience and time spent in the operating theater. Familiarity with surgical instruments and with various tissues and their responses together with a tactile sensibility achieved by practice produces expertise in surgical dissection. The major principle of dissection is the distraction of tissues by the application of traction and counter-traction so that a plane of separation can be identified and entered by the dissection instrument (**Figs. 1–3**).

SUMMARY

A considerable thought has been given to writing this article which the authors feel compelled to educate the novice surgeon on the importance of the knowledge and application of the thoracic surgical instruments and the requirement of professional behavior in the operating theater. The lessons pertaining to this can only be taught to the junior staff by thoughtful approach by the senior surgeon who must understand the dire need for this particular education, unfortunately frequently ignored, which is as important as the technique of the operation itself.

CLINICS CARE POINTS

- Technical considerations – patient position on the operating table, instruments – bone instruments, retractors, special scissors and needle holders, forceps, clamps, haemostats, rib resection, special instruments for general use and for surgery of the great vessels and drainage system for chest operations.
- History of the renowned thoracic surgeons.
- Arrangement of the operating suite, operating theatre rules and guidance, and the conduct of the operation.
- Familiarity and knowledge of surgical instruments.

REFERENCES

1. James K, editor. Pye's surgical handicraft. A John Wright & Sons LTD Publication; 1977.
2. Ailawadi G, Nagji AS, Jones DR. The Legends Behind Cardiothoracic Surgical Instruments. Ann Thorac Surg 2010;89:1693–700.
3. Kirkup JR. The history and evolution of surgical instruments Part I Introduction. Ann R Coll Surg Engl 1981; 63:279–85.
4. Kirkup JR. The history and evolution of surgical instruments Part II Origins: function: carriage: manufacture. Ann R Coll Surgeons Engl 1982;64:125–32.
5. Panchabhai TS, Mehta AC. Historical Perspectives of Bronchoscopy – Connecting the Dots. Ann Am Thorac Soc 2015;12(5):631–41.
6. Sweet RH. Thoracic surgery. 2nd edition. W.B. Saunders Company; 1954.
7. Obdeijn MC, de Lange MY, Lichtendahl DH, et al. Vacuum-assisted closure in the treatment of poststernotomy mediastinitis. Ann Thorac Surg 1999;68:2358-2360.
8. Agarwal JP, Ogilvie M, Wu LC, et al. Vacuum-assisted closure for sternal wounds: a first-line therapeutic management approach. Plast Reconstr Surg 2005; 116:1035-1040.

Superior Vena Cava Resection and Reconstruction with Resection of Primary Lung Cancer and Mediastinal Tumor

Robert James Cusimano, MD, FRCSC, FACS[a],*,
Farid M. Shamji, MBBS, FRCSC, FACS[b]

KEYWORDS

- Superior vena cava • Reconstruction • Lung cancer

KEY POINTS

- Embryologically, there are 2 superior vena cavas (SVCs), with the left regressing. If not, it drains into the coronary sinus, which enlarges out of proportion to the SVC size and may or may not be attached to the right SVC via a bridging vein.
- The SVC is about 7 to 8 cm long and 2 cm wide with the vast majority outside or abutting the pericardium.
- Eighty-five percent of SVC obstruction is caused by malignancy, with two-thirds being advanced lung cancer, most commonly small cell cancer.
- Reconstruction can be simple or with small diameter ring reinforced polytetrafluoroethylene to allow rapid flow of blood to reduce thrombus risk.

REGIONAL AND APPLIED ANATOMY OF THE SUPERIOR VENA CAVA

The superior vena cava (SVC) is a mediastinal structure in the middle mediastinum. Embryologically, there are bilateral venae cavae, with the left being in continuity with the coronary sinus. Usually the left side regresses and typically there is an isolated SVC, found on the right side of the body. A persistent left SVC (LSVC) is not uncommon, and rarely, the right-sided SVC is absent.[1] When present, a persistent LSVC is associated with an abnormally large coronary sinus and often (but not always) has a "bridging vein," the left brachiocephalic vein, of varying size. In fact, when a small or nonexistent brachiocephalic vein is found, a persistent LSVC must be considered. When isolated, the SVC is a wide vessel, about 7 cm long (6–8 cm), and its transverse diameter is usually 20 to 22 mm.[2–4] It is formed by the confluence of the 2 brachiocephalic veins as they join deep to the lower border of the first right costal cartilage near the border of the manubrium. It descends vertically behind the manubrium and body of the sternum to enter the right atrium at the level of the third right costal cartilage. Its upper half is outside the pericardial sac; its lower half is inside the fibrous pericardium, where it pierces level with the second costal cartilage. Within the pericardium, only a very small portion is completely intrapericardial (from the inferior portion of the pulmonary artery to the heart). The pericardium needs to be divided to isolate the more superior portions, which have the posterior and lateral portions outside the pericardium. It possesses no valves.

[a] University of Toronto, Peter Munk Cardiac Centre, Toronto General Hospital, 4n468. 200 Elizabeth Street, Toronto, Ontario M5G 2C4, Canada; [b] University of Ottawa, General Campus, Ottawa Hospital, 501 Smyth Road, Ottawa, Ontario K1H 8L6, Canada
* Corresponding author.
E-mail address: robert.cusimano@uhn.ca

Thorac Surg Clin 31 (2021) 463–468
https://doi.org/10.1016/j.thorsurg.2021.07.006
1547-4127/21/© 2021 Elsevier Inc. All rights reserved.

The right and left brachiocephalic veins receive the ipsilateral internal jugular and subclavian veins. The internal jugular vein collects blood from the head and deep sections of the neck, whereas the subclavian veins drain the upper limbs, superior chest, and superficial head and neck regions. Several other veins from the cervical region, chest wall, and mediastinum drain directly into the brachiocephalic veins.

The blood pressure in the SVC normally ranges from −5 to +5 mm Hg, depending on the body position and cardiac valvular and fluid status of the individual, and its flow is discontinuous depending on the cardiac cycle.

Relationship: in its lower half it is covered by the pericardium. Anterior are the thymus gland, right lung and pleura, and the manubrium. Posterior is the right lung root, right laterotracheal lymphatic chain, the pulmonary artery, and superior pulmonary vein. Medial are the ascending aorta and the right brachiocephalic artery. Lateral are the right pleura, phrenic nerve, and the lung. The right pulmonary artery passes to the hilum of the right lung deep to the ascending aorta and SVC. The azygous vein is its only tributary, entering it posteriorly. At the level of the fourth thoracic vertebra, it arches forward superior to the hilum of the right lung to enter the SVC superior to the pulmonary artery. The Azygous vein drains the ascending lumbar veins and the subcostal veins on the right side. In this way, it connects the SVC and inferior vena cava (IVC) and thus can provide an important alternative path for blood to the *right atrium* when either of the venae cavae is blocked. Anterior chest wall drainage also occurs via the internal thoracic veins, which drain into the subclavian veins bilaterally. Thus, SVC or IVC obstruction may cause extensive venous engorgement of surface and mediastinal veins.

There are no valves in either the SVC or the brachiocephalic veins. The azygos vein contains a valve halfway along the azygos.

SUPERIOR VENA CAVA OBSTRUCTION

More than 85% of all cases of SVC obstruction are caused by tumor. Cancer of the lung is responsible for more than 60% of cases, about 20% being accounted for by other tumors, such as lymphoma, thymoma, thymic carcinoma, germ cell tumors, and metastatic mediastinal lymphadenopathy. The few remaining cases are caused by rare benign conditions including fungal or tuberculous granulomatous disease, cryptogenic mediastinal fibrosis, intrathoracic goiter, thoracic aortic aneurysm, and venous thrombosis from descending necrotizing mediastinitis or instrumentation by pacemaker wires.

In the case of lung cancer, the histologic type most commonly involved is small cell lung cancer followed by squamous cell carcinoma. The tumor is nearly always right sided and often situated in the right upper lobe. The tumor usually compresses the vessel from without by direct mediastinal invasion and bulkiness but occasionally invades its wall. Bulky metastatic lymph node disease in the paratracheal area may compress the SVC.

Obstruction of the SVC produces the clinical manifestation of SVC syndrome (**Table 1**).

CLINICAL MANIFESTATION OF SUPERIOR VENA CAVA OBSTRUCTION SYNDROME

The patient notices swelling of the face and neck with tightness about the collar, which may progress to gross edema. The arms may also become edematous and the veins over the upper part of the body become distended. The distension continues even when the arms are raised above the level of the heart. The earliest and most common sign, however, is bilateral jugular venous engorgement. There is loss of jugular venous pulsation. Postural persistent flushing of the face may be produced by asking the patient to bend down and straighten up again. Symptoms of intracranial venous hypertension may be present, especially when the patient bends forward, for instance to tie shoes, with the patient complaining of headaches, nausea, blurred vision, and ultimately serious neurologic sequelae.

The diagnosis is usually obvious from the symptoms and signs, and the next step is to obtain radiographic and histologic confirmation of the inciting cause. Between 5% and 10% of patients with primary lung cancer may present with symptoms and signs due to SVC obstruction. Often, it is the small cell cancer of the lung, which is the cause, nearly always in the right upper lobe.

Diagnosis

SVC obstruction, although unpleasant, is itself unlikely to result in mortality but the underlying cause is, and it is therefore important to determine this cause as accurately as possible.

The investigations that are helpful include computed tomography with contrast venography in determining the extent of the disease. Intravenous bilateral arm venography to produce SVC grams is necessary to produce a "road map" in those very few cases where bypass surgery is contemplated.

Histologic diagnosis is usually obtained by bronchoscopy, endobronchial ultrasound, and needle aspiration biopsy and infrequently requires

Table 1 Causes of superior vena cava obstruction syndrome	
Malignant Cause: • Most common cause	Benign Cause: • 5%–25%
Primary • Bronchogenic carcinoma	Inflammatory • Mediastinal granulomatosis • Fibrosing mediastinitis • Pericardial adhesions
Secondary metastatic carcinoma from: • Breast • Thyroid • Lymphoma • Melanoma	Neoplastic • Substernal mediastinal goiter Traumatic • Fibrosing mediastinitis secondary to blunt chest trauma • Secondary to prolonged catherization for hyperalimentation • Indwelling cardiac pacemaker wire • Following palliative procedures for cyanotic congestive heart disease
	Vascular • Aortic aneurysmal compression • SVC thrombosis ○ Secondary to prolonged catherization for hyperalimentation ○ Indwelling cardiac pacemaker wire
	Idiopathic • Thrombosis of undetermined cause
	Congenital • Pericardial bands • Secondary to total anomalous pulmonary venous drainage

Data from Tyson RR, Grosh JD. Superior Vena Cava Syndrome. In: Rhoads JE, Hardy JD, eds. RHOADS Textbook of Surgery: Principles and Practice. 5th ed. Lippincott; 1977: 1900-1903.

mediastinoscopy or anterior mediastinotomy. Fine-needle aspiration biopsy of a palpable ipsilateral cervical lymph gland (scalene lymph node) will often yield histologic confirmation.

Evidence of extrapulmonary dissemination of the cancer other than SVC obstruction is common in this group of patients. Frequently, recurrent laryngeal nerve palsy producing hoarseness is present as an indication of mediastinal invasion.

Treatment

Treatment in cases due to cancer of the lung depends on whether the histology is consistent with small cell carcinoma or not. In a patient with small cell carcinoma a decision to use chemotherapy as primary treatment should be undertaken. There is evidence that where chemotherapy is being used as the primary treatment of small cell carcinoma, SVC obstruction is satisfactorily relieved, and radiotherapy confers no additional benefit. There is no need to add radiotherapy to chemotherapy, which will involve extra burden of toxicity.

In non–small cell carcinoma, chemotherapy has not been shown to produce any relief over and above that resulting from treatment with radiotherapy but is attended by greater morbidity and mortality.

Surgical treatment

Surgical treatment specifically for SVC obstruction is very seldom indicated when cancer of the lung is the cause. It is almost always an unresectable advanced lung cancer. This type of procedure is usually only resorted to when symptoms and signs persist and are severe in patients in whom investigation has failed to achieve a histologic diagnosis. Clearly such operative intervention is unjustified in patients in whom the prognosis is short. Extended resection for SVC invasion (by T4 disease and often with N2 mediastinal lymphatic spread) of non–small cell lung cancer and anterior mediastinal neoplasms (frequently mediastinal lymphoma, advanced invasive thymoma, and giant germ cell tumors) often evokes controversy about its long-term benefit. Recent published series

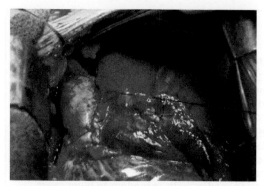

Fig. 1. Autologous pericardial reconstruction of the anterior wall of the SVC.

indicate favourable reports with acceptable morbidity and survival. The reported 5-year survival rate after SVC resection and reconstruction for lung cancer is 21% to 31%, and for anterior mediastinal neoplasms it is 45% to 53%.

TECHNIQUE OF SUPERIOR VENA CAVA RESECTION AND RECONSTRUCTION

Partial resections of the SVC can be performed with autologous or bovine pericardium (**Fig. 1**). However, if the whole cava is resected, reconstruction may be undertaken by numerous methods, the most common form being with ringed polytetrafluoroethylene (PTFE)[5–12] (**Fig. 2**). Reconstruction can be solely of the SVC or of both the left brachiocephalic vein and SVC, either individually or as a Y graft of the 2 superior systems draining into a confluent vein into the right atrium. The reconstruction details depend largely on which portion of the SVC is involved with the disease process. With low-lying malignancies, where the confluence of the left and right brachiocephalic veins is in continuity, a simple tube to the

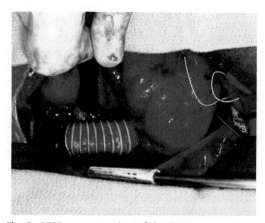

Fig. 2. PTFE reconstruction of the SVC.

right atrium suffices but when the confluence is involved, either a Y graft joining the 2 or, more commonly, separate grafts from each site are constructed. Grafts are to be kept short, and on the smaller side, generally a 12 to 14 mm ringed PTFE graft is used to allow for rapid flow in order to reduce stasis and thus thrombosis. Patients are treated with Warfarin postoperatively for a period of 3 to 6 months. Cardiopulmonary bypass is not usually required. A shunt can be used[13] but not necessary, especially if the occlusion is complete. If not, most investigators suggest clamp times of 30 minutes or less to avoid the ill consequences of cerebral venous hypertension. If 2 grafts are used, the left brachiocephalic to right atrial bypass is done first in order to reduce cerebral venous pressures.

Insertion of the graft into the right atrium can be anatomic or to the right atrial chamber directly, depending on the level of resection and if there is a separate graft to the left-sided brachiocephalic vein. If there are separate grafts to the upper venous systems, smaller grafts can be used and the left-sided graft can be placed to the right atrial free wall, notably the atrial appendage. If so, a partial occluding clamp is placed on the atrial appendage and the internal trabeculae removed to allow clear flow into the right atrium. The ends can be beveled to reduce the risk of stenosis at the 2 anastomoses. The typical size for the left vein would be 8 to 10 mm and the right side 10 to 14 mm. When a single graft is placed (the confluence of the left and right brachiocephalic veins is intact), the superior incision can be placed either on the undersurface of the brachiocephalic vein or the SVC proper if enough room. A short 12 to 14 mm ringed graft is usually used but constructed biological grafts have also shown good patency.[6] If impossible to reconstruct, at least one graft to a superior vessel would help with venous drainage from the head and arms given the rich collateral venous connections in the head.

The SVC can be unilateral or bilateral and is sometimes involved by malignancy, requiring resection for complete control of the malignancy. Resection is possible, likely will not require cardiopulmonary bypass to carry out, and is safe, either performed by simple clamp or with a shunt. Reconstruction can be with biological material but most commonly ring reinforced PTFE is used. Long-term results are related to the underlying disease process. Long-term patency is good.

COMMENT

There have been several single-center experiences reported on the management of non–small cell lung cancer that has involved SVC. It may be by direct extension into the mediastinum from the anterior segment of the right upper lobe, making it a T4 descriptor. Lymphatic spread of lung cancer to the mediastinal lymph nodes (N2 descriptor) by abutting the SVC can involve this great vessel by compression and adhesion or possibly by invading the vessel wall.

By definition this local extent of the cancer in the mediastinum by direct extension and/or lymphatic spread makes it stage IIIB, as T4 descriptor with possibly N2 lymphatic metastasis.

The prognosis is guarded, and assessment is performed for surgical treatment if the likelihood of complete resection seems promising. In a single-center experience from the Toronto General Hospital by Shargall and colleagues in 2004 of 15 patients with direct SVC invasion by tumor, 7 patients had confirmed N2 lymphatic metastases, and 1 patient had bulky right upper lobe tumor. These patients received induction therapy. Eight patients required lobectomy (3 sleeve) and 7 had pneumonectomies (2 carinal). The SVC was replaced by interposition graft in 9 patients and 6 had partial resection. There were 2 postoperative deaths (14%) and 3 major morbidities (23%). There was 1 late graft thrombosis. Overall, 1- and 3-year survival was 68% and 57% and disease-free survival was 55% and 27%, respectively. Induction therapy seemed to delay recurrence.[14]

The report by Suzuki and colleagues from Japan in 2004 was about 40 patients who underwent combined resection of the SVC for lung cancer. Lobectomy and pneumonectomy were performed in 19 and 21 patients, respectively. Eleven patients had complete SVC resection with graft reconstruction and 29 patients had partial resection. Thirty-day mortality was 10%. The 5-year survival rate was 24%, with the median follow-up of 67 months for living patients (actual 5-year survivors were 7). The prognosis was better in those patients with SVC invasion by direct tumor extension (n = 25) with 5-year survival at 36% compared with those patients (n = 15) with SVC invasion by metastatic nodes with 5-year survival at 6.6%.[15]

The report from Paris by Yildizeli and colleagues in 2008 was on 39 of the 271 patients who required SVC replacement. Operative mortality and morbidity rates were 4% and 35%, respectively. The overall 5-year survival rate was 38.4%; for the SVC replacement it was 29.4%.[16]

SUMMARY

SVC or one of the innominate veins may be obstructed by compression due to direct pressure, by invasion, or by secondary venous thrombosis. In most cases of causative lung cancer, surgical treatment of SVC obstruction is not an option, and survival is limited to less than 6 months. Treatment with chemotherapy or radiotherapy for advanced cancer is indicated for rapid symptomatic relief or in ideal case, resection and reconstruction of the large veins in the mediastinum.

The SVC is one of the so many important structures in the mediastinum lying in close proximity to each other and any expanding or invasive lesion developing among them or from the adjoining right upper lobe of the lung has potential for interfering with their functions by simple irritation, compression, or direct invasion, aptly described as "mediastinal compression syndrome."

CLINICS CARE POINTS

- Look for persistent left SVC if the coronary sinus is very large or there is a very small or no bridging/brachiocephalic vein.
- The azygous vein may allow for collaterals from either SVC or IVC.
- Malignant SVC obstruction carries a poor prognosis and represents advanced stage.
- If resectable, survival may be reasonable even in advanced cancer.
- Replacement by grafts should be with small caliber tubes to allow for rapid blood flow, thus reducing the risk of thrombosis.
- Replacement is followed by anticoagulation for at least 3 months.

REFERENCES

1. Uemura M, Suwa F, Takemura A, et al. Classification of persistent left superior vena cava considering presence and development of both superior venae cavae, the anastomotic ramus between superior venae cavae, and the azygos venous system. Anat Sci Int 2012;87(4):212–22.
2. Last RJ. Anatomy: regional and applied. 5th edition. Churchill, Livingstone, 1972. p.343–53.
3. TJ Kent. Rhoads textbook of surgery. 5th edition. Superior Vena Cava Anat. p.1482.
4. TR Robert, Grosh JD. Rhoads textbook of surgery. 5th edition. Superior Vena Cava Syndrome. J B Lippincott Co, 1977. p. 1900–3.

5. Oizumi H, Suzuki K, Banno T, et al. Patency of grafts after total resection and reconstruction of the superior vena cava for thoracic malignancy. Surg Today 2016;46:1421–6.

6. D'Andrilli A, De Cecco CN, Maurizi G, et al. Reconstruction of the superior vena cava by biologic conduit: assessment of long-term patency by magnetic resonance imaging. Ann Thorac Surg 2013; 96:1039–45.

7. Odell DD, Liao K. Superior vena cava and innominate vein reconstruction in thoracic malignancies: double-vein reconstruction. Semin Thorac Cardiovasc Surg 2011;23(4):326–9.

8. Maurizi G, Poggi C, D'Andrilli A, et al. Superior vena cava replacement for thymic malignancies. Ann Thorac Surg 2019;107:386–92.

9. Dong-Seok L, Flores RM. Management of NSCLC invading the superior vena cava. Oper Tech Thorac Cardiovasc Surg 2017;22:224–34.

10. Sekine Y, Suzuki H, Saitoh Y, et al. Prosthetic reconstruction of the superior vena cava for malignant disease: surgical techniques and outcomes. Ann Thorac Surg 2010;90:223–8.

11. Nakano T, Endo S, Kanai Y, et al. Surgical outcomes after superior vena cava reconstruction with expanded polytetrafluoroethylene grafts. Ann Thorac Cardiovasc Surg 2014;20:310–5.

12. Venuta F, Rendina E, Coloni GF. Lung resections combined with vena cava replacement. Multimed Man Cardiothorac Surg 2017;18:2017.

13. Yotsukura M, Kinoshita T, Kamiyama I, et al. Temporary extravascular shunt for reconstruction of a superior vena cava invaded by a lung tumor. Ann Thorac Surg 2014;98:2242–3.

14. Shargall Y, de Perrot KS, Keshavjee S, et al. 15 years single center experience with surgical resection of the superior vena cava for non-small lung cancer. Lung Cancer 2004;45:357–63.

15. Suzuki K, Asamura H, Watanabe S, et al. Combined resection of superior vena cava for lung carcinoma: prognostic significance of patterns of superior vena cava invasion. Ann Thorac Surg 2004;78:1184–9.

16. Yildizeli B, Dartevelle PG, Fadel E, et al. Results of primary surgery with T4 non-small cell lung cancer during a 25-year period in a single center: the benefit is worth the risk. Ann Thorac Surg 2008;86: 1065–75.

Neuroendocrine Tumors of the Lung

Simran Randhawa, MD[a],*, Nikolaos Trikalinos, MD[b], G. Alexander Patterson, MD[a]

KEYWORDS

- Neuroendocrine tumors • Carcinoid • Bronchoscopy • Sleeve lobectomy

KEY POINTS

- Pulmonary neuroendocrine tumors (NETs) are a group of rare tumors arising from neuroendocrine cells.
- Anatomic resection with nodal sampling and/or dissection is the mainstay in management of these patients.
- Grade I NET has an excellent prognosis with surgical resection.
- Patients with grade II NETs are significantly more likely to develop recurrent disease.
- Grade III NETs are aggressive lung cancers with poor prognosis.

DEFINITION

Neuroendocrine tumors (NETs) are a heterogeneous group of uncommon cancers that arise from specialized, peptide- and amine-producing cells dispersed throughout the diffuse endocrine system. They are broadly categorized into foregut (bronchial, gastric, duodenal, and pancreas), midgut (jejunal, ileal, appendiceal, and ascending/transverse colon), and hindgut (distal colon and rectum) tumors.

Because of their rarity, heterogeneity, and variable natural history, NETs remain a poorly understood disease. An SEER database analysis suggested that the incidence of some NETs (including lung) in the United States is steadily increasing, and currently 2000 to 4500 patients are diagnosed with a lung NET every year,[1] which amounts to 1% to 2% of all lung cancers. This is likely attributable to an improvement in diagnostic tools, including the dramatic diffusion of lung cancer screening programs worldwide. Moreover, because of the commonly indolent nature of this disease, the prevalence of individuals with NETs is also increasing and is currently greater than 170,000 for all-comers. This also applies to the lung subcategory, as median survivals for patients with localized or low-grade disease can be in excess of 15 years.

Lung NETs are the second most common site for NETs after the gastrointestinal (GI) system, accounting for 30.6% of all NETs.[2] Most of them are sporadic lesions with poorly understood risk factors; smoking does not seem to be a risk factor, in contrary to the more common bronchogenic counterparts. Hereditary NETs can be associated with familial syndromes, some of which include multiple endocrine neoplasia types 1 (MEN1) and 2 (MEN2), von Hippel-Lindau disease, tuberous sclerosis complex, and neurofibromatosis.

Some patients with lung NETs may have symptoms attributable to hormonal hypersecretion, and these tumors are considered to be "functional," whereas those without any associated hormonal symptoms are considered "nonfunctional" tumors. In contrast to the GI counterparts, serotonin hypersecretion and the classic "carcinoid syndrome" are not very common, even in metastatic disease. Functional tumors, however, can be associated with severe, prolonged flushing or adrenocorticotrophin hormone (ACTH) hypersecretion that can cause Cushing syndrome.[3] There is also a

---

[a] Division of Thoracic Surgery, Department of Surgery, Washington University School of Medicine, 1 Barnes Jewish Hospital, St Louis, MO 63110, USA; [b] Division of Medical Oncology, Department of Internal Medicine, Washington University School of Medicine, 1 Barnes Jewish Hospital, St Louis, MO 63110, USA
* Corresponding author.
E-mail address: srandhawa@wustl.edu

pathologic entity called diffuse intrapulmonary neuroendocrine cell hyperplasia (DIPNECH) that is considered a premalignant form of the disease and can be associated with chronic cough and episodic shortness of breath.

Most patients with lung NETs have proximal tumors and nonspecific presentation symptoms that can result in delayed diagnosis. These include shortness of breath, cough, and hemoptysis or recurrent pneumonia in the same lung segment. Timely diagnosis and appropriate management of primitive neuroectodermal tumors (PNETs) can be achieved using a multidisciplinary approach comprising specialized pathologists, endocrinologists, pulmonologists, and medical, radiation, and thoracic surgical oncologists.

CLASSIFICATION AND PATHOLOGY

According to the 2015 World Health Organization (WHO) classification of lung, NETs fall into 3 categories: low-grade (typical carcinoid), intermediate-grade (atypical carcinoid), and high-grade (large-cell neuroendocrine and small-cell carcinoma) (Fig. 1). The higher grade counterparts usually denote a more aggressive disease and carry a worse prognosis.

Well-differentiated NETs of the lung are subcategorized into typical or atypical using histologic criteria. Typical carcinoid tumors have fewer than 2 mitoses/10 per high-power field (HPF) and lack any evidence of necrosis. Atypical carcinoid tumors have 2 to 10 mitoses/10 HPF with necrotic features or architectural disruption. High-grade, poorly differentiated NETs have greater than 10 mitoses/10 HPF and extensive foci of necrosis. NETs of the lung and bronchi follow the tumor-node-metastasis (TNM) staging system as for lung carcinomas. As in squamous and adenocarcinoma lung cancer, the prognosis becomes poorer with increasing stage at diagnosis.

IMAGING AND ADDITIONAL TESTING

Pulmonary NETs are traditionally divided into central and peripheral lesions based on their origin with respect to the bronchial tree. Patients with DIPNECH will complain of chronic cough spanning multiple years in the setting of negative standard chest radiographs. Most patients with peripheral tumors will be diagnosed incidentally on imaging

	Histology	Cytology
Grade I (Typical) 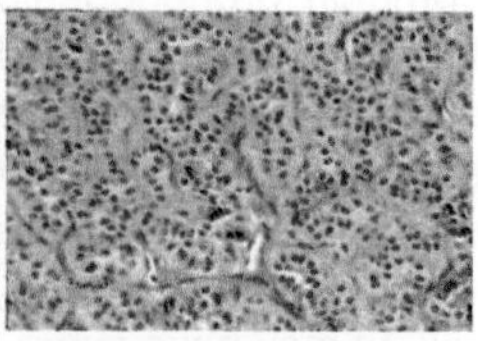	Nested growth pattern Absent mitoses	Monomorphic Eosinophilic cytoplasm
Grade II (Atypical) 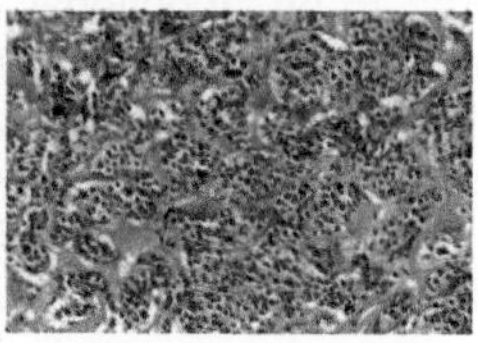	Presence of necrosis Loss of nested growth Mitotic activity (> 5/ 10 HPF)	Pleomorphic Variation in nuclear size
Grade III (Large cell) 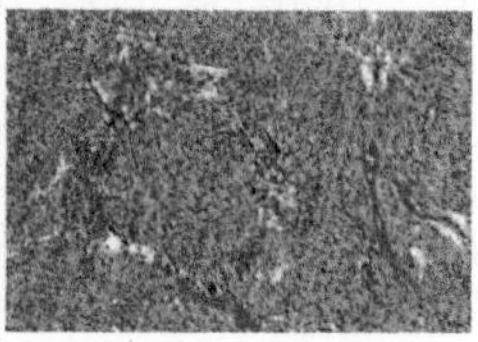	Extensive necrosis Mitotic activity (> 10/ 10 HPF)	Hyperchromatic nuclei Large cell (4-6 X lymphocyte) Small cell (1-3 X lymphocyte)

Fig. 1. Pulmonary NETs grading system.

performed for other reasons. However, patients with central tumors can be symptomatic and will complain of obstructive respiratory symptoms such as recurrent chest infections, cough, hemoptysis, chest pain, dyspnea, and wheezing. Patients who present with symptoms suspicious of lung NETs should be discussed within a multidisciplinary tumor board and undergo evaluation with both biochemical testing as well as imaging studies to assess disease burden.

BIOCHEMICAL TESTING

Those who have clinical symptoms that suggest hormonal hyper secretion such as Cushing or flushing/diarrhea should undergo testing for serum cortisol, ACTH, serum serotonin levels, or urine 5-hydroxyindoleacetic acid as indicated. Patients presenting with Cushing syndrome must undergo a complete evaluation and workup with input from endocrinology,[4] as some of the diagnostic tests for ectopic ACTH secretion might be inconclusive. Screening for hormone hypersecretion in asymptomatic individuals is not routinely recommended; however, obtaining a baseline serum chromogranin-A is sometimes recommended in nonfunctioning tumors and can be followed during treatment if abnormal.[5]

DIAGNOSTIC IMAGING
Computed Tomography of the Chest

The most commonly used imaging modality for diagnosis of lung NETs is multiphase contrast-enhanced computed tomography (CT) of the chest. These tumors frequently seem as a smooth, rounded, homogenous nodule or mass within the lung parenchyma or in an endobronchial location with an associated postobstructive process (**Fig. 2**A, B). NETs of the lung are characterized by good blood flow that leads to higher uptake of contrast medium; this allows a differentiation of benign round nodules, which mostly show only a low-contrast medium uptake.

For DIPNECH, high-resolution CT with an expiration study shows mosaic attenuation or air trapping along with multiple nodules due to multiple tumorlets and carcinoid tumors.

PET-Computed Tomography

Most patients with a lung lesion will at some point undergo a PET with fludeoxyglucose F 18 (FDG-PET) as part of their evaluation. Bronchial NETs can present as either central lesions (suggesting lung adenocarcinoma) or peripheral solitary nodules on chest imaging and are included in a wide range of differentials such as lung carcinoma, hamartoma, inflammatory, or infectious lesions. FDG-PET-CT, however, is unreliable for diagnosis of low-grade tumors such as DIPNECH, tumorlets, and typical carcinoid due to their low metabolic activity and FDG uptake. Most of the slow-growing tumors do not take up FDG and thus seem "cold" on imaging. Conversely, aggressive varieties such as large and small cell lung cancer will demonstrate significant FDG uptake.

About 80% of low-grade and 60% of intermediate-grade lung NETs express somatostatin receptors on their surfaces, making them eligible for functional imaging using somatostatin analogues. These imagings include radiolabeled octreotide imaging (a relatively older modality), as well as the newer somatostatin receptor PET/CT scans.

The current Food and Drug Administration–approved tracers are 68-Gallium dotatate and 68-Ga dotatoc. Somatostatin receptor PET can provide useful information on overall tumor burden, as well as confirm the presence of somatostatin receptors, which can have therapeutic implications (somatostatin receptor positive disease carries usually a better prognosis and can be associated with response to somatostatin analogue treatments). A meta-analysis of 22 studies determined that 68-Ga dotatate had a

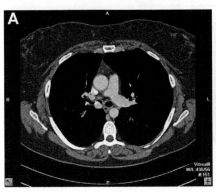
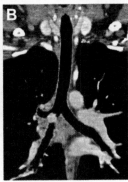

Fig. 2. CT imaging. CT chest showing a solitary well-defined, round, homogeneous mass in the right main stem bronchus (A) seen extending to the BI in sagittal views (B).

pooled sensitivity and specificity of 91% and 94%, respectively, for the initial diagnosis of NETs.[6] There are limited data on whether long-acting somatostatin receptor inhibition in the therapeutic setting can interfere with 68-Ga Dotatate PET/CT scans, one study showed that timing did not make a difference.[7] 68-Ga dotatate PET/CT or PET/MRI is currently preferred over radiolabeled octreotide scanning, as it is more sensitive than SSR scintigraphy for determining somatostatin receptor status.

Luminal Imaging

Imaging is no substitute for tissue sampling in the setting of lung NETs and flexible bronchoscopy, and biopsy is the most important diagnostic test for central lesions. On bronchoscopy, these tumors are pathognomonically characterized by a strongly vascularized mass covered by bronchial epithelium (**Fig. 3**). They are mostly broad-based and grow intraluminally as well as extraluminally—the so-called iceberg phenomenon. For more peripheral lesions, navigational bronchoscopy or percutaneous techniques may be used to establish diagnosis. In spite of vascularization, serious problems with hemorrhage are rare during the biopsy procedure (<1%). In the event of hemorrhage, endobronchial interventions such as cryotherapy, injection of dilute epinephrine, or occasionally, use of the neodymium:yttrium-aluminum-garnet (Nd:YAG) laser can be helpful with hemostasis.

Endobronchial ultrasound-guided transbronchial needle aspiration (EPBUS-TBNA) or mediastinoscopy is also recommended for the purpose of staging according to the TNM classification for lung cancer. EBUS-TBNA is unlikely to differentiate typical from atypical carcinoids, and hence its utility is primarily in detection of nodal involvement.

Echocardiography

Carcinoid heart disease is a feared complication of almost half of the patients with long-standing carcinoid syndrome and can be particularly debilitating in its later stages. Affected patients have pathognomonic plaquelike deposits of fibrous tissue on cardiac valves, leaflets, and papillary muscles. Most commonly affected areas are the tricuspid and pulmonic valve leading to right-sided heart failure. For those diagnosed with bronchial carcinoid, echocardiography and evaluation of left- and right-sided heart valves is recommended to assess the presence of carcinoid heart disease; this is particularly important as part of preoperative evaluation.

Therapeutic Options and Treatment Guidelines

Management of lung NETs depends on tumor size, stage, and the general condition of the patient. As a general rule, patients with asymptomatic, nonfunctional, slow-growing disease have the option of observation, whereas all others should consider surgery or systemic treatments. Unfortunately, most approaches are based on low-quality data and medium-strength evidence with the exception of small cell lung cancer (SCLC). Current consensus supports surgical resection as the primary treatment of choice and the only curative option for localized, resectable disease.

For patients with locoregional or metastatic, unresectable disease and symptoms of hormone hyper secretion, symptom control with somatostatin analogues such as octreotide or lanreotide is of paramount importance. Somatostatin analogues are also suggested perioperatively in surgical patients in whom there is concern for hormone hypersecretion from tumor manipulation during resection, also known as carcinoid crisis.

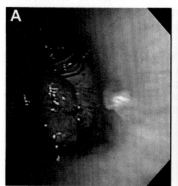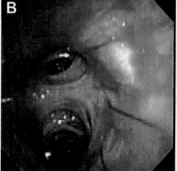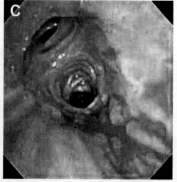

Fig. 3. Bronchoscopic features. Bronchoscopy images showing round, smooth mass covered by bronchial epithelium in the left upper lobe orifice highly suspicious for typical carcinoid (*A*). Postoperative bronchoscopy after left upper lobe sleeve resection (*B*) and subsequent bronchoscopy months later showing completely healed anastomotic sites (*C*).

Surgery for localized disease

For patients with peripheral lung tumors, the surgical extent of choice is complete anatomic resection (lobectomy and segmentectomy) with hilar/mediastinal lymph node dissection or sampling. The most important objective is a microscopically tumor-free resection margin (R0), which is associated with a good prognosis and best outcomes. Small (<2 cm), peripheral typical carcinoid tumors with clinically negative lymph nodes can be successfully treated with sublobar resection with frozen section confirmation of negative margins. There are multiple retrospective database studies comparing the survival difference between wedge resections and segmentectomies for stage I typical carcinoids. Although some report a survival advantage with anatomic resections,[8] others have shown no difference in cancer-specific or disease-free survival with wedge resections for stage I typical carcinoids.[9,10] A randomized clinical trial is the only tool capable of providing an accurate answer, but it is difficult to conduct such a study for a rare disease as this.

For larger or central typical carcinoids, atypical carcinoids, or tumors with clinically positive lymph nodes, lobar resection is preferred along with lymph node assessment. An important tenet of surgical treatment of lung NETs is the sparing of normal lung parenchyma especially due to the low malignant and recurrence potential. Where possible, bronchial sleeve resection or a sleeve lobectomy should be carried out in preference to pneumonectomy (ideally with intraoperative frozen section of the resection margins).[11] Achieving a negative margin should suffice from an oncologic standpoint, and there is no current consensus on a specific distance or margin associated with improved long-term outcomes.[12]

There is little evidence to guide on surgical resection as part of management of recurrent locoregional disease or isolated distant metastatic disease.[13] Surgery is considered in selected patients with adequate performance status, with limited disease and curative intent after a multidisciplinary discussion.

Where possible, surgical resection of liver metastases can be considered with curative intent, to aid symptom control or for debulking when greater than 90% of tumor can be removed. Complete resection of liver metastases can increase 5-year overall survival rates to greater than 70%.[14]

Endobronchial

Inoperable tumors requiring palliative treatment can be resected bronchoscopically, in order to alleviate symptoms such as retention pneumonia. Even in case of the rare endobronchial growth without expansion through the cartilage, bronchoscopic resection should not be undertaken due to the increased risk of local recurrence. Endobronchial resection should hence only be reserved for patients unable to tolerate formal surgical resection.

Cryotherapy is a safe and effective adjunct to endobronchial resection to decrease local recurrence rates with lower risks of bronchial stenosis.[15] Laser bronchoscopy is another option that can also be used along with other therapies and offers the advantages of being rapid, immediately effective, and repeatable.[16]

Endobronchial resection can also be used as a potential bridge to surgery in cases of central PNETs presenting with postobstructive pneumonitis and destroyed lung parenchyma. An initial local endobronchial resection can be performed to open the airway and enable drainage before reassessment for lung parenchymal-sparing surgery.

On occasion, small carcinoid tumorlets (<5 mm) are observed on bronchoscopy or cross-sectional imaging. In this case, a diagnosis of diffuse idiopathic pulmonary neuroendocrine cell hyperplasia (DIPNECH) can be made. This condition is thought to be generally indolent, and such tumorlets should not be routinely resected. These patients can be observed with chest CT scans every 12 to 24 months or as clinically indicated. The use of somatostatin analogues for symptom control is debatable and currently investigated.

Locoregional therapy

Current National Comprehensive Cancer Network (NCCN) guidelines recommend use of stereotactic body radiation therapy as an option for patients who are not medically fit for surgery, and thermal ablation can be recommended in cases where both surgery and radiation therapy are contraindicated.[17]

Adjuvant radiation is recommended in atypical and high-grade carcinoids with mediastinal N2 or greater disease[18] but the survival benefit has not been established in a high-quality randomized study. For patients with localized unresectable disease, definitive radiation can be offered, with chemotherapy, but the optimal dose and sequence is yet unclear. Common practice has been modeled after the regimens used in similar settings for either non–small-cell or small-cell cancers.

For metastatic lung NETs, palliative radiation is considered for symptomatic lesions. Radiofrequency ablation can be considered in cases of liver, lung, or bone metastasis.

Systemic therapy

Metastatic or unresectable disease is generally considered incurable, thus management is palliative and requires a multidisciplinary evaluation. The treatment goals are to both control hormone-related symptoms (if any) as well as prevent tumor growth. Systemic therapy options depend on the histology and functional status of the tumor and include somatostatin analogues, mTOR inhibitors (everolimus), peptide receptor radionuclide therapy, and chemotherapy. As in every rare tumor, participation in clinical trials is highly encouraged.

As in the GI counterparts, somatostatin analogues such as octreotide or lanreotide have the potential to control the carcinoid syndrome and inhibit tumor growth; cytoreduction is less common. The NCCN guidelines recommend initiation of somatostatin analogues for advanced low- and intermediate-grade and all functional tumors. Additional options include initiation of everolimus based on results of phase III RADIANT-4 study, which included about 30% lung NETs and showed a 52% reduction in the estimated risk of progression or death.[19] Other oral pathway inhibitors are currently being studied in large clinical trials.

Chemotherapy has been generally somewhat effective in high-grade tumors with a good amount of randomized data in the SCLC pathology. Much less is known for atypical carcinoids and large-cell lung neuroendocrine neoplasms. Regimens are borrowed from the SCLC literature and include cisplatin with etoposide, carboplatin with etoposide, or temozolomide. Its role in the adjuvant treatment of resected, high-grade tumors is debatable and currently studied. Some small studies have shown a 19% to 22% response rate in patients with atypical NETs treated with chemotherapeutic agents.[20,21]

Immunotherapy with checkpoint inhibitors such as nivolumab, pembrolizumab, or CTL4 inhibitors such as ipilimumab has shown positive results in high-grade tumors such as SCLC but its efficacy is limited in well-differentiated, slow-growing histologies (consistent with the experience in GI NETs).

As previously mentioned, lung NETs can express somatostatin receptors on their surface, and this has led to a growing interest in the use of peptide receptor radionuclide therapy (PRRT) with (177)Lu-DOTATATE. PRRT attaches radiolabeled ligands to somatostatin analogues to deliver a radiation dose to somatostatin receptor positive tumors and has been particularly successful in GI NETs.[22] Several studies[23–26] have reported the use of PRRT as a potential therapeutic option in advanced lung NETs. Overall response rates ranged from 13% to 30%, whereas progression-free survival ranged from 19 to 28 months and overall survival ranged from 32 to 59 months. Data are mostly retrospective and of average quality, but large studies are being planned to effectively answer that question.

In general, results with systemic therapy have been largely disappointing, and survival data have to be interpreted with caution due to the small numbers of patients and data from retrospective single-institutional series, with several limitations. As such, benefits of systemic therapy are at best, modest, with no clear benefits in overall survival.

Prognosis and Follow-Up

The prognosis of PNETs is significantly associated with the degree of differentiation and lymph node metastases. Long-term results from numerous surgical series suggest that the histologic subtype of a bronchial carcinoid is the most important prognostic factor. Tumor-node-metastasis (TNM) stage seems less critical.

After complete resection, typical carcinoids have the best prognosis, with a 10-year survival rate of more than 80%. The 5-year survival rate in atypical carcinoid without lymph node metastases is 80% and with lymph node metastases is 60%.

Because recurrences and distant metastases can develop years after resection of the primary tumor, prolonged follow-up care is indicated. For patients with typical carcinoid, conventional CT can be performed at 3 and 6 months and then annually. For atypical carcinoids, closer monitoring is recommended: first at 3 and 6 months and then at 6-month intervals. After 10 years, surveillance should be considered as clinically indicated. Chromogranin-A levels can be used as a tumor marker and elevated levels, although not diagnostic, can be associated with recurrence.[27,28] Their use is not encouraged after curative resection, and the levels can be affected by certain medications, making the interpretation difficult.

CLINICS CARE POINTS

Pearls:

- Pulmonary NETs are the second most common NETs after the GI system.

- Most patients are asymptomatic; however, some patients can have symptoms related to hormone overproduction (most commonly Cushing syndrome) and should be worked up accordingly.

- CT chest is the most commonly used imaging modality; however, bronchoscopy and biopsy are pertinent to diagnosing and classifying pulmonary NET.

- Small (<2 cm), peripheral typical carcinoid tumors with clinically negative lymph nodes can be successfully treated with sublobar resection with frozen section confirmation of negative margins.
- For larger or central typical carcinoids, atypical carcinoids, or tumors with clinically positive lymph nodes, lobar resection is preferred along with lymph node dissection. R0 resection is key.

Pitfalls:

- Despite the vascularity, chances of hemorrhage with biopsy of these tumors is less than 1%. Any bleeding can be controlled by endoscopic interventions such as cryotherapy, epinephrine, or Nd:YAG laser.
- Carcinoid heart disease is a feared complication in patients with long-standing carcinoid syndrome related to NETs, and preoperative ECHO of the heart is important to assess the valves.
- Even in a case of endobronchial growth without expansion through the cartilage, bronchoscopic resection should not be undertaken due to the increased risk of local recurrence. Endobronchial resection should only be reserved for symptomatic patients unable to tolerate formal surgical resection.
- Results with use of systemic therapy for pulmonary NETs have been largely disappointing in terms of overall survival.

DISCLOSURE

The authors have nothing to disclose.

REFERENCES

1. Dasari A, Shen C, Halperin D, et al. Trends in the Incidence, Prevalence, and Survival Outcomes in Patients With Neuroendocrine Tumors in the United States. JAMA Oncol 2017;3(10):1335–42.
2. Man D, Wu J, Shen Z, et al. Prognosis of patients with neuroendocrine tumor: a SEER database analysis. Cancer Manag Res 2018;10:5629–38.
3. Melmon KL, Sjoerdsma A, Mason DT. Distinctive clinical and therapeutic aspects of the syndrome associated with bronchial carcinoid tumors. Am J Med 1965;39(4):568–81.
4. Florez JC, Shepard J-AO, Kradin RL. Case records of the Massachusetts General Hospital. Case 17-2013. A 56-year-old woman with poorly controlled diabetes mellitus and fatigue. N Engl J Med 2013; 368(22):2126–36.
5. Yang X, Yang Y, Li Z, et al. Diagnostic value of circulating chromogranin a for neuroendocrine tumors: a systematic review and meta-analysis. PLoS One 2015;10(4):e0124884.
6. Singh S, Poon R, Wong R, et al. 68Ga PET Imaging in Patients With Neuroendocrine Tumors: A Systematic Review and Meta-analysis. Clin Nucl Med 2018; 43(11):802–10.
7. Ayati N, Lee ST, Zakavi R, et al. Long-Acting Somatostatin Analog Therapy Differentially Alters 68Ga-DOTATATE Uptake in Normal Tissues Compared with Primary Tumors and Metastatic Lesions. J Nucl Med 2018;59(2):223–7.
8. Filosso PL, Guerrera F, Falco NR, et al. Anatomical resections are superior to wedge resections for overall survival in patients with Stage 1 typical carcinoids. Eur J Cardiothorac Surg 2019;55(2):273–9.
9. Rahouma M, Kamel M, Narula N, et al. Role of wedge resection in bronchial carcinoid (BC) tumors: SEER database analysis. J Thorac Dis 2019;11(4): 1355–62.
10. Brown LM, Cooke DT, Jett JR, et al. Extent of Resection and Lymph Node Assessment for Clinical Stage T1aN0M0 Typical Carcinoid Tumors. Ann Thorac Surg 2018;105(1):207–13.
11. Caplin ME, Baudin E, Ferolla P, et al. Pulmonary neuroendocrine (carcinoid) tumors: European Neuroendocrine Tumor Society expert consensus and recommendations for best practice for typical and atypical pulmonary carcinoids. Ann Oncol 2015;26(8):1604–20.
12. Schmid S, Aicher M, Csanadi A, et al. Significance of the resection margin in bronchopulmonary carcinoids. J Surg Res 2016;201(1):53–8.
13. Stamatis G, Freitag L, Greschuchna D. Limited and radical resection for tracheal and bronchopulmonary carcinoid tumour. Report on 227 cases. Eur J Cardiothorac Surg 1990;4(10):527–32 [discussion 533].
14. Glazer ES, Tseng JF, Al-Refaie W, et al. Long-term survival after surgical management of neuroendocrine hepatic metastases. HPB (Oxford) 2010; 12(6):427–33.
15. Bertoletti L, Elleuch R, Kaczmarek D, et al. Bronchoscopic cryotherapy treatment of isolated endoluminal typical carcinoid tumor. Chest 2006;130(5): 1405–11.
16. Cavaliere S, Foccoli P, Farina PL. Nd:YAG laser bronchoscopy. A five-year experience with 1,396 applications in 1,000 patients. Chest 1988;94(1): 15–21. https://doi.org/10.1378/chest.94.1.15.
17. National Comprehensive Cancer Network. NCCN clinical practice guidelines in oncology (NCCN Guidelines Version 2.2020): neuroendocrine tumors of the Gastrointestinal Tract, Lung, and Thymus.
18. Mackley HB, Videtic GMM. Primary carcinoid tumors of the lung: a role for radiotherapy. Oncology (Williston Park) 2006;20(12):1537–43 [discussion 1544-1545, 1549].

19. Yao JC, Fazio N, Singh S, et al. Everolimus for the treatment of advanced, non-functional neuroendocrine tumours of the lung or gastrointestinal tract (RADIANT-4): a randomised, placebo-controlled, phase 3 study. Lancet 2016;387(10022):968–77.

20. Wirth LJ, Carter MR, Jänne PA, et al. Outcome of patients with pulmonary carcinoid tumors receiving chemotherapy or chemoradiotherapy. Lung Cancer 2004;44(2):213–20.

21. Fazio N, Granberg D, Grossman A, et al. Everolimus plus octreotide long-acting repeatable in patients with advanced lung neuroendocrine tumors: analysis of the phase 3, randomized, placebo-controlled RADIANT-2 study. Chest 2013;143(4): 955–62.

22. Strosberg J, El-Haddad G, Wolin E, et al. Phase 3 Trial of 177 Lu-Dotatate for Midgut Neuroendocrine Tumors. N Engl J Med 2017;376(2):125–35.

23. Mariniello A, Bodei L, Tinelli C, et al. Long-term results of PRRT in advanced bronchopulmonary carcinoid. Eur J Nucl Med Mol Imaging 2016;43(3): 441–52.

24. Sabet A, Haug AR, Eiden C, et al. Efficacy of peptide receptor radionuclide therapy with 177Lu-octreotate in metastatic pulmonary neuroendocrine tumors: a dual-centre analysis. Am J Nucl Med Mol Imaging 2017;7(2):74–83.

25. Parghane RV, Talole S, Prabhash K, et al. Clinical Response Profile of Metastatic/Advanced Pulmonary Neuroendocrine Tumors to Peptide Receptor Radionuclide Therapy with 177Lu-DOTATATE. Clin Nucl Med 2017;42(6):428–35.

26. Ianniello A, Sansovini M, Severi S, et al. Peptide receptor radionuclide therapy with (177)Lu-DOTATATE in advanced bronchial carcinoids: prognostic role of thyroid transcription factor 1 and (18)F-FDG PET. Eur J Nucl Med Mol Imaging 2016;43(6):1040–6.

27. Massironi S, Rossi RE, Casazza G, et al. Chromogranin A in diagnosing and monitoring patients with gastroenteropancreatic neuroendocrine neoplasms: a large series from a single institution. Neuroendocrinology 2014;100(2–3):240–9.

28. Rossi RE, Ciafardini C, Sciola V, et al. Chromogranin A in the Follow-up of Gastroenteropancreatic Neuroendocrine Neoplasms: Is It Really Game Over? A Systematic Review and Meta-analysis. Pancreas 2018;47(10):1249–55.

Aerogenous Metastasis and Spread Through the Air Spaces – Distinct Entities or Spectrum of the Same Process?

Carolina A. Souza, MD, PhD, FRCPC[a],*, Marcio M. Gomes, MD, PhD, FRCPC[b]

KEYWORDS

- Computed tomography • Chest computed tomography • Lung cancer
- Spread through the air spaces • Aerogenous metastasis • Lung adenocarcinoma

KEY POINTS

- Metastatic spread of cancer cells from the primary tumor through the airways may occur in primary lung cancers.
- The concept of spread through the airspaces (STAS) was introduced in the current World Health Organization classification. The term aerogenous metastasis was proposed years before STAS.
- The pathogenesis of aerogenous metastasis and STAS is not fully elucidated, but these entities share similarities and may be part of the same phenomenon.
- Presence of STAS has been shown to be a negative prognostic factor in early lung cancers.
- Further studies are required to better define the pathogenesis and clinicopathological features of aerogenous metastasis and STAS, as well as their impact on prognosis and management.

The presence of metastases is the most important factor in the staging and management of lung cancer. There are 3 established mechanisms of metastatic spread in lung cancer: hematogenous, lymphatic, and transcoelomic (pleural) metastases. Clinicopathological and imaging observations suggest that an additional mechanism of metastatic spread characterized by discontinuous spread of cancer cells from the primary tumor through the airways to adjacent or distant lung parenchyma may occur, and the term aerogenous metastasis has been proposed.

Local invasion in primary lung cancers has been traditionally defined as infiltration of the stroma, vessels, or pleura on pathologic specimen. More recently, the concept of airspace invasion has been proposed as a novel mechanism of invasion and tumor spread in lung cancer,[1,2] named spread through the airspaces (STAS). STAS was first mentioned in the 2015 World Health Organization (WHO) Classification of Lung Tumors,[3] defined histologically as tumor cells, including 1 or more micropapillary structures, solid nests, or single cells, spreading beyond the edge of the tumor into airspaces in the surrounding lung parenchyma. The concept of STAS captured the attention of the scientific community, and several studies were published since the 2015 WHO classification. However, there are important areas of uncertainty and relatively little evidence to support the current definition of STAS.

PROPOSED MECHANISMS OF AIRWAY SPREAD

Aerogenous metastasis and STAS are described primarily in lung adenocarcinomas. Histologic characteristics of specific patterns of adenocarcinoma

[a] Division of Thoracic Imaging, Department of Medical Imaging, Ottawa Hospital Research Institute, University of Ottawa, 501 Smyth Road, Ottawa K1H 8M2, Canada; [b] Department of Pathology and Laboratory Medicine, Ottawa Hospital Research Institute, University of Ottawa, 501 Smyth Road, Ottawa K1H 8M2, Canada
* Corresponding author.
E-mail address: csouza@toh.ca

Thorac Surg Clin 31 (2021) 477–483
https://doi.org/10.1016/j.thorsurg.2021.05.006
1547-4127/21/© 2021 Elsevier Inc. All rights reserved.

seem to correlate with the risk of airway spread. Lepidic adenocarcinoma is characterized by growth of cancer cells along the alveolar walls with no evidence of stromal invasion. Papillary and micropapillary patterns also frequently show growth within the airspaces albeit with destructive and invasive behavior. These 3 patterns of adenocarcinoma have an abundance of neoplastic cells in direct contact with the airspace that are theoretically more likely to shed and spread through the airways. Another important histologic concept is the presence of 2 main cytologic phenotypes of adenocarcinoma, regardless of growth patterns, namely mucinous and nonmucinous adenocarcinoma. Invasive mucinous adenocarcinomas account for approximately 5% to 10% of lung adenocarcinomas and are characterized by the presence of intracellular mucin, which is frequently accompanied by abundant extracellular mucin production that fills the alveoli and often contains viable detached neoplastic cells. These floating cells are potentially prone to spread through the airways. It has been shown that discontinuous neoplastic foci are more commonly seen in mucinous neoplasms.[4] In addition, the concept of papillary or micropapillary cell clusters floating within mucin is an accepted pattern of invasive biologic behavior in mucinous adenocarcinoma, even in the absence of stromal invasion.

Although the pathogenesis of STAS has not been fully elucidated, the mechanisms likely parallel those postulated for aerogenous metastases.[5] For both STAS and aerogenous metastases to occur, cancer cells growing at the primary site need to detach from the main tumor, spread through the airways, and re-attach to the lung parenchyma away from the primary tumor. Normally, survival, growth, and differentiation of cancer cells depend on cell basement membrane attachment or anchorage. Detachment of the basal membrane invariably causes anoikis, a form of programmed cell death. Thus, to spread through the airways, neoplastic cells need to overcome natural biologic obstacles and require, among other properties, cell discohesiveness and anchorage-free survival. Previous studies have shown the occurrence of anchorage-independent survival and growth, supporting the occurrence of airway spread.[6]

The current definition of STAS is controversial and deserves critical appraisal. First, lung cancer epithelial cells are frequently in direct contact with the airspaces. Therefore, when growing within the airspaces, tumor cells do not invade but rather spread, a term and definition deemed more appropriate than invasion. Secondly, the concept of continuous and discontinuous spread needs to be considered. To support the current definition of STAS, authors described direct continuity of tumor cells with the main tumor using 3-dimensional techniques. However, presence of single cells is considered a histologic feature of STAS, and the presence of tumor islands beyond the growing edge of the tumor is one of the diagnostic criteria, both implying discontinuity from the primary tumor. Discontinuity is also evidenced by detection of tumor cells in the lung parenchyma away from the main tumor or in bronchial secretions, features that allegedly support the concept of STAS.[7] Continuous spread through the airways likely coexists, but it would correspond to continuous tumor growth through the path of least resistance rather than invasion of airspaces. The distinction between continuous and discontinuous growth in STAS and its clinical implications has not been studied and might represent the missing link in contradictory clinicopathological and molecular findings in the STAS literature.

The 2 putative forms of STAS might share a common initial pathogenetic mechanism leading to intra-alveolar growth, but with distinct evolution depending on the characteristics of the primary tumor. Such characteristics would involve several factors, including tumor-specific intra-alveolar environment that can be less or more favorable to survival and spread of viable floating cancer cells, as is described in mucinous adenocarcinomas. The continuous spread could therefore relate to local tumor growth, whereas the discontinuous spread would be associated with metastatic potential. Importantly, understanding the mechanisms involved in aerogenous metastasis and STAS is not semantical or purely academic. The underlying cellular and molecular pathways required for the continuous and discontinuous spread of tumor cells are different, and their elucidation is crucial to determine the clinical and potential therapeutic implications of airway tumor spread.

CLINICOPATHOLOGICAL FEATURES AND CLINICAL RELEVANCE

An increased risk of aerogenous metastases is described in patients with adenocarcinoma of mucinous phenotype, tumors with papillary and lepidic subtypes, and those with primary lesions manifesting on imaging as predominant airspace disease and/or poorly defined margins.[5,8–10] The clinicopathological characteristics of aerogeneous metastases, however, have not been studied at length. The diagnosis of aerogenous spread is based on the presence of intrapulmonary lesions away from the primary tumor that must be differentiated from other forms of metastatic spread and multicentric tumors. Aerogenous metastasis can typically be differentiated from hematogenous or lymphatic metastases on computed tomography (CT) and pathology. The issue of multifocal adenocarcinomas, however, is more controversial, specifically whether multiple lesions originate from one primary site (intrapulmonary metastasis) or develop de novo at multiple sites (synchronous primary cancers). It is accepted that both phenomena occur,[5,11] and distinction is crucial, because it influences tumor staging and treatment. Molecular analysis of tumor DNA has the potential for characterizing multicentric tumors as either metastatic or synchronous primaries.[12,13] A polyclonal basis and the coexistence of different histologic subtypes (including preinvasive lesions and invasive adenocarcinoma) support the diagnosis of synchronous primary malignancies. In contrast, immunohistochemical[14] and genetic[13,15] studies demonstrating monoclonal origin support the occurrence of intrapulmonary spread from a primary lung lesion. Although a definitive distinction between metastasis and synchronous primary may require tumor genotyping, comprehensive histologic assessment has been shown to have similar accuracy.[5,16] The authors' group has previously described the radiological and pathologic criteria to make such distinction using comprehensive histologic assessment, [17] and molecular studies are being conducted to support it.

The clinical relevance of STAS was proposed in 2015 by 2 large cohorts of patients with early adenocarcinomas. Kadota and colleagues[1] described STAS in 38% of 411 resected small (<2 cm) stage I lung adenocarcinomas and observed a significant association with lymphovascular invasion and high-grade histologic pattern. In the study of 569 adenocarcinomas described by Warth and colleagues,[2] STAS was associated with male sex, lymph node and distant metastasis, tumor stage, and high-grade histologic patterns, and there was a correlation with KRAS and BRAF mutations. In subsequent studies, the reported incidence of STAS ranged from 14.8% to 60.5% in adenocarcinomas and was consistently associated with worse prognosis.[18–22] The association of STAS with smoking history and male gender has been suggested by some, but not confirmed in other studies.[19,23] Interestingly, contrary to the findings by Warth and colleagues, an association with higher rate of ALK rearrangement has been described.[24,25] STAS has been identified more frequently in adenocarcinomas with micropapillary, papillary, and solid subtypes and seems to be uncommon in tumors with lepidic histology.[24]

Most of the available data on STAS thus far come from studies of nonmucinous adenocarcinomas.

Recently, the occurrence of STAS was investigated in a cohort of 132 resected solitary mucinous adenocarcinomas and was identified in 72.2% of cases, a higher incidence than that reported for nonmucinous tumors. The presence of STAS correlated with older age, presence of nodal metastases, and poor differentiation on histology.[26] STAS has been also recently described in histologic subtypes of lung cancer other than adenocarcinomas. In 2017, Lu and colleagues described for the first time the occurrence of STAS in 30% of 445 resected stage I to III squamous cell carcinomas (SCCs), followed by subsequent studies showing similar association in up to 40% of cases.[20,27] STAS was shown to be one of the most significant prognostic histologic findings in SCC and was associated with increased risk of locoregional and distant metastases. STAS has also been described in lung neuroendocrine tumors, more commonly large cell and small cell lung cancer, but also in typical and atypical carcinoids. In the largest study of 487 patients with neuroendocrine tumors, the reported overall incidence of STAS was 26%; it was associated with early distant metastasis and recurrence, and it was an independent poor prognostic factor in patients with large cell and small cell lung cancers.[28]

PROGNOSTIC SIGNIFICANCE OF AIRWAY SPREAD

The prognostic significance of aerogenous metastasis remains to be determined. Factors such as the extent of intrapulmonary spread and whether spread is limited to one or both lungs or associated with systemic metastases are expected to influence prognosis. It is not known how the prognosis of aerogenous spread compares to hematogenous or lymphatic metastases limited to the lungs. In the study by Aokage and colleagues,[29] the presence of isolated intrapulmonary metastases, presumed to be aerogenous spread, had a better prognosis than similar stage disease with nodal metastasis or vascular invasion. It is also known that mucinous adenocarcinomas with contralateral pulmonary metastases tend to have a better outcome than those with systemic spread.

Differentiation between aerogenous metastases and synchronous lesions in the adenocarcinoma spectrum is important for prognosis and management. Synchronous primary adenocarcinomas (clonally unrelated tumors) tend to have a more indolent course and are often treated with surgical resection with favorable results, including sublobar resection. This cannot be extrapolated to primary adenocarcinoma with multifocal intrapulmonary involvement and presumed aerogenous metastasis. Lobectomy may be considered for selected patients with disease limited to 1 lobe, but the presence of multilobar and bilateral disease may preclude curative-intent surgery.

STAS has been shown to be an independent negative prognostic factor regardless of tumor staging.[18,20,30] In a meta-analysis including 14 studies and 3754 patients, pooled results demonstrated an association with worse recurrence-free survival and overall survival in patients with NSCLC.[31] In the study by Kadota and colleagues,[1] STAS was a significant risk factor for locoregional and distant recurrence in patients with limited resection but not in those treated with lobectomy. Similar findings were found in subsequent studies,[32–34] highlighting the potential impact on management. Shiono and colleagues[35] reported a higher rate of pulmonary metastases in patients with STAS treated with sublobar resection compared to those treated with lobectomy. In another study, risk of recurrence following sublobar resection was independently associated with STAS and tumor margins less than 1 cm. Worth noting, when resection margin was greater than 2 cm, no local recurrence was observed in this cohort, even in patients with STAS.[32] It has been therefore suggested that lobectomy may arguably be preferred when STAS is present in early stage adenocarcinoma, even for potential candidates for sublobar resection. If sublobar resection is performed, wide surgical margins would be advised. Similarly, for nonsurgical ablative treatments such as stereotactic body radiation and imaging-guided percutaneous ablation, wider treatment margins would be warranted should STAS be present. Furthermore, given the association of STAS with lymphovascular invasion and metastasis, adjuvant treatment might benefit patients with early stage adenocarcinoma and STAS.

An important issue is that the diagnosis of STAS requires surgical resection. Thus far, STAS cannot be diagnosed preoperatively in small biopsy specimens, and the role of frozen section remains to be defined. While pathologists were able to diagnose STAS on intraoperative frozen section specimens with acceptable sensitivity (71%) and high specificity (92%) in a recent study,[36] earlier studies reported unacceptable low sensitivity and negative predictive values.[37,38] Importantly, the distinction between artifacts and STAS is of utmost clinical importance to avoid false-positive diagnosis. Standardized procedures for tissue handling and processing are crucial as well as familiarity with potential diagnostic pitfalls. In an interesting study, diagnosis of STAS was obtained in bronchial washing cytology and formalin-fixed paraffin-embedded secretions from resected specimens of mucinous adenocarcinoma,[7] but this remains to be validated.

IMAGING FINDINGS OF AEROGENOUS METASTASIS AND SPREAD THROUGH THE AIRSPACES

The CT features of aerogenous metastasis have been described and share striking imaging similarities to small airways and airspace diseases such as seen in inflammatory bronchiolitis and bronchopneumonia, presumably reflecting cancer cells lining the small airways and alveolar spaces with variable amounts of intra-alveolar secretions and tumor cells.[5,14,39] CT findings include persistent centrilobular nodules and branching opacities (tree-in-bud nodules), typically with ill-defined margins and ground glass attenuation. Nodules tend to be clustered and invariably grow on serial CT, occasionally progressing to confluent airspace disease. When remote from the primary lesion, nodules tend to have a lower lobe and dependent distribution.[5,40] CT features of the primary lesion that seem to be associated with aerogenous metastasis include nodular or mass-like appearance, consolidation with air bronchograms, poorly defined margins, and presence of ground glass (**Fig. 1**).

Aerogenous metastasis must be differentiated from synchronous primary adenocarcinomas on CT. The latter typically manifest with randomly distributed nodules rather than clustered centrilobular lesions and tend to have more variable sizes, often associated with part-solid lesions. Synchronous lung primaries manifesting as ground glass nodules are indolent and demonstrate slow growth in serial CT in contrast to the relatively rapid growth and further spread expected in aerogenous metastases.[5,14,40,41]

The current definition and diagnosis of STAS is based on microscopic analysis of small resected lung cancers and detection of abnormal clusters of cells. These cells are below the resolution of the human eye and cannot be visualized on CT studies. Although the imaging manifestations of STAS per se cannot be assessed using current definition, studies have assessed the role of CT in predicting the presence of STAS based on the characteristics of the primary tumor. In a study comparing the CT features of resected STAS-positive and STAS-negative adenocarcinomas, the primary lesion in STAS-positive cases was more commonly solid (71/92%, 77%) than part-solid (21/92%, 23%), and STAS was not seen in primary pure ground-glass nodules (P<.001). STAS was more common in lesions with central

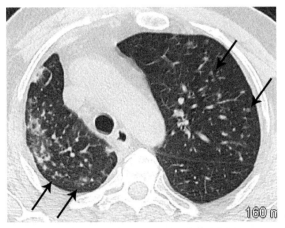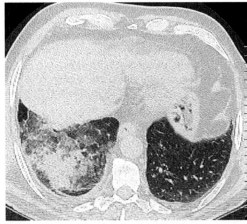

Fig. 1. 74-year-old man with biopsy-proven invasive mucinous lung adenocarcinoma and presumed aerogenous metastasis. Axial CT image shows the primary lesion in the right lower lobe manifesting as air space disease with surrounding ground glass opacities. Image through the upper lobes demonstrates centrilobular ground glass nodules and branching opacities involving both lungs (*arrows*), consistent with aerogenous metastases.

low attenuation, ill-defined peripheral opacities and absence of air bronchograms, but was not associated with size of the primary lesion. Small solid tumors were more likely to spread through the airspaces than larger part-solid lesions. For part-solid adenocarcinomas, the percentage of solid component was an independent predictor of STAS.[24] In another study of 327 resected adenocarcinomas, 191 with STAS, part-solid lesions accounted for 36% of STAS-positive cases; the absence of ground-glass component on CT was the most significant finding associated with STAS in univariate and multivariate analysis. In the same study, STAS was significantly associated with lesion diameter greater than 2 cm.[19,42] Although further studies are required to validate the role of CT in prognosis, these findings support current guidelines for sublobar resection of small (<2 cm) peripheral lesions with 50% or greater ground glass component on CT.

AEROGENOUS METASTASIS AND SPREAD THROUGH THE AIRSPACES S – DISTINCT ENTITIES OR SPECTRUM OF THE SAME PROCESS?

As discussed previously, aerogenous metastasis and STAS reflect patterns of tumor spread in primary lung cancer, particularly adenocarcinomas, and seem to share common pathogenetic mechanisms. It can be argued that aerogenous metastasis and STAS might be part of the spectrum of tumor spread through the airways. The current definition of STAS likely incorporates 2 distinct but related phenomena: (1) the growth of tumor cells within airspaces, in direct continuity with the growing edge of the main tumor mass, described as a microscopic form of invasion, and (2) the shed of neoplastic cells from the growing edge with discontinuous spread through adjacent airspaces. Aerogenous metastasis in turn is defined as the discontinuous spread and seeding of tumor cells through the airways to the lung parenchyma situated away from the main tumor with subsequent grow of focal metastatic lesions. Therefore, the mechanisms involved in aerogenous metastasis and the discontinuous form of STAS seem to be a related phenomenon. Discontinuous spread is a necessary initial step for aerogenous metastasis to occur. Therefore, one may argue that aerogenous metastasis may reflect the progression of STAS, eventually manifesting as macroscopic lesions detectable on imaging studies. To determine the potential link and clarify the pathways of STAS and aerogenous metastasis, pathologic studies of resected specimens are required but may be difficult to be performed because advanced lung cancers are usually not resected. Aerogenous metastases can spread to any pulmonary lobe and often to the contralateral lung, limiting pathologic assessment of potential metastatic lesions.

Although areas of uncertainty remain, STAS has been shown to be an independent prognostic finding and may need to be included in the staging and possibly in the treatment algorithm of patients with early adenocarcinoma. Active search for STAS on resected specimens and inclusion in pathology reports is advocated by some. A better understanding of the clinical and pathologic features of STAS and tools for preoperative diagnosis are necessary to assist in treatment decision making.

Further studies are required to better define the pathogenetic mechanisms and clinicopathological features of aerogenous metastasis and STAS, as well as their impact on prognosis. This will hopefully allow more clear classifications and guidelines for management and open research venues for exploring suitable therapeutic interventions.

CLINICS CARE POINTS

- Airway spread is more common in certain subtypes of lung cancers, notably adenocarcinomas

- STAS, as defined in the current WHO classification, has been shown to be an independent negative prognostic factor regardless of tumor staging.

- Presence of STAS may need to be included in the staging and possibly in the treatment algorithm of patients with early adenocarcinoma, including surgical decision making.

- Tools for preoperative diagnosis are necessary to diagnose STAS, currently limited to detection in resection specimens.

- The prognostic significance of aerogenous metastasis remains to be determined. Factors such as the extent of intrapulmonary spread and whether spread is limited to one or both lungs or associated with systemic metastases are expected to influence prognosis.

DISCLOSURE

C.A. Souza: Consultant fees and honorarium: Pfizer, Boehringer-Ingelheim, AstraZeneca, Hoffmann-La Roche. Advisory board: AstraZeneca, Boehringer-Ingelheim. Educational Grant: Boehringer-Ingelheim. M.M. Gomes: Educational Grants: Pfizer, BMS, Merck, AstraZeneca, Roche, Eli Lilly, Boehringer-Ingelheim. Honoraria: AstraZeneca, Hoffmann-La Roche.

REFERENCES

1. Kadota K, Nitadori JI, Sima CS, et al. Tumor spread through air spaces is an important pattern of invasion and impacts the frequency and location of recurrences after limited resection for small stage I lung adenocarcinomas. J Thorac Oncol 2015; 10(5):806–14.

2. Warth A, Muley T, Kossakowski CA, et al. Prognostic impact of intra-alveolar tumor spread in pulmonary adenocarcinoma. Am J Surg Pathol 2015;39(6): 793–801.

3. Travis WD, Brambilla E, Nicholson AG, et al. The 2015 World Health Organization classification of lung tumors: impact of genetic, clinical and radiologic advances since the 2004 classification. J Thorac Oncol 2015;10(9):1243–60.

4. Lakshmanan I, Ponnusamy MP, Macha MA, et al. Mucins in lung cancer: diagnostic, prognostic, and therapeutic implications. J Thorac Oncol 2015;10(1):19–27.

5. Gaikwad A, Souza CA, Inacio JR, et al. Aerogenous metastases: a potential game changer in the diagnosis and management of primary lung adenocarcinoma. AJR Am J Roentgenol 2014;203(6):W570–82.

6. (5–9).

7. Isaka T, Yokose T, Miyagi Y, et al. Detection of tumor spread through airspaces by airway secretion cytology from resected lung cancer specimens. Pathol Int 2017;67(10):487–94.

8. Miyake H, Matsumoto A, Terada A, et al. Mucin-producing tumor of the lung: CT findings. J Thorac Imaging 1995;10(2):96–8.

9. Wislez M, Massiani MA, Milleron B, et al. Clinical characteristics of pneumonic-type adenocarcinoma of the lung. Chest 2003;123(6):1868–77.

10. Epstein DM, Gefter WB, Miller WT. Lobar bronchioloalveolar cell carcinoma. AJR Am J Roentgenol 1982;139(3):463–8.

11. Gazdar AF, Minna JD. Multifocal lung cancers–clonality vs field cancerization and does it matter? J Natl Cancer Inst 2009;101(8):541–3.

12. Girard N, Ostrovnaya I, Lau C, et al. Genomic and mutational profiling to assess clonal relationships between multiple non-small cell lung cancers. Clin Cancer Res 2009;15(16):5184–90.

13. Warth A, Macher-Goeppinger S, Muley T, et al. Clonality of multifocal nonsmall cell lung cancer: implications for staging and therapy. Eur Respir J 2012; 39(6):1437–42.

14. Gaeta M, Blandino A, Pergolizzi S, et al. Patterns of recurrence of bronchioloalveolar cell carcinoma after surgical resection: a radiological, histological, and immunohistochemical study. Lung Cancer 2003;42(3):319–26.

15. Wang X, Wang M, MacLennan GT, et al. Evidence for common clonal origin of multifocal lung cancers. J Natl Cancer Inst 2009;101(8):560–70.

16. Chang NIJ, Lai C, Gupta A, et al. Lung adenocarcinomas with aerogenous spread: description of histologic features and radiologic-pathologic correlation. Arch Pathol Lab Med 2016;140(3):263.

17. Brownell R, Moua T, Henry TS, et al. The use of pretest probability increases the value of high-resolution CT in diagnosing usual interstitial pneumonia. Thorax 2017;72(5):424–9.

18. Shiono S, Yanagawa N. Spread through air spaces is a predictive factor of recurrence and a prognostic

factor in stage I lung adenocarcinoma. Interact Cardiovasc Thorac Surg 2016;23(4):567–72.

19. Toyokawa G, Yamada Y, Tagawa T, et al. Significance of spread through air spaces in resected pathological stage I lung adenocarcinoma. Ann Thorac Surg 2018;105(6):1655–63.

20. Kadota K, Kushida Y, Katsuki N, et al. Tumor spread through air spaces is an independent predictor of recurrence-free survival in patients with resected lung squamous cell carcinoma. Am J Surg Pathol 2017;41(8):1077–86.

21. Uruga H, Fujii T, Fujimori S, et al. Semiquantitative assessment of tumor spread through air spaces (STAS) in early-stage lung adenocarcinomas. J Thorac Oncol 2017;12(7):1046–51.

22. Shiono S, Endo M, Suzuki K, et al. Spread through air spaces is a prognostic factor in Sublobar resection of non-small cell lung cancer. Ann Thorac Surg 2018;106(2):354–60.

23. Lee JS, Kim EK, Kim M, et al. Genetic and clinicopathologic characteristics of lung adenocarcinoma with tumor spread through air spaces. Lung Cancer 2018;123:121–6.

24. Kim SK, Kim TJ, Chung MJ, et al. Lung adenocarcinoma: CT features associated with spread through air spaces. Radiology 2018;289(3):831–40.

25. Onozato ML, Kovach AE, Yeap BY, et al. Tumor islands in resected early-stage lung adenocarcinomas are associated with unique clinicopathologic and molecular characteristics and worse prognosis. Am J Surg Pathol 2013;37(2):287–94.

26. Lee MA, Kang J, Lee HY, et al. Spread through air spaces (STAS) in invasive mucinous adenocarcinoma of the lung: Incidence, prognostic impact, and prediction based on clinicoradiologic factors. Thorac Cancer 2020;11(11):3145–54.

27. Lu S, Tan KS, Kadota K, et al. Spread through air spaces (STAS) is an independent predictor of recurrence and lung cancer-specific death in squamous cell carcinoma. J Thorac Oncol 2017;12(2):223–34.

28. Aly RG, Rekhtman N, Li X, et al. Spread through air spaces (STAS) is prognostic in atypical carcinoid, large cell neuroendocrine carcinoma, and small cell carcinoma of the lung. J Thorac Oncol 2019; 14(9):1583–93.

29. Aokage K, Ishii G, Nagai K, et al. Intrapulmonary metastasis in resected pathologic stage IIIB non-small cell lung cancer: possible contribution of aerogenous metastasis to the favorable outcome. J Thorac Cardiovasc Surg 2007;134(2):386–91.

30. Yokoyama S, Murakami T, Tao H, et al. Tumor spread through air spaces identifies a distinct subgroup with poor prognosis in surgically resected lung pleomorphic carcinoma. Chest 2018;154(4):838–47.

31. Chen D, Mao Y, Wen J, et al. Tumor spread through air spaces in non-small cell lung cancer: a systematic review and meta-analysis. Ann Thorac Surg 2019;108(3):945–54.

32. Masai K, Sakurai H, Sukeda A, et al. Prognostic impact of margin distance and tumor spread through air spaces in limited resection for primary lung cancer. J Thorac Oncol 2017;12(12):1788–97.

33. Eguchi T, Kameda K, Lu S, et al. Lobectomy is associated with better outcomes than sublobar resection in spread through air spaces (STAS)-positive T1 lung adenocarcinoma: a propensity score-matched analysis. J Thorac Oncol 2019;14(1):87–98.

34. Kadota K, Kushida Y, Kagawa S, et al. Limited resection is associated with a higher risk of locoregional recurrence than lobectomy in stage I lung adenocarcinoma with tumor spread through air spaces. Am J Surg Pathol 2019;43(8):1033–41.

35. Shiono S, Endo M, Suzuki K, et al. Spread through air spaces in lung cancer patients is a risk factor for pulmonary metastasis after surgery. J Thorac Dis 2019;11(1):177–87.

36. Eguchi T, Adusumilli PS. Competing risks analysis in the prognostic assessment of patients undergoing lung resection. J Thorac Dis 2017;9(4):E395–7.

37. Yeh YC, Nitadori J, Kadota K, et al. Using frozen section to identify histological patterns in stage I lung adenocarcinoma of </= 3 cm: accuracy and interobserver agreement. Histopathology 2015; 66(7):922–38.

38. Walts AE, Marchevsky AM. Current evidence does not warrant frozen section evaluation for the presence of tumor spread through alveolar spaces. Arch Pathol Lab Med 2018;142(1):59–63.

39. Gaeta M, Caruso R, Barone M, et al. Ground-glass attenuation in nodular bronchioloalveolar carcinoma: CT patterns and prognostic value. J Comput Assist Tomogr 1998;22(2):215–9.

40. Akira M, Atagi S, Kawahara M, et al. High-resolution CT findings of diffuse bronchioloalveolar carcinoma in 38 patients. AJR Am J Roentgenol 1999;173(6): 1623–9.

41. Tateishi U, Muller NL, Johkoh T, et al. Mucin-producing adenocarcinoma of the lung: thin-section computed tomography findings in 48 patients and their effect on prognosis. J Comput Assist Tomogr 2005;29(3):361–8.

42. Koezuka S, Mikami T, Tochigi N, et al. Toward improving prognosis prediction in patients undergoing small lung adenocarcinoma resection: radiological and pathological assessment of diversity and intratumor heterogeneity. Lung Cancer 2019;135: 40–6.

Controversies in Lung Cancer
When to Resect with Compromised Pulmonary Function

Farid M. Shamji, MBBS, FRCSC, FACS

KEYWORDS

- Lung cancer • Compromised lung function • Clinical assessment • Spirometry FEV_1/FVC
- Diffusion capacity • Quantitative V/Q scan cardiopulmonary exercise testing • Vo_2max

KEY POINTS

- Operative risk factors in pulmonary resection need to be assessed from the clinical assessment.
- Exercise tests, pulmonary function tests and preoperative evaluation are essential.
- Major risk factors, intermediate risk factors, and minor risk factors must be assessed.

INTRODUCTION

Patients with lung cancer frequently have impaired pulmonary function, usually secondary to smoking-related chronic obstructive lung disease. If these patients are referred for possible curative surgery, they are at increased risk of developing postoperative complications, and some have such poor respiratory reserve that a pneumonectomy may result in an unacceptable quality of life or fatality. Numerous techniques have been used to evaluate the postsurgical risk. These techniques include preoperative pulmonary function test (PFTs), 6-minute walk test (6MWT), stage 1 cardiopulmonary exercise test (CPET), 2D echocardiography (ECHO), and quantitative ventilation-perfusion (V/Q) scintigraphy.

Preexisting chronic obstructive pulmonary disease (COPD) is the most common limiting factor in resectional surgery of the lung because it relates directly to postoperative morbidity and mortality. The purpose of preoperative assessment of the respiratory function is the identification of the high-risk patient. In this group, resection is not necessarily prohibited, but the type of operation should be carefully selected and prophylactic measures applied to decrease the incidence of postoperative complications.

It is well recognized that patients with heart disease and chronic lung disease, both limiting cardiopulmonary functional reserve, undergoing noncardiac thoracic surgery are at special risk, which varies according to

- The patient's functional status and general health: risk increases proportionately with impaired function
- The increasing age of the patient: those older than 80 years are at high risk
- The type of surgical procedure: highest risk with pneumonectomy
- The skill of the anesthetist and surgeon: competency is essential

Identification of the Operative Risk Relating to Mortality and Morbidity by Evaluation of Total Function of Both Lungs

Preoperative assessment should aim to fulfill 3 objectives. The first is to understand the implications of the disease for which surgery has been recommended and the consequences of the procedure that is planned. The second is to confirm that optimum preoperative preparation has been achieved, and the third is to recognize and make allowance for any coexistent disease or idiosyncrasy of physique or personality. The aims should be to highlight those anatomic and functional features that are of particular relevance to noncardiac

University of Ottawa, General Campus, Ottawa Hospital, 501 Smyth Road, Ottawa, Ontario K1H 8L6, Canada
E-mail address: faridshamji@hotmail.com

Thorac Surg Clin 31 (2021) 485–495
https://doi.org/10.1016/j.thorsurg.2021.07.004
1547-4127/21/© 2021 Elsevier Inc. All rights reserved.

thoracic surgery and to outline preoperative measures that can be used to create the best possible conditions for a successful outcome.

CLINICAL EVALUATION
Clinical Assessment

The patient's clinical status is an important consideration in deciding whether the patient is a candidate for pulmonary resection. Comorbidity is common in patients with lung cancer. Lack of clinical abnormalities does not rule out pulmonary illness.

History of present illness to identify pulmonary risk factors

1. Dyspnea at rest or on exertion.
2. Daily amount and color of phlegm produced.
3. Frequent use of bronchodilators for relief of asthmatic bronchitis.
4. Declining exercise capacity and tolerance.
5. Smoking history: active or ex-smoker, duration of smoking.
6. General condition: increasing age (>80 years), impaired nutritional status (amount of weight loss), obesity (increased body mass index).
7. Continuous or periodic use of supplemental oxygen.
8. Documented heart disease: ischemic, valvular, cardiomyopathy, congestive heart failure, chronic atrial fibrillation responsible for dyspnea.
9. Occupational history: exposure to asbestos, mining (uranium, nickel, iron ore, coal, crystalline silica), and dust (pneumoconiosis).

Major cardiac risk factors for increased perioperative cardiac morbidity and mortality

1. Unstable coronary artery syndromes
   a. Acute or recent myocardial infarction with evidence of threatening myocardial ischemia by clinical symptoms or noninvasive radionuclide study
   b. Unstable or severe angina
2. Decompensated heart failure
3. Significant cardiac arrhythmias
   a. High-grade atrioventricular block
   b. Symptomatic ventricular arrhythmias in the presence of underlying heart disease
   c. Supraventricular arrhythmias with uncontrolled ventricular rate
4. Severe valvular heart disease
   a. Significant and critical aortic valve stenosis
   b. Severe mitral valve stenosis

Past medical history
Generalized lung disease at the level of the alveoli due to

1. Pulmonary fibrosis from recurrent pneumonia
2. Diffuse bronchiectasis with complicating recurrent lung infections
3. Idiopathic interstitial pulmonary fibrosis
4. Significant pulmonary fibrosis caused by advanced pulmonary sarcoidosis
5. Fibrosing alveolitis
6. COPD: diffuse panacinar emphysema (the vanishing lung syndrome)
7. Pulmonary asbestosis from industrial exposure

Physical examination

- *General:* Assessing for nutritional status, anemia, jaundice, cyanosis, clubbing, pedal edema, cervical lymphadenopathy, superior vena cava obstruction syndrome (SVCO), mouth for cancer and dental caries (tongue and the state of teeth), hoarseness, and recent skin nodules if any.
- *Chest examination* for symmetric chest expansion, bilateral air entry, and breath sounds. Rule out atelectasis, pleural effusion, previous thoracotomy incision, median sternotomy incision
- *Cardiac examination* for cardiac rhythm, heart rate, heart sounds, cardiac murmur, congestive heart failure, and carotid arterial stenosis
- *Abdomen examination* for liver enlargement, ascites, splenomegaly, abdominal artery aneurysm, and any abnormal mass
- *Neurologic examination* for integrity of the cranial nerves and the peripheral nervous system for neurologic deficit

Simple exercise tests for measuring functional capacity: exercise testing stresses the cardiopulmonary and oxygen delivery system and provides a good indication of cardiopulmonary reserve
Stair climbing test is the simplest screening test: can the patient walk briskly up 2 flights of stairs without stopping while maintaining a conversation?
a. Record heart rate, respiratory rate, and oxygen saturation before stair climbing and immediately after at the top of the stairs.
b. This test is an exercise tolerance test with rough estimation of the cardiopulmonary reserve.
c. This test is an acceptable rough-and-ready guide to fitness for surgery in uncomplicated cases

6-Minute walk test is a standardized test The 6MWT is a cost-effective and well-documented field test for assessing functional exercise capacity and response to medical interventions in diverse patient groups and predicting cardiorespiratory fitness among healthy people. 6MWT is a tool for predicting maximal aerobic power (oxygen consumption [Vo_2max]) in healthy adults, and it can be used for preoperative assessment.[1]

The patient is asked to walk as far as possible along a corridor in 6 minutes. The test should be performed indoors along a long, flat, straight, enclosed corridor. The result is expressed in meters covered. The course is 30 m in length with cones at either end to act as turnaround points. The advantage is that the test simulates real-life conditions. The 6MWT performed along a 15-m track is a valid field test for predicting Vo_2max of healthy adults with accuracy of about 1 MET.

For men, the best predictors for Vo_2max are walking distance, age, body mass index, heart rate at the end of 6MWT, and height, and for women, the predictors are walking distance, age, and height.

Shuttle walk test is a standardized test The patient walks around 2 marker cones placed 10 m apart. The course is 10 m in length. The subject aims to walk around the 10-m course and turn around the first marker cone when the first audio signal is given, and so on. The walking speed is controlled by the audio signal that "beeps," and the walking speed is successively increased. The test stops when the patient is too breathless to maintain the speed required or after 12 min, and the number of cones reached is recorded.

Tests of Pulmonary Function

The normal lung has enormous reserves of function at rest. When a normal subject exercises, the O_2 uptake and CO_2 output can be increased 10-fold, and these increases occur without decrease in arterial Po_2 or increase in Pco_2. Therefore, to reveal minor dysfunction, the stress of exercise is often useful.

1. *Exercise testing* is done to assess disability as an objective measurement of performance because patients vary considerably in their own assessment of the amount of activity they can do. Less formal exercise tests by stair climbing test and 6MWT can also be informative.[1] More objective and reliable and reproducible measurement of exercise capacity is from CPET.
2. *Pulmonary function testing* is an important practical application of respiratory physiology. Spirometric studies are of value because they give objective data on lung function and help to screen the high-risk patients. These studies should be done routinely on every patient

before pulmonary resection. Diament and Palmer[2] showed that 30% of patients undergoing elective surgery have unequivocal evidence of increased airway resistance, although 15% admitted to a productive cough. Stein and Cassara[3] correlated preoperative spirometry to postoperative complications and found that one of 33 patients with normal tests had pulmonary complications, whereas 23 of 30 with abnormal tests had complications.

3. *Lung volumes and capacities* are 2 distinct terms in spirometry. Volume changes are brought about by inspiratory and expiratory efforts and are termed *volumes*. Volumes that are determined by the size of the lungs and thorax are termed *capacities*. Lung volumes and lung capacities of a subject are recorded on a spirometer.[4,5]

Definition of lung volumes measured with a simple spirometer

1. *Tidal volume:* With quiet breathing the lung volume increases from the resting respiratory level of 3 L to between 3.4 and 3.5 L, and it is measured; this gives a tidal volume of 400 to 500 mL.
2. *Forced vital capacity (FVC):* It is a measure of the ability to ventilate during which maximal inspiration is followed by maximal expiration — the total amount of air the subject can exhale after maximum inspiration. The best value after optimal bronchodilator therapy is used.
3. *Forced expiratory volume in first second (FEV_1) is timed forced vital capacity:* FEV_1 is a particularly useful and simple test of pulmonary function; it is the measurement of a single forced expiration. FEV_1 is the volume of air expelled in the first second of a maximal forced expiration from a position of full inspiration. The best value after optimal bronchodilator therapy is used.

The subject makes a maximal inspiration and then exhales as rapidly and as fully as possible. The volume of air expired after 1, 2, and 3 seconds is measured and related to the total volume of air expired (FVC). The total volume of air expired in the first second is the *timed forced vital capacity* denoted by the term FEV_1. The result is expressed as a percentage of this volume. A normal subject will expel over 83% of the FVC in 1 second, 91% in 2 seconds, and 97% in 3 seconds. In a normal subject, at least 80% of the FVC can be expelled in the first second; the FEV_1 is about 80% of the FVC.[4,5]

There are 2 defects recognized from the measurements of

a. FEV_1 timed forced vital capacity
b. FVC

These 2 defects are as follows

a. *Obstructive defect* in which there is diffuse airway obstruction seen in asthma and COPD. In this situation FEV_1 is affected to a greater extent than the FVC and the ratio of FEV_1/FVC is reduced less than 0.7; this pattern is referred to as *obstructive defect*.
b. *Restrictive defect* is recognized when lung volume is restricted as in reduced lung compliance, chest wall deformity, or thoracic muscle weakness. The FVC is reduced and the FEV_1 is also reduced roughly in proportion so that the ratio FEV_1/FVC is essentially normal. This pattern of ventilatory impairment is referred to as the *restrictive defect*.

4. *Maximum ventilation volume (MVV)* is another test of lung function to determine the maximum breathing capacity of the subject. It is an overall performance test that requires optimal cooperation from the subject. As rapid deep breathing cannot be kept up for a whole minute, the subject is asked to breathe as rapidly and as deeply as possible for 15 seconds and the results are multiplied by 4. The pulmonary ventilation per minute calculated on the recording spirometer is termed the maximum ventilation volume. Normal subjects can exceed 100 L/min.

Correlations

Gaensler and colleagues[6] reported in 1955 that postoperative disability correlated well with the type of operation performed, the degree of preoperative disability, and preoperative function studies.

There will be patients who are considered not to be surgical candidates from clinical assessment only and these include arriving for consultation in a wheel chair, on supplemental oxygen for extended periods, inability to maintain conversation due to monosyllabic speech, or being unable to walk long distance or climb stairs or walk uphill.

Eight early postoperative deaths due to respiratory insufficiency occurred in patients with MVV less than 50%. Boushy and colleagues[7] showed that 40% of patients older than 60 years with borderline lung function with FEV_1 less than 2.0 L did not tolerate surgery. Gerson[8] also found a correlation between peak flow rates, FEV_1, and immediate operative survival. Lockwood[9] identified a very-high-risk group (vital capacity < 1.85 L, FVC < 1.70 L, FEV_1 < 1.2 L, and MVV < 28 L/min). In Deslauriers series, 61 of 498 consecutive patients had a preoperative FEV_1 less than 1.2 L.[9] The operative mortality was not higher in this group, but there was a significant increase in the rate of major pulmonary complications. To obtain the best possible value, the patient should have maximum preparation before testing.

Spirometry

This technique should be repeated in chronic obstructive lung disease to assess response after a trial of bronchodilators. The response is considered favorable and encouraging when improvement in FEV_1 is noted in response to bronchodilation; it reflects the possibility of relieving some of the dynamic airway obstruction by bronchodilator aerosol, and is especially helpful in making a wise surgical decision.

Pulmonary resection for lung cancer is considered safe with an acceptable low operative risk when a thoughtful surgical decision for complete resection of lung cancer is made from FEV_1 measurement:

An acceptable operative risk with a low mortality can be achieved for pneumonectomy if the preoperative FEV_1 is >2.0 L. For lobectomy, the preoperative FEV_1 >1.5 L is the minimum necessary for the pulmonary resection.

Arterial Blood Gases Analysis

Arterial Po_2, O_2 saturation, Pco_2, HCO_3, and pH are most commonly measured on a sample of arterial blood obtained by puncture of radial artery and analyzed by Po_2, Pco_2, and pH blood gas electrodes. All 3 electrodes are arranged to give their outputs on the same meter (**Table 1**).

Arterial $Paco_2$ greater than 45 mm Hg does not seem to be an independent predictor of poor outcome. However, preoperative hypoxemia with oxygen saturations less than 90% and desaturation greater than 4% with exercise has been associated with an increased risk of complications.

There are 4 recognized causes of hypoxemia: (1) hypoventilation with reduced alveolar ventilation, (2) impaired gaseous diffusion in the lungs, (3) true intrapulmonary or intracardiac right to left

Table 1	
Normal values for arterial blood gases while breathing normal room air at sea level	
Arterial Blood Gases	**Normal Values**
pH	7.35–7.45
Pco_2	33–45 mm Hg
Po_2	90–105 mm Hg
Actual bicarbonate	22–26 mmol/L
Base excess	−3 to +3 mmol/L
Oxygen saturation	96%–99%

shunt, and (4) V/Q mismatch from lung parenchymal disease. Hypoventilation is always associated with a raised arterial P_{CO_2}. However, persistent hypercapnia (>45 mm Hg) indicates advanced lung parenchymal disease with minimal reserve and a high risk of postoperative morbidity and mortality.

Preoperative hypoxemia (low arterial P_{O_2} <70 mm Hg) is not an absolute contraindication to pulmonary resection because the lung to be resected may be the contributing factor to hypoxemia from parenchymal lung disease or atelectasis. It is recognized that patient with diffuse pulmonary emphysema seen on chest computed tomographic scan (the so-called vanishing lung syndrome of the pink puffer) is worse with prohibitively high operative risk than the patient with chronic bronchitis (the blue bloater) who has favourable bronchodilation response to preoperative bronchodilators and improved measured lung function after a trial of pulmonary rehabilitation and smoking cessation for 6 weeks.

Cardiac Pulmonary Exercise Testing

Formal testing of cardiopulmonary exercise capability seems to give the most accurate indication of postoperative complications. The normal lung has enormous reserves of function at rest. The O_2 uptake and CO_2 output can be increased 10-fold when a normal subject exercises, and these increases occur without any decrease in arterial P_{O_2} or increase in Pa_{CO_2}.[10]

CPET is a noninvasive technique that involves submaximal and maximal treadmill or bicycle exercise with continuous electrocardiography monitoring and breath-by-breath determination of oxygen uptake and carbon dioxide output, and spirometry, maximum oxygen consumption V_{O_2}max, peak heart rate, exercise capacity, anaerobic threshold, and respiratory gas exchange ratio can be calculated.[9] V_{O_2}max is the highest oxygen consumption achieved at maximal work before stopping the test and is reported in units of mL/kg/min. The predicted normal V_{O_2}max for the patient is derived from charts and expressed as the percent of predicted normal (% V_{O_2}max predicted).

Either progressive or steady-state exercise on cycle ergometer, while recording heart rate and minute ventilation, can be used to document the cardiac and respiratory responses to exercise with greater precision than the stair climbing test or supervised 6MWT.[9]

The exercise test measures the ability of the subject to perform work. Reichel[11] demonstrated that it was the only objective measurement of cardiopulmonary reserve that showed a statistically significant difference between groups of patients who had a benign postoperative course and groups who had cardiac or ventilatory complications.[12] The important measurements are the heart rate and respiratory rate during exercise and the recovery time. The arterial P_{O_2}, P_{CO_2}, O_2 percent saturation, and V_{O_2}max are objectively measured before and after exercise.

Value of measured V_{O_2}max:

1. Patients with a normal preoperative V_{O_2}max greater than 20 mL/kg/min are not at increased risk of complications or death and are acceptable for safe pulmonary resections.
2. Patients with a low preoperative V_{O_2}max less than 15 mL/kg/min are at an increased risk of complications and worrisome for pulmonary resections.
3. Patients with significant reduction in preoperative V_{O_2}max less than 10 mL/kg/min have an extremely high risk of postoperative complications with operative mortality rates of 40% to 50% and are considered unacceptable for pulmonary resection.

Preoperative V_{O_2}max % predicted is more sensitive than absolute V_{O_2}max.

1. V_{O_2}max % predicted greater than 75% indicates a low risk of complications.
2. V_{O_2}max % predicted less than 43% indicates a high risk of complications.
3. V_{O_2}max % predicted of 60% or more acceptable for lobectomy

Check that the arterial P_{O_2}, P_{CO_2}, O_2 percent saturation, and V_{O_2}max are also measured before and after exercise.

Regional Lung Function Studies

In an ideal pair of lungs all the alveoli would be supplied with equal amount of air of uniform gas composition during inspiration. Also, all the alveoli would be ideally supplied with the same flow of mixed venous blood. This condition would permit optimal gas exchange between the blood in pulmonary circulation and the air in the alveoli. The pulmonary distribution of ventilation and perfusion tends to be optimally matched for most of the lung tissue allowing for differences at the base compared with the apices; this means that the ratio of ventilation to blood flow, the ventilation/perfusion ratio (V/Q ratio), varies by a small amount throughout normal lungs. Spirometric tests may fail to accurately reflect pulmonary function because excision of destroyed lung with no function may not affect postoperative status (medical lobectomy) or may even correct preoperative hypoxemia (because resected lung may be the site of abnormal V/Q ratios).

Quantitative V/Q scanning calculates the percentage function of each lung; this is achieved by the inhalation of radioactive xenon (xenon 133) and the intravenous administration of technetium-labeled macroaggregates (technetium 99m macroaggregated albumin).[13–17] A gamma camera and computer calculate the uptake of radioactive ions by the lung or the perfusion of technetium. The percentage of radioactivity taken up by each lung correlates with the contribution of that lung to overall function.

Using the measured radioactive uptake of the lung that will not be operated on, the predicted FEV_1 of the residual lung after pneumonectomy or lobectomy can be calculated by the following simple equations:

- Postpneumonectomy pulmonary function:

Postop FEV_1 (L) = Preop FEV_1 (L) × % radioactivity of nonoperated lung

- Postlobectomy pulmonary function:

Expected loss of function = preop FEV_1 × % function of affected lung × number of segments in lobe to be resected ÷ total number of segments in whole lung

Radionuclide ventilation (xenon 133) and perfusion (technetium 99m macroaggregated albumin) studies gives 2 types of information:

1. *Qualitative:* analysis of patterns of regional V/Q relationship.
2. *Quantitative:* measurements of predicted postoperative values

Burrows and Earle[12] showed that when FEV_1 decreases less than 1.0 L, there is CO_2 retention and the mortality from COPD increases significantly (several investigators have combined spirometry and radionuclide studies to predict postoperative FEV_1 and reject resection if the predicted value is less than 0.8–1.0 L). Wirmly and DeMeester have shown that a postoperative FEV_1 greater than 1.0 L is associated with low surgical mortality and acceptable quality of life.[14]

The acceptable operative risk for pneumonectomy is when FEV_1 is measured at 2.0 L or more and for lobectomy when FEV_1 is measured to be 1.5 L or more. Pneumonectomy is physiologically considered to be a disease because it will remove the entire lung function (normal right lung function is 55% and left lung function is 45% of the total lung function measured on radionuclide scanning). It must be remembered that any lung cancer operation, lobectomy or pneumonectomy, must leave behind after pulmonary resection adequate lung function with FEV_1 of 0.8 L or greater for quality of life and to be able to cough effectively, which is the most important defense mechanism for the patient.[13–17]

The results of PFTs and radionuclide scintigraphy (V/Q ratio) before the operation and 1 month after the operation are correlated and provide reliable information about the functional capability of the subject.

Calculation of postoperative pulmonary function

1. Predicted postoperative pulmonary function after pneumonectomy: calculation from spirometry and radionuclide scan
   a. Preoperative FEV_1 (L) × % perfusion (Q) contralateral lung
2. Predicted postoperative pulmonary function after lobectomy:
   Postoperative FEV_1 (L) "ppo-FEV_1 (L)":
   a. Preoperative FEV_1 (L) × number of segments remaining after resection (19 − number of segments removed) ÷ total number of segments[18]
   b. Postoperative FEV_1 % (ppo- FEV_1%) = Preoperative FEV_1 % × number of segments remaining after resection (19 − number of segments removed) ÷ total number of segments[18]

Bronchospirometry

Bronchospirometry allows evaluation of one lung compared with the other by inserting a double-lumen tube in the tracheobronchial tree and measuring the O_2 consumption, CO_2 elimination, FVC, and its subdivisions. The test is now seldom used because it is unpleasant for the patient and requires skilled personnel. The same information is obtained from isotope studies.

Unilateral Pulmonary Artery Occlusion (±Bronchial Obstruction)

This test is valuable in older patients with a decreased pulmonary capillary bed who may develop postoperative pulmonary hypertension. However, it is now seldom used today. Combining insertions of double-lumen tube for single-lung ventilation of unaffected lung and Swan-Ganz catheter in the main pulmonary artery on the diseased side under fluoroscopy for split

Table 2
Preoperative evaluation of pulmonary function

Clinical: Function of Both Lungs	Low Risk	High Risk	Prohibitively High Risk
Dyspnea scale (0–4) *	0–1	2–3	3–4
Smoking	0	+	++
General condition, age, obesity, weight loss	1: age 75–80 y; no weight loss; normal BMI	2–3: age 80–85 y; moderate weight loss; not cachectic; high BMI	3–4: age >85 y; cachexia; significant weight loss; variable BMI
Stairs climbing	Return to normal	Maximum 5 min	<5 min
Spirometry			
Forced vital capacity	>3–4 L	2–3L	<1.85 L
FEV_1	>2–2.5 L	1.2–2.0 L	<1.2 L
FEV_1/FVC ratio	>70%	<70%	<50%
Diffusion capacity	> 80% low operative risk	< 80% associated with increased pulmonary complications	<60% poor lung function and increased mortality
MVV	>60%	50%–60%	<50%
Bronchodilation	Positive response with improvement	Minimal improvement	Unchanged
ABG			
Po_2 (mm Hg)	80–90	70–80	<70
Pco_2 (mm Hg)	35–40 Low operative risk	40–45 Arterial $Paco_2$ > 45 mm Hg does not seem to be an independent predictor of poor outcome but preoperative hypoxemia with low oxygen saturations < 90% and desaturation > 4% with exercise have all been associated with an increased risk of complications	>45
% O_2 saturation	95%–98%	85%–95%	<85%
Exercise tolerance (CPET)			
Po_2 (mm Hg)	80–90	<70	<50; limited capacity and cannot exercise
Pco_2 (mm Hg)	35–40	40–45	>45; limited capacity and cannot exercise
% O_2 saturation	>90%	85–90	<85%
Vo_2 maximum	>20 mL/kg/min	<15 mL/kg/min	<10 mL/kg/min
Regional lung function studies			
Predicted postoperative FEV_1	>1.0 L	0.8–1.0	<0.8 L
Pulmonary artery occlusion PA pressure (mm Hg)	<30	30–35	>35

(continued on next page)

Table 2 (continued)			
Clinical: Function of Both Lungs	**Low Risk**	**High Risk**	**Prohibitively High Risk**
Pulmonary resection	Resection up to pneumonectomy	Resection up to lobectomy or limited resection	Pulmonary resection not recommended; consider other options
EF calculated from 2D ECHO	Normal range for EF is 55% to 80% (mean 67%)	EF <55% indicates depressed myocardial contractility	EF <35% indicates high surgical risk

Abbreviations: ABG, arterial blood gases; BMI, body mass index; EF, ejection fraction.

lung function measurement used to be done as a split lung function test in high-risk patients. The parameters measured were oxygen saturation and cardiac output at different levels of fraction of inspired oxygen and pulmonary artery pressure over 30 minutes. The test helped in determining whether the patient could tolerate pneumonectomy.

Sloan and colleagues17 showed that an increase in pulmonary artery pressure (PA) pressure, an increase in arterio-venous oxygen difference (AV O_2) difference, or a failure to increase the cardiac output may indicate that the patient will not tolerate resection. PA mean pressure of 30 to 35 mm Hg during exercise is accepted as the upper limit of normal, and valuable information is today now easily obtained from 2D ECHO. Fixed pulmonary vascular resistance will result in unacceptable level of worsening pulmonary hypertension after pulmonary resection and consequent right-sided heart failure and cor pulmonale from increase in pulmonary blood flow to the remaining lung.

Lateral Position Test

The lateral position test (LPT) estimates the percent of ventilation of each lung when compared with the overall function. Marion and colleagues[19] have shown that the LPT seems to be a valid procedure for evaluating unilateral function. The advantages are that it is technically simple and well tolerated by patients.

2D ECHO

This noninvasive test is performed to evaluate heart function and pulmonary circulation, which is important in the planning of the extent of pulmonary resection for lung cancer.

The following are the measurements required:

1. Right and left ventricular function
2. Functional integrity of the heart valves
3. Pulmonary artery pressures
4. Intracardiac shunt through patent foramen ovale
5. Ejection fraction

The normal pulmonary arterial pressure is 25/8 mm Hg and the mean is approximately 15 mm Hg. If the mean pulmonary artery pressure is elevated more than 15 mm Hg, then pulmonary arterial hypertension is considered to be present and preoperative consultation with the cardiologist should be requested before undertaking pulmonary resection. In the presence of pulmonary arterial hypertension and high fixed pulmonary vascular resistance, pulmonary resection, if extensive, carries a risk for developing right-sided heart failure and cor pulmonale.

Normal reference ejection fraction is 50% to 75%

Less than 35% ejection fraction carries a high risk for sudden death during intrathoracic operation.

Prophylactic measures

The identification of pulmonary risk factors permits the institution of preventive measures to

1. Allow resection in the compromised patient
2. Decrease the postoperative complication rate in poor risk individuals
3. Insure acceptable quantity and quality of life following resection

Preoperative

Prophylactic measures include cessation of smoking for minimum of 4 to 6 weeks, maintenance of adequate nutrition, and bronchodilator and antibiotic therapy if necessary. The most important aspects of preoperative preparation are based on

Table 3
Clinical predictors of risk for lung surgery: cardiac and pulmonary risk factors in lung cancer surgery

Predictors	Examples
Major risk factors	
Major risk category	Increasing age >80 y
	Reduced functional capacity by CPET: MVO_2 <10 mL·kg·min
	Low FEV_1 <1.2 L
	Calculated ppo FEV_1 <0.8 L
	Low diffusion capacity (DLCO) at rest <25 mL·min·mm Hg (<75%); as low as 5 mL·min·mm Hg in pulmonary fibrosis
	mMRC dyspnea scale: 0–4
	3. Breathlessness, stops walking after ~100 m or a few minutes
	4. Breathless when dressing or not able to leave the house
	Type of elective operation
	Standard pneumonectomy
	Carinal pneumonectomy
	Tracheal carinal resection
	En bloc lung and chest wall resection
	En bloc SVC resection with pulmonary resection
	Continuous supplemental O_2
	Unstable coronary artery syndrome
	Low ejection fraction <35 (normal from 55% to 80%)
	Decompensated congestive heart failure
	Severe valvular aortic stenosis usual definition criteria:
	• Mean transvalvular gradient >40 mm Hg.
	• AVA <1 cm²
	• Peak aortic jet velocity >4.0 m/s
	Critical valvular aortic stenosis usual definition criteria:
	• High fixed cardiac output
	• Mean transvalvular gradient > 80 mm Hg.
	• AVA < 0.5 cm²
	Assessment of aortic stenosis severity should integrate the flow-gradient pattern to the classic measurement of AVA:
	NF/HG and AVA <1 cm²: benefit from AVR
	LF/ HG and AVA <1 cm² benefit from AVR
	Pulmonary arterial hypertension: mean PAP >24 mm Hg.
	BMI >30
	Low arterial blood gases Pao_2 <70 mm Hg
	Low oxygen saturation <70%
Intermediate risk factors	
Intermediate risk category	Chronic lung disease: panacinar emphysema, interstitial pulmonary fibrosis, pulmonary sarcoidosis, asbestosis, silicosis, recurrent pneumonia, fibrosing alveolitis
	Diffuse bronchiectasis
	Age 70–79 y
	Active cigarette smoker ≥1 ppd for 20 y
	Reduced functional capacity by CPET: MVO_2 <15 mL·kg·min
	FEV_1 1.2–1.5 L
	Ejection fraction <50
	BMI 25–29.9
	Significant cardiac arrhythmias: >5 PVCs documented before the operation, bundle branch block, uncontrolled atrial fibrillation
Minor risk factors	

(*continued on next page*)

Table 3 (continued)	
Predictors	**Examples**
Minor risk category	mMRC dyspnea scale: 0–4
	0. No breathlessness
	1. Breathless when hurrying or walking up a hill
	Age 60–69 y
	Ex-smoker
	Normal functional capacity MVO_2 >20 mL·kg·min
	FEV_1 >1.5 L for lobectomy
	FEV_1 >2.0 L for pneumonectomy
	BMI 18.5–24.9
	Ejection fraction >55% (55%–80%) and mean 67%
	Diffusion capacity (DLCO) at rest 25–30 mL·min·mm Hg. (>90%)
	Type of elective operation:
	Standard lobectomy
	Sleeve lobectomy
	Segmental resection
	Wedge resection
	Normal pulmonary artery pressure: 25/8 mm Hg and mean pulmonary arterial pressure 15 mm Hg

Abbreviations: AVA, aortic valve area; AVR, aortic valve replacement; BMI, body mass index; HG, high gradient; LF, low flow; mMRC, Modified Medical Research Council; NF, normal flow; ppo, postoperative; DLCO, diffusion capacity for carbon monoxide as gas transfer factor; PAP, pulmonary artery pressure; PVC, pulmonary vascular capacity.

chest physiotherapy and *teaching* of required respiratory maneuvers.

Intraoperative

Limited resections whenever possible (segmental resection, standard lobectomy, or lung preserving sleeve resection) are desirable.

Postoperative

Postoperative care is based on adequate chest physiotherapy and early ambulation, provision of supplemental oxygen, broad spectrum antibiotic coverage depending on bacteriologic culture and sensitivity result of sputum specimen, postural drainage, early mobilization and diagnosis, and treatment of pulmonary complications. Sustained inspiratory (yawn maneuver, incentive spirometry) and expiratory maneuvers are variably effective in preventing postoperative atelectasis. Late reeducation (3–20 weeks after operation) with controlled exercise program seems helpful in rehabilitation (**Table 2**).

Modified Medical Research Council dyspnea scale

The severity of breathlessness on exertion reported by modified Medical Research Council score was 0 (no breathlessness) in 33 (13%), 1 (breathless when hurrying or walking up a hill) in 88 (35%), 2 (breathless when walking slower than people of same age or has to stop when walking) in 75 (30%), 3 (breathlessness, stops walking after ~100 m or a few minutes) in 34

(13%), and 4 (breathless when dressing or not able to leave the house) in 23 (9%) of the patients[18] (**Table 3**).

SUMMARY

Lung cancer is the most common cause of cancer-related death worldwide among both men and women. Most patients with lung cancer have a history of chronic cigarette smoking, which often causes associated COPD and thereby compromises lung function and exercise capacity and increasing operative risk for pulmonary resection.[20–22]

Despite advances in radiation therapy and chemotherapy, surgical resection remains the choice of treatment of patients with resectable non–small cell cancer.[6,23,24] Only complete resection cures; incomplete resection does not cure.[25] Nevertheless, it is estimated that only 20% to 25% of patients, with stage I, stage II, and stage IIIa lung cancer undergo complete resection. Limited resection by segmentectomy has more favourable outcome than wedge resection, which has higher local recurrence rate and reduced survival.

REFERENCES

1. Mänttäri A, Suni J, Sievänen H, et al. Six-minute walk test: a tool for predicting maximal aerobic power (VO₂ Max) in healthy adults. Clin Physiol Funct Imaging 2018;38:1038–45.

2. Diament ML, Palmer KN. Spirometry for preoperative assessment of airways resistance. Lancet 1966;2:180.

3. Stein M, Cassara EL. Preoperative pulmonary evaluation, and therapy for surgery patients. JAMA 1970; 211:787.

4. West JB. Respiratory physiology - the essentials. In: Chapter 10. Tests of pulmonary functione. 7th edition; 2004. p. 153–67.

5. West JB. Pulmonary pathophysiology – the essentials. In: Part one – Chapters 1,2, and 3. 6th edition; 2003. p. 3–48.

6. Gaensler EA, Cugwell DW, et al. The role of pulmonary insufficiency in mortality and invalidism following surgery for pulmonary tuberculosis. J Thorac Surg 1955;29:163.

7. Boushy SF, Billig DM, et al. Clinical course related to preoperative and postoperative pulmonary function in patients with bronchogenic carcinoma. Chest 1971;59:383.

8. Gerson G. preoperative respiratory function tests and postoperative mortality. Br J Anaesth 1969;41:967.

9. Lockwood P. The principles of predicting the risk of post thoracotomy function related to complication of bronchial carcinoma. Respiration 1973;30:329.

10. Voduc N. Physiology and clinical applications of cardiopulmonary exercise testing in lung surgery. Thor Surg Clin 2013;23(2):233–45.

11. Reichel J. Assessment of operative risk of pneumonectomy. Chest 1972;62:570.

12. Burrows B, Earle RH. Course and prognosis of chronic obstructive lung disease – a prospective study of 200 patients. N Engl J Med 1969;280:397–404.

13. Olsen GN, Block AJ, et al. Prediction of post-pneumonectomy function using quantitative macro-aggregate lung scanning. Chest 1974;66:13.

14. Wirmly JA, DeMeester TR, et al. Clinical use of quantitative ventilation-perfusion lung scans in the surgical management of bronchogenic carcinoma. J Thorac Cardiovasc Surg 1980;80:535.

15. Boysen PG, Hains JO, Block AJ, et al. Prospective evaluation for pneumonectomy using perfusion scanning. Chest 1981;80:163.

16. Boysen PG, Block AJ, Olsen GN, et al. Prospective evaluation for pneumonectomy using the 99mTechnetium quantitative perfusion lung scan. Chest 1977;72:442.

17. Sloan H, Morris JD, et al. Temporary unilateral occlusion of the PA in the preoperative evaluation of thoracic patients. J Thorac Surg 1955;30:591.

18. Hsu KY, Lin JR, Lin MS, et al. The modified Medical Research Council dyspnoea scale is a good indicator of health-related quality of life in patients with chronic obstructive pulmonary disease. Singapore Med J 2013;54(6):321–7.

19. Marion JM, Alderson PO, Lefrak SS, et al. Unilateral lung function. Comparison of the lateral position test with radionuclide ventilation-perfusion studies. Chest 1976;69(1):5–9.

20. Burrows B, Kettel LJ, Niden AH, et al. Patterns of cardiovascular dysfunction in chronic obstructive lung disease. N Engl J Med 1972;286:912–8.

21. Bourke SJ, Burns GP. Respiratory medicine. In: Chapter 3; pulmonary function tests. 8th edition; 2011. p. 23–36.

22. Gould G, Pearce. Assessment of suitability for lung resection. Contin Educ Anaesth Crit Care Pain 2006;6(3):97–100.

23. DeMeester TR, Van Heertum RL, Karas JR, et al. Preoperative Evaluation with Differential Pulmonary Function. Ann Thorac Surg 1974;18(1):61–71.

24. Stein M, Kosta GM, et al. Pulmonary evaluation of surgical patients. JAMA 1962;181:103.

25. Armstrong P, Congleton J, Fountain SW, et al. Guidelines on the selection of patients with lung cancer for surgery. Thorax 2001;56:89–108.

Medical Audit to Improve the Quality of Patient Care in Thoracic Surgery

Farid M. Shamji, MBBS, FRCSC, FACS[a,*], Joel Cooper, MD, FRCSC, FACS[b],
Gilles Beauchamp, MD, FRCSC[c]

KEYWORDS

- Medical audit • Structure-process-outcome of audit • Template for medical data collection
- Adverse events • Historical legends • Thoracic diseases

KEY POINTS

- Historical pioneers and historical perspectives on surgical lessons.
- Current definitions and conduct of medical audit.
- Basis of the medical audit and quality of clinical care.
- Audit in Thoracic Surgery.
- Requirements and surgical guidance on the conduct of elective operation.
- Template for medical data collection.

INTRODUCTION OF MEDICAL AUDIT

The audit of medical practice is neither a new concept nor a new activity. All medical practitioners have examined the effects of their treatment and have assessed outcome for centuries. It became a formal process of observing and assessing the effects of treatment regimens as a major advancement in medical practice during the twentieth century. The need for a formal basis to audit first recognized in 1981 began linking medical care to the need for the cost-effective use of resources.[1]

The formal basis of audit required first to describe the philosophy of medical audit. From this evolved the second component of the audit, which was to establish the type of information required in different specialties. The third component was to outline the methods of audit activity. A coherent pattern for audit and acquisition of and storage of clinical data and medical information was the fourth component of the audit process.[2,3]

The medical audit must have a defined focus and a target to meet, that has as its most important mandate to enhance the standard of clinical care for the patients. This requires medical education of the quality that teaches the 4 most essential ingredients, which are hearing, listening, understanding, and communicating.

LESSONS IN AUDIT LEARNED FROM THE PAST TEACHERS

The concept of audit was first introduced in 1867 by Professor Joseph Lister, the British Surgeon, by his analysis of the therapeutic effects of phenol in compound fractures. He was a pioneer of antiseptic surgery, whose research into bacteriology and infection in wounds, raised his skillful operative technique and operative outcomes, to a new plane where his observations, deductions, and practices revolutionized surgery throughout the world. Lister promoted the idea of sterile surgery while working at the Glasgow Royal Infirmary. Lister successfully introduced carbolic acid (now

[a] University of Ottawa, General Campus, Ottawa Hospital, 501 Smyth Road, Ottawa, Ontario K1H 8L6, Canada;
[b] Hospital of the University of Pennsylvania, Ravdin 6, 3400 Spruce Street, Philadelphia, PA 19104, USA;
[c] Thoracic Surgery Unit, Department of Surgery, Maisonneuve-Rosemount Hospital, University of Montreal, 5415, L'Assomption Boulevard, Montreal, Quebec H1T 2M4, Canada
* Corresponding author.
E-mail address: faridshamji@hotmail.com

Thorac Surg Clin 31 (2021) 497–508
https://doi.org/10.1016/j.thorsurg.2021.07.001
1547-4127/21/© 2021 Published by Elsevier Inc.

known as phenol) to sterilize surgical instruments and to clean wounds. Statistics, now recognized to be important in medical audit, began as a science of births and deaths in 1833.[1,4]

Applying Professor Louis Pasteur's advances in microbiology, Lister championed the use of carbolic acid as an antiseptic, so that it became the first widely used antiseptic in surgery. He first suspected it would prove an adequate disinfectant because it was used to ease the stench from fields irrigated with sewage waste. Lister's work led to a decrease in postoperative infections and made surgery safer for patients, distinguishing him as the "father of modern surgery."[5–7]

HISTORICAL PIONEERS AND ADVANCES IN THE MEDICAL AUDIT IN THORACIC SURGERY: THE IMPORTANCE OF SURGICAL EDUCATION

Surgery is an art as well as a science, and it is timely to remind the young doctor that although he or she can cure sometimes, alleviate frequently, the young doctor must at times be compassionate and accept that the art of caring is difficult. In 1884, surgery was in its infancy and regarded as a hazardous undertaking. During the next 85 years, developments in all branches of medicine occurred at an ever-increasing rate.[8] Major contributions were made by 3 British Surgeons, namely, Professor John Hunter, Sir Astley Cooper, and Professor Joseph Lister, who educated young doctors on the necessity of acquiring knowledge in 3 important basic sciences: anatomy, physiology, and pathology.

The guidance on the practical application of the new beginning in the auditing process to the patient care evolved gradually later in the medical profession. Ever since the beginning, medical and patient-centered clinical audits have concentrated efforts to deliver consistently higher standards of care. The medical profession has done much to embrace medical audit as part of its regular responsibilities.

- Ernest Codman, originally from Harvard, was the first surgeon to advocate auditing of cases.[9] More than a century ago, Codman wrote, "We believe it is the duty of every hospital to establish a follow-up system, so that as far as possible the result of every case will be available at all times for investigations by members of the staff, the trustees, or administration, or by other authorized investigators or statisticians." Codman joined the surgical staff of Massachusetts General Hospital and became a member of the Harvard Faculty. While there, he instituted the first morbidity and mortality conferences the study of medical outcomes.[9–18] In 1910 Codman, helped to start the American College of Surgeons and he chaired its Committee for Hospital Standardization, which studied hospital outcomes (end results) and how they could be improved. Eventually the committee led to the creation of the Joint Commission. Codman was an advocate of hospital reform and is the acknowledged founder of what today is known as outcomes management in patient care.

The importance of surgical education, as a lifelong teaching and learning process, must be regularly enforced to improve understanding of its importance in the life and well-being of the patients.[19–24] It begins with a desire to learn and to progress and to improve and to avoid errors of omission and commission. Too often, the terms used in the medical profession are on morbidity and mortality, and now it is more about the "adverse events." It begins with an adequate knowledge in anatomy to which is knowledge of physiology. A thorough knowledge of human anatomy is the real groundwork of all surgical sciences.

- Sir Astley Cooper, the British Surgeon in 1841, stressed that "anatomy" likewise teaches us how to discriminate diseases in which lies more than one-half of the cure. A lack of anatomic knowledge is a reason for litigation against the medical and surgical practitioners. As well, "physiologic knowledge" is of the utmost importance in surgery—a knowledge of the healthy functions enables you to better understand the nature of diseased action.[25–30] Sir Astley Cooper insisted that to be a good judge of surgical cases is essential in the making of a good surgeon. Students must understand that the "study of medicine is important to the surgeon." Surgery is an art as well as a science. Surgery is an art of science, whereas an operation is only a technique. The learner must first learn the art of science. It is opportune time to revisit what the legends of the remote past believed to be true, taught the keen learners to impart their wisdom to them, and emphasize on learning more from experiments than from hypothesis.
- The famous Scottish surgeon Professor John Hunter, "the Master of Surgery and Research," stood, admired by the wise. John Hunter was a one of the most distinguished scientists and surgeons of his day. He was an early advocate of careful

observation and scientific method in medicine. He was a teacher of, and collaborator with, Edward Jenner, the pioneer of the smallpox vaccine. In 1753, John Hunter was elected a master of anatomy at Surgeon's Hall, responsible for reading lectures. In 1776 he was named surgeon extraordinary to King George III.

HISTORICAL PERSPECTIVES ON SURGICAL LESSONS TAUGHT BY THE LEGENDS: LESSONS TO REMEMBER IN THORACIC SURGICAL AUDIT

It is an opportune time to revisit what the legends of the remote past believed to be true, taught the keen learners to impart their wisdom to them, and emphasize on learning more from experiments than from hypothesis.

Surgery is an art as well as a science, whereas operation is only a technique. It will be the worst mistake for all trainees to concentrate on learning only the technical aspect of the operation. This culture of the art is the direct responsibility of a surgical teacher who must have good understanding on the art of teaching, on what to teach and how to teach and how to impart that teaching with words of wisdom in all aspects of teaching and learning. To respect surgery as an art of science is of immense value and to continuously acquire knowledge of the basic sciences is essential—learning anatomy, physiology, anatomic pathology, and chemical pathology and microbiology—will go into the making of a complete and competent surgeon and in surgical auditing.

Surgery is as old as man, and its evolution has been molded in every age by current technical and scientific advances, and not forgetting the its demands both an art and a science, whereas its practice largely depends on the human relations between doctor and patient. A knowledge of the development of surgery is of much significance in understanding its art and science as practiced today.

The British surgeon and anatomist Sir Astley Cooper highlighted the importance of surgical education in his 19th century Introductory Lecture, stressing that "operations cannot be safely undertaken by any man, unless he possesses a thorough knowledge of anatomy" and that "physiologic knowledge is of the utmost importance to the profession of surgery."[4] To prevent complications, he stated that "it is the duty of the surgeon never to advise an operation unless there is a probability that it will be attended with success."[4]

About Qualities of Surgeons

Guy de Chauliac stated in 1360 in his "Chirurgia Magna" on the "Qualities of Surgeons": "Let the surgeon be *bold* in all sure things, and *fearful* in dangerous things; let him *avoid* all faulty treatments and practices. He ought to be *gracious* to the sick, *considerate* to his associates, *cautious* in his prognostications. Let him be modest, dignified, pitiful, and merciful, not covetous nor extortionist of money; but rather let his reward be according to his work, to the means of the patient, to the quality of issue, and to his own dignity."

The important qualities of surgeons described by Guy de Chauliac have been summarized as follows to help the learner of surgery:

A good surgeon knows how to operate.

A better surgeon knows when to operate.

The best surgeon knows when not to operate.

As Professor Edward Churchill, former professor of surgery at Harvard, once said, "Surgery is not a single applied science; it is the application of many sciences to the management of disease and injury. Of these sciences, none outranks pathology in importance."

The 3 renowned pathologists who exemplified this philosophy and always to be remembered Giovanni Battista Morgagni (1682–1771), who was an Italian Anatomist, in the mid-eighteenth century directed attention to diseased organs. Marie Francois Xavier Bichat (1771–1802), who was a French anatomist and pathologist, in the early nineteenth century was concerned with diseased tissues. Rudolf Ludwig Carl Virchow (1821–1902) later led the development of cellular pathology. He was a German physician, anthropologist, and pathologist.

CURRENT DEFINITIONS AND THE CONDUCT OF MEDICAL AUDIT

The audit in thoracic surgery must be thoughtful and follow specific requirements. These requirements are in the recording of case histories and findings on physical examination for clinical decision in the planning of treatment. The selection of special investigations to support clinical diagnosis is considered essential. The preoperative management must consider patient-related risk factors, the disease-related factors, and the treatment-related factors. The recording of the operation, intraoperative adverse events, postoperative management, and complications is essential. The course of the postoperative care must be with diligent documentation of all happenstances. All the documentation should be on prepared templates and to be used in the audit for a formal discussion within the division.[18,31–39]

The audit processes that are recognized in 3 definitions are the medical audit, clinical audit, and patient care audit.

1. The medical audit defined as the review of the clinical care of patients provided by the medical staff only. It ignores the effects of resources on the review process.
2. The clinical audit is the review of the activity of all aspects of the clinical care of patients by the medical and paramedical staff. It ignores the effects of resources on the review process.
3. The patient care audit maintains the vital link between clinical practice and resource management. This requires the audit by medical profession to consider the effects of resource changes on their clinical practice. The patient care audit is defined as a review of all activity within the health service that has a direct effect on patient care.

By proper teaching and education and making progress, the absolute requirement from the surgical and medical leadership is for complete medical and surgical data collection on every patient. The information collected on adverse events must be subjected for critical review for productive discussion and corrective action. The data resources include patient chart, incident reporting, electronic databases, interviews of clinical staff and examination of patients. Unfortunately, this is all subjective and not objective that would permit measurements. The 4 essential ingredients of the audit to be kept in the forefront of the mind in the audit process are hearing, listening, understanding, and communicating.

It must be kept in mind that an adverse event is harmful, and its occurrence has detrimental effects on both patients and families and health care workers including physical and/or psychological harm and suffering, a loss of trust in the health care system, reduced staff morale, and the possible legal consequences of making errors and litigation against the responsible medical profession and the hospital.

The absolute requirement to be honored by the responsible clinician is the complete well-being of the patient, who has come as a quest in the hospital expecting to be treated with respect and by competency in the medical profession. Clinicians are expected to provide an efficient and cost-effective service.

THE BASIS OF THE MEDICAL AUDIT

For the medical audit to be successful and meet its defined mandate, there has to a clear understanding of the structure of the audit, the process of the audit, and the outcome of the audit in various specialties. In so doing, the reasons for the audit to be conducted, the defined objectives of the audit, requirement of the audit, and educated active participation of the interested clinicians and hospital administration staff become important.[2]

The success of the audit is related to the attention given to 3 important components of the audit. These are:

1. The structure that takes into the consideration the resources within the hospital for staff hospital facilities, in-patient beds, equipment, technology, operating rooms, laboratories, human resources, and allocation of financial resources for optimal functioning.
2. The process takes into the consideration the efficiency in the medical treatment of patients by timely diagnosis and appropriateness of medical care with focus on proper utilization of resources.
3. The output (outcome) is global effect of the process on the patients, the treating clinicians, the patient advocacy group, the community, individual patients, and the legal counseling. The expectations of the patient have to be considered and appropriately addressed. An intrinsic part of audit in medical practice is the ability to measure outcome. This part is difficult, because most outcome measures are subjective, such as patient satisfaction and quality of care. Objective outcome measures are difficult to define, except death rates, revision of rates for major hip replacement surgery, and rate of nonunion fractures. There is the expectation of maintaining an acceptable standard of medical care, which requires achieving an excellent or good result with a minimum of complications for each individual patient. It is necessary to accept a degree of subjectivity in assessing outcomes and accept that statistical methods cannot be applied with any degree of accuracy to compare one unit's outcome with another.

Understanding the terminology used in the audit (from *The Webster's Third New International Dictionary*)

- Audit: This is defined as a hearing; a methodical examination and review of a situation or condition concluding with a detailed report of findings; a judicial examination (as in court); an official examination of accounts. The emphasis is on critical evaluation.

- Auditor: This refers to a person who hears or listens and learns by aural instruction and listens intently; one that audits a course of study in a college or university.
- Quality assurance: This is the quality of a person, taking into consideration character, capacity, and skills reflecting on the grading of excellence; something that inspires confidence; the quality or state of being sure or safe.
- Assurance: This reflects on commitment to improving in all important matters; is a guarantee or pledge of safety or peace; tends to inspire confidence.

The audit has been defined as a "systematic appraisal of implementation and outcome of any process in the context of prescribed targets and standards. Clinical audit is a process by which medical staff collectively review, evaluate and improve their practice." Although deaths and complications traditionally have been considered, the quality of life after surgery and the degree of patient satisfaction should also be assessed as far as possible.

Medical Audit and Quality of Clinical Care

A medical audit is defined as a systematic critical analysis of the quality of medical care, including the procedures used for diagnosis and treatment, the use of resources and the resulting outcome for patients.

Hospital-based Care

This definition of medical audit has become widely accepted in hospital-based care. Consideration of resources is not and should never be the prime purpose of audit; however, it is inevitable that the resources should be considered if optimum care is to be given to a population within the resources that will always be finite. Doctors working in a publicly funded health service that attempts to provide comprehensive and equitable care to the population it serves have a duty to provide the highest possible standard of care within the available resources.

The requirements for medical audit, determined by the hospital by-laws, are as follows.

- Every consultant should participate in a form of medical audit agreed between the hospital administration and the profession locally.
- The audit should be conducted by the local medical audit advisory committee chaired by a senior clinician.
- The hospital administration should be responsible for ensuring that an effective system of

medical audit is in place and that the clinical work of each medical team is reviewed at predetermined regular intervals.

- Peer review findings in individual cases should be confidential.
- The hospital management should be able to initiate an independent professional audit when there is a cause to question the quality or cost effectiveness of a service.
- Local activity and central support with coordination:
    A medical audit must be done primarily at a local level. This is where data are collected, and where most doctors will compare their performance in terms of process and outcome with that of their immediate peers. There should exist a proper quality assurance programs for clinical performance. The reports of the audit committee should not identify individual patients or doctors.
- Audit, continuing education, and research:
    An audit of clinical practice is not a new idea; audit, integrity, and service to patients are the bedrock of the Western medical ethics. Now that more formalized audit has been introduced into clinical practice, it allows systematic review of the clinical work for ongoing improvement to achieve uniform, high-quality, clinical care. The audit is a responsible reaction by the medical profession. Audits and quality assurance endeavor to improve good practice equitably to the care of each patient.

Audit in Thoracic in Surgery

For a medical audit in thoracic surgery to be effective it must be carried out in an atmosphere of mutual trust and respect, if it is to achieve its primary aim of improving, through self-education or peer group education, the quality of clinical care provided by thoracic surgeons. Doctors are likely to be most frank in their discussions of patient management if those discussions are kept completely confidential.

Thoracic nurses, physiotherapists, radiologists, pharmacists, and social workers all have a legitimate interest in how patients are treated, and should, where appropriate, be involved in interdisciplinary clinical audit. It should not underestimate the difficulties of having a frank and constructive discussion about the way patients are treated, when the outcome, including death or major disability, is being considered.

The audit cycle

Audit is a biofeedback mechanism.[2] Standards and clinical guidelines are set, practice observed, variation of practice from standard assessed and then action taken to improve the clinical practice or to alter the standards if they prove incorrect in use.

Stage one of an audit is to set and write the standard of practice by reviewing the relevant medical research literature, by consensus among colleagues, or by formal consensus conferences.

Stage two of n audit is applying the standard to everyday clinical activity and measuring how practice varies from the standard.

Stage 3 of an audit is closing the audit loop—feedback. Direct feedback, particularly of adverse comments, has to be achieved confidentially if it is to be helpful and constructive. The aim of the audit is to improve the clinical care of patients and clinical practices.

Information needs of audit

It is now a prerequisite that a minimum dataset must be collected for each patient to meet the standard of properly conducted audit.

A thoracic surgical audit must have regular review of the surgical results to find out the outcome in the thoracic surgical unit both in achievement and shortcomings. It is meant to be undertaken with the objective of using all the information necessary to achieve higher levels of practice. Once collected, the data will be subject to meaningful analysis and the results reviewed regularly by the thoracic surgical team. As a result of this review, recommendations for improvement will need to be implemented and recorded.

1. Demographic data analysis
   The computer software should be designed for data entry so that it is possible to retrieve the stored facts on any patient through a variety of "index" fields. These will include the following items:
   a. Patient hospital registration number
   b. Admission date
   c. Discharge date
   d. Date of birth
   e. Admitting diagnosis
   f. Comorbid illnesses
   g. Admitting diagnosis
   h. Type of operation performed
   i. Postoperative complications
   j. Duration of hospital stay
   k. Number of days in the intensive care unit
   l. Cause and date of death
2. The operation performed
   a. The responsible surgeon

   b. The anesthetist
   c. The type of operation
   d. Complication during administration of anesthesia
   e. Duration of the operating time
   f. Intraoperative complications: hypotension, hypoxemia, cardiac arrhythmias, myocardial infarction, significant bleeding, and organ or tissue injury
   g. Need for blood transfusion
   h. Prophylaxis for venous thrombosis
   i. Prophylactic antibiotic coverage
3. Data collection

The thoracic surgical audit will collect the relevant clinical data on daily basis from the surgery residents, nursing, and from the patient's clinical notes and entered directly into a computer. It is the outcome measures, which will include morbidity, mortality, complication rates, and patient satisfaction, that are clearly the most useful in determining whether the clinical care has been adequate. The information will be collected and discussed on a monthly basis. This will include postoperative complications categorized according to the Clavien-Dindo Morbidity Classification order to rank a complication in an objective and reproducible manner.[24] The therapy used to correct a specific complication is the basis of this classification to rank a complication in an objective and reproducible manner. It consists of 5 grades (I, II, III, III, IV, and V).

Clavien–Dindo Morbidity Classification

Grade I: Any deviation from the normal postoperative course without the need for pharmacologic treatment or surgical, endoscopic, and radiologic interventions.

Grade II: Requiring pharmacologic treatment with drugs, blood transfusion, and total parenteral nutrition.

Grade III: Requiring surgical, endoscopic, or radiologic intervention.

Grade IV: Life-threatening complication including central nervous system complications requiring management in the intensive care unit.

Grade V: Death of a patient.

Audit cycle and audit meetings

To fulfill all the criteria needed for presentation at the audit meeting, accuracy in data collection is essential. The audit cycle describes the process by which the audit is supposed to improve clinical care. Surgical practice is to be monitored first by diligently collecting the data. The next stage is to analyze the data and compare the results with a standard to define areas that need further attention. When these have been defined, recommendations are made that are designed to implement changes and improve clinical practice. A regular audit will provide a good means of monitoring set standards and prevent the level of care from decreasing.

An essential feature of the thoracic surgical audit will be the regular review and discussion of the results under strict confidentiality with the relevant peer group within the hospital. It will be at these meetings that the results achieved will be compared with the standards that are available.

Responsibility of the thoracic surgery program

Thoracic surgery program is required to have a mandate to provide excellence in clinical care for the patients afflicted with the following diseases and clinical problems:

1. Thoracic oncology: For lung cancers, esophageal cancers, mediastinal tumors, chest wall sarcomas, malignant mesotheliomas, lymphoma, and secondary lung cancers.
2. Chest injuries: For both immediately life-threatening and relatively life-threatening conditions.
3. Benign esophageal disorders: These disorders are common and require management of gastroesophageal reflux disorders, giant hiatus hernias, potentially life-threatening esophageal perforations, eosinophilic esophagitis, and non–life-threatening esophageal motility disorders.
4. Proximal airway diseases: These diseases are uncommon and complex, and demand excellence in diagnosis and surgical management for including idiopathic tracheal stenosis, tracheal tumors, and complications of tracheostomy.
5. Infections in the mediastinum: Mediastinal infections in the form of descending necrotizing mediastinitis from oropharyngeal infections, which is life-threatening. Mortality without surgical intervention is 100% and requires urgent operation to save the patient's life. Suppurative necrotizing mediastinitis is a manifestation of esophageal perforation and demands urgent surgical intervention to prevent sepsis syndrome, septic pericarditis, and empyema.
6. Infections in the pleural space: Pleural space infections in the form of acute empyema, which occurs in a variety of clinical settings, include percutaneous drainage of a pleural effusion, pneumothorax, all types of chest operations, esophageal perforation, open heart surgery, pneumonia, extension of subphrenic abscess, and bronchopleural fistula complicating pulmonary resection and necrotizing pneumonia. Delayed treatment or a lack of proper treatment results in chronic empyema and fibrothorax.
7. Pleural and pulmonary complications of tuberculosis: These complications include aspergilloma in a tuberculous cavity, bronchiectasis, destroyed lung from bronchostenosis and superimposed chronic infection, tuberculous empyema, and calcific fibrothorax.
8. Life-threatening massive hemoptysis is frequently due to inflammatory lung disease, such as bronchiectasis, lung abscess, aspergilloma, necrotizing pneumonia, and tuberculosis.
9. Pulmonary and mediastinal complications of the fungal infections of the lung can be due to histoplasmosis, blastomycosis, coccidioidomycosis, mucormycosis and, aspergillosis.

The responsibility must reflect in the process of auditing beginning with a desire for a change in the clinical care and defining the terms of a mandate, fiscal and clinical responsibility, and accountability.

Surgical audit governed by clinical information and data

The surgical audit has been defined as the "systematic critical analysis of the quality of surgical care," including the procedures used for diagnosis and treatment, the use of resources and the resulting outcome for patients. Once this is carried out, it is a tool with which levels of care can be both maintained and improved. Central to the process of auditing is the necessity of obtaining reliable clinical information and data.

The logical process of data collection requires templates that must be prepared for data collection to ensure uniformity in gathering important and precise clinical information without ambiguity for the clinical care and for a thoracic surgical audit. To achieve not only success in the audit, but importantly to make it a tool for enhancing education and learning for improving patient care, demands precision in obtaining clinical information from the patient and family members, the results of the investigations performed, the diagnosis, preoperative risk assessment, and finally the decision for treatment.

REQUIREMENTS AND SURGICAL GUIDANCE ON THE CONDUCT OF AN ELECTIVE OPERATION

Preoperative Care: Clinical Information and Data Collection for Audit of Preoperative Health and Diagnosis

The clinician must ask himself or herself the following questions before every operation, which must only be performed once each question has been answered satisfactorily.

A. Has the diagnosis been firmly established?
  1. With modern techniques, this can be done in the vast majority of cases.
  2. Occasionally an exploratory operation is necessary if the possibility of serious disease cannot be confidentially ruled out, but this must be an exception.
B. Is an operation necessary?
  1. Operations have certain indications that must be present before an operation is justified.
  2. An operation is potentially dangerous and is only indicated if the risks of the disease are greater than the risks of the operation. For this one must know:
    a. Natural history of the disease
    b. Risk of the operation
  3. Would you have the operation if you were in the patient's position? If in doubt:
    a. Seek a second opinion or
    b. Reevaluate the case later
  4. It is not justifiable to perform an operation merely on the possibility that it may be necessary; there must be a reasonable probability, or preferably a certainty that it is required.
C. Is the patient fit for the operation and anesthetic? If not, make him fit and make use of appropriate investigations according to the system review for functional assessment.
  1. Age
    a. Advanced age is not an absolute contraindication to operation by itself; a patient's physical and physiologic health are more important.
    b. Advancing age does increase the risk of an operation.
    c. Be more selective after 70 years and careful after 80 years.
  2. Cardiac function
  3. Pulmonary function
  4. Renal function
  5. Liver function
  6. Laboratory tests
    Hemoglobin level
    Serum electrolytes
    Coagulogram
  7. Medications
  8. Results of investigations
    a. Computed tomography scan of the chest and abdomen
    b. MRI of the head
    c. PET scan
    d. Pulmonary function test
    e. Arterial blood gas analysis
    f. Two-dimensional echocardiogram
    g. Cardiopulmonary exercise testing
    h. Esophagogastroscopy
    i. Endobronchial ultrasound lymph node biopsy
    j. Staging cervical mediastinoscopy and/or left anterior mediastinotomy
    k. Video thoracoscopy
    l. Nuclear cardiac stress test
    m. Radionuclide V/Q lung scan
D. When is the best time for the operation?
  1. In general, if an operation is well indicated, it should be done without undue delay.
  2. Reasons for postponing an operation.
    a. To improve the patient's state of fitness – operate as soon as maximal improvement has taken place .
    b. To allow inflammatory reaction to subside and so make operation easier – operate when maximal improvement has taken place .
    c. The benefits of delay must be judged against the possible harm of progression of the disease – careful judgment and possible compromise required to balance out these 2 factors .
E. Who should perform the operation?
  1. Someone with the adequate training to perform the operation competently.
  2. In emergencies, this may have to be compromised.
F. Postoperative care: Data collection for audit of adverse postoperative events
    The process of thoracic surgical audit to be structured according to the:
  1. Collection of clinical and surgical data
  2. Coding and validation
  3. Audit cycle
  4. Data analysis
  5. Review of results
  6. Recommendations for implementing changes
  7. Comparative audit by comparisons with other centers
  8. Confidential enquiry into adverse events

Once collected, the data will be subject to meaningful and proper analysis and the results reviewed on a regular basis by the thoracic surgical team without bias. As a result of this review, recommendations for improvement will be made and recorded. These will be reviewed again, later in time, to ensure that these have been implemented.

G. Early recognition and prompt treatment of postoperative complications

1. Careful clinical examination of the patient at least once per day.
2. Fever: Temperature chart should be examined daily.
   a. Elevated temperature during the first 72 hours not above 101 °F (38 °C), probably owing to inflammatory response to the operation.
   b. Elevated temperature outside this range must be investigated.
      Think of 4 Ws: wind (lungs), water (urosepsis), wound, work (legs).
      i. With early onset of fever on first, second, or third postoperative day suspect atelectasis.
      ii. Intermediate (about third day to fifth postoperative days) is probably due to a surgical wound infection or urosepsis.
      iii. Late (about ninth postoperative day) is probably due to venous thrombosis.
   c. If these causes are excluded, further investigations are needed to elucidate the cause of the elevated temperature.
3. Pulmonary atelectasis
   a. Diagnosis made from
      i. Abnormal pyrexia.
      ii. Thick viscid yellowish sputum.
      iii. Impaired aeration of portion of a lung, usually the posterior basal segment.
      iv. Minimal radiologic signs unless atelectasis is extensive.
   b. Vigorous treatment is always successful.
      i. Postural drainage.
      ii. Inhalations.
      iii. Breathing exercises.
      iv. Induced coughing.
      v. Ambulation.
      vi. Bronchoscopy only if there is massive atelectasis, which does not quickly aerate on treatment above.
      vii. Antibiotics usually not necessary unless sputum cultures reveal infection.
4. Deep vein thrombosis
   a. Diagnosis must be made early before pulmonary embolism occurs.
      i. Consider all risk factors and precautions taken in the early stage when symptoms and signs are minimal, and diagnosis is only made if it is deliberately looked for localized calf tenderness, minimal ankle edema; gross symptoms and signs only found at a later stage owing to proximal extension of venous thrombosis to involve iliofemoral veins.
      ii. Venous Doppler studies
      iii. Computed tomography scan/pulmonary embolism protocol if pulmonary a embolism suspected from clinical assessment: hypoxia, tachyarrhythmias, hypotension, and dyspnea.
      iv. At this early stage before a pulmonary embolism develops, symptoms and signs in the legs are minimal, and diagnosis only made if it is deliberately looked for. A clinical diagnosis of a deep vein thrombosis is made on tthe basis of: treatment should be immediate requiring intravenous anticoagulation with heparin.
5. Fluid and electrolyte imbalance
   Early recognition and management require:
      i. Careful evaluation of daily intake and output chart.
      ii. Careful clinical examination.
      iii. Serum electrolyte estimations must be interpreted with caution.
6. Wound infection
   a. First evidence usually an abnormal pyrexia starting about the fifth postoperative day.
   b. Confirmation requires
      i. No other cause of postoperative fever.
      ii. Wound inspection is abnormal for pain in the incision, swelling, tenderness, redness from cellulitis, and drainage of offensive smelling fluid.
      iii. Diligently search for the 5 cardinal signs of acute inflammation from wound sepsis.
   c. Early and aggressive management is necessary to decrease morbidity: establish urgent drainage by reopening the incision, wound debridement, and obtain wound culture, intravenous antibiotic, and establish negative pressure wound treatment.
7. Cardiac complications
   a. Myocardial infarction: Precordial chest pain, dyspnea, hypotension, cardiac arrhythmias, congestive heart failure, elevated serum troponin level, and an

abnormal electrocardiogram; consider anticoagulation.

b. Cardiac arrhythmias: Frequently atrial fibrillation needs immediate treatment.

c. Appropriate treatment and consult cardiology.

8. Urinary retention
   i. Early diagnosis is essential from the intake and output chart.
   ii. Urinary retention with overflow may be missed and should be looked for.
   iii. Urinary bladder catheterization to differentiate between retention and anuria.
   iv. If it is urinary retention or it recurs, then reinsert the catheter and consult urology.

9. Constipation and fecal impaction
   a. Readily recognized.
   b. Treat by following the standard constipation protocol and saline enemas.

10. Sudden postoperative collapse may be due to
   a. Complications of the operation:
      i. Hemorrhage.
      ii. Infection–septicemia and sepsis syndrome with septic shock.
      iii. Massive pulmonary embolism.
      iv. Acute coronary thrombosis.
      v. Metabolic disturbances, such as hypocalcemia, hypokalemia, and hypoglycemia.
   b. Cerebrovascular accident.

11. Complications of esophagectomy
   a. Cardiac arrhythmias
   b. Respiratory failure
   c. Pneumonia and pulmonary aspiration
   d. Anastomotic leak and empyema
   e. Necrosis of interposed conduit
   f. Chylothorax
   g. Recurrent laryngeal nerve palsy
   h. Venous thrombosis and pulmonary thromboembolism
   i. Empyema
   j. Tracheobronchial injury
   k. Mediastinitis and pericarditis with pericardial effusion
   l. incomplete resection of cancer and positive resection margins

12. Complications of pneumonectomy
   a. Respiratory failure
   b. Bleeding
   c. Recurrent nerve palsy
   d. Esophagopleural fistula
   e. Empyema
   f. Bronchopleural fistula and empyema
   g. Postpneumonectomy syndrome
   h. Cardiac herniation
   i. Postpneumonectomy pulmonary edema
   j. Refractory hypoxemia
   k. Venous thrombosis and pulmonary embolism
   l. Chylothorax

13. Complications of lobectomy
   a. Prolonged air leak
   b. Empyema
   c. Cardiac arrhythmias
   d. Deep vein thrombosis and pulmonary embolism
   e. Bronchopleural fistula and empyema
   f. Respiratory failure

14. Complications of mediastinoscopy
   a. Hemorrhage from injury to azygous vein, right main pulmonary artery, bronchial artery, superior vena cava, pulmonary vein, and roof of left atrium
   b. Left recurrent laryngeal nerve injury
   c. Esophageal injury and necrotizing mediastinitis
   d. Bronchial injury and bronchomediastinal fistula
   e. Pneumothorax

15. Abdomen compartment syndrome
   Abdomen compartment syndrome is a serious complication of surgery in the abdomen and prompt clinical recognition is necessary and diagnosis confirmed by measurement of pressure in the urinary bladder. If not quickly rectified, then the intestinal viability is threatened by ischemia.

SUMMARY

The purpose and conduct of medical audit, from educational perspective, is a means of quality control for medical practice by which the profession shall regulate its activities with the intention of improving overall patient care. The quality assurance depends on patient satisfaction, as well as the doctors. The medical profession needs to be educated about the structure, the process, and the outcome of an audit. The structure equates to resources found within the hospital. The outcome, which concerns the patient, not only the patient's outcome from surgery, but also the surgeon's expectation, the patient's expectation, the community's expectation through community health councils and any legal means. The outcome is when quality of care becomes preeminent. The requirements for medical audit, determined by the hospital bylaws, are that:

- Every consultant should participate in a form of medical audit agreed between the hospital administration and the profession locally.
- The audit should be conducted by the local medical audit advisory committee chaired by a senior clinician.
- The hospital administration should be responsible for ensuring that an effective system of medical audit is in place and that the clinical work of each medical team is reviewed at pre-determined regular intervals.
- Peer review findings in individual cases should be confidential.
- The hospital management should be able to initiate an independent professional audit when there is a cause to question about the quality or cost effectiveness of a service.

CLINICS CARE POINTS

- Historical pioneers in medicine and surgery.
- The importance of surgical education as a life-long teaching and learning process.
- Current definitions and conduct of the medical audit.
- Historical perspectives on surgical education taught by the legends.
- The current definitions and basis of the medical audit.
- Audit in Thoracic in Surgery.
- Clavien-Dindo Morbidity Classification.

REFERENCES

1. Burdett HC. The relative mortality, after amputations, of large and small hospitals and the influence of the antiseptic (listerian) system upon mortality. J Stat Soc 1882;45:444–83.
2. Frostick SP, Radford PJ, Angus Wallace W. Medical Audit Rationale, and practicalities. Cambridge University Press, 1993.
3. Pollock A, Evans M. Surgical audit. London: Butterworths; 1989.
4. Hey Groves EW. Surgical statistics: a plea for a uniform registration of operation and results. Br Med J 1908;2:1008–9.
5. Lister J. An address on the antiseptic system of treatment in surgery. Br Med J 1868;2(394):53–6.
6. Lister J. On the antiseptic principle in the practice of surgery. Lancet 1867;90(2299):353–6.
7. Lister J. On the effects of the antiseptic system of treatment upon the salubrity of a surgical hospital. Lancet 1870;95(2418):2–4.
8. Roberts FH. Joseph Bell – the origins of paediatric surgery in Edinburgh. J R Coll Surg Edinb 1969;14:304–7.
9. Berwick DM. E. A. Codman and the rhetoric of battle: a commentary. Milbank Q 1989;67(2):262–7.
10. Codman EA. Committee for Standardization of Hospitals [of the American College of Surgeons]. Minimum standard for hospitals. Bull Am Coll Surg 1924;8:4.
11. Codman EA. A study in hospital efficiency. As demonstrated by the case report of the first five years of a private hospital. Boston: Thomas Todd Co.; 1918-1920.
12. Codman EA. Bone sarcoma: an interpretation of the nomenclature used by the Committee on the Registry of Bone Sarcoma of the American College of Surgeons. New York: Paul B. Hoeber, Inc.; 1925.
13. Codman EA. The shoulder: rupture of the supraspinatus tendon and other lesions in or about the subacromial bursa. Boston: Thomas Todd Co.; 1934.
14. Donabedian A. "The end results of health care: Ernest Codman's contribution to quality assessment and beyond. Milbank Q 1989;67(2):233–56. Mallon, Bill.
15. Mallon B. Ernest Amory Codman: the end result of a life in medicine. Philadelphia: W. B. Saunders (Elsevier); 1999.
16. Neuhauser D. Ernest Amory Codman, M.D., and end results of medical care. Int J Tech Assess Health Care 1990;6:307–25.
17. Reverby S. Stealing the golden eggs: Ernest Amory Codman and the science and management of medicine. Bull Hist Med 1981;55:156–71.
18. Ernest Amory Codman, 1869-1940. N Engl J Med 1941;224:296–9.
19. Allison PR, Leslie J, Temple. The future of thoracic surgery. Thorax 1966;21:99–103.
20. Henry Ellis F. Education of thoracic surgeon. Thorax 1980;35:405–14.
21. Cox M, Irby DM. Educational strategies to promote clinical reasoning. N Engl J Med 2006;355(21):2217–25.
22. Alexander J. The training of a surgeon who expects to specialize in Thoracic Surgery. AATS; 1936. p. 579–82.
23. W Halstead. The training of the surgeon. Bulletin of John Hopkins Hospital Vol XV 1904; 162:267-276.
24. Murray GM. "Though medicine can be learned, it cannot be taught"—the first 100 years: Flexneran competency 2010. Ann Thorac Surg 2010;90:1–10.
25. Gupta A, Gupta R, Singal R, et al. Sir Astley Paston Cooper: life and work on anatomy, science and surgery. Acta Chir Belg 2011;111(1):51–4.
26. Hutchison RL, Rayan GM. Astley Cooper: his life and surgical contributions. J Hand Surg Am 2011;36(2):316–20.

27. Doganay E. Sir Astley Paston Cooper (1768-1841): the man and his personality. J Med Biogr 2015; 23(4):209–16.

28. Schoenberg DG, Schoenberg BS. Eponym: Sir Astley Paston Cooper: good sense, good surgery, and good science. South Med J 1979;72(9):1193–4.

29. Ellis H. Sir Astley Cooper: pioneering surgeon, anatomist, and teacher. Br J Hosp Med (Lond) 2018; 79(8):474.

30. de Chauliac, G. Chirurgia magna. (1363).

31. Dindo D, Demartines N, Clavien PA. Classification of surgical complications: a new proposal with evaluation in a cohort of 6336 patients and results of a survey. Ann Surg 2004;240(2):205–13.

32. du Plessis DJ. Principles of surgery. Bristol: John Wright & Sons LTD; 1976.

33. Cohen IB. Foreword", in the Dover edition (1957) of: Bernard, Claude, an introduction to the study of experimental medicine. Introduction to the study of experimental medicine (originally published in 1865; first English translation by Henry Copley Greene). Macmillan & Co., Ltd.; 1927.

34. Olmsted JM, Harris E. Claude Bernard and the experimental method in medicine. New York: Henry Schuman; 1952.

35. Cannon WB. Bodily changes in pain, hunger, fear and rage. New York: D. Appleton & Company; 1915.

36. Cannon WB. The way of an investigator: a scientist's experiences in medical research. New York: W. W. Norton; 1945. p. 130–45.

37. Cannon WB. The role of emotions in disease. Ann Intern Med 1936;9:1453–65.

38. Brieger GH. The development of surgery. Historical aspects important in the origin and development of modern surgical practice. 12th edition. Davis-Christopher Textbook of Surgery; 1981. p. 1–22.

39. Sabiston DC, JR. Milestones in surgery. Essentials of surgery. 1st Edition. Philadelphia: W.B. Saunders Company, Elsevier; 1987: 1-9.

Anesthetic Management for Pulmonary Resection
Current Concepts and Improving Safety of Anesthesia

Daniel Ankeny, MD, PhD, Hovig Chitilian, MD*, Xiaodong Bao, MD, PhD

KEYWORDS

- Thoracic anesthesia • Lung resection • Thoracic ERAS • Non-intubated VATS • Anesthesia safety

KEY POINTS

- Perioperative management of the pulmonary resection candidate is evolving to incorporate prehabilitation as well as enhanced recovery after surgery (ERAS) pathways to facilitate recovery.
- With a shift toward less invasive surgical procedures, the avoidance of general anesthesia through approaches incorporating regional anesthesia and spontaneous ventilation are being explored.
- ERAS protocols to improve patient recovery and minimize hospital length of stay are being developed and adopted more broadly.

INTRODUCTION

Lung resection surgery presents a unique set of challenges for anesthesiologists. Significant advances in surgical techniques have dramatically increased the scope and complexity of the patients presenting for surgery. This article provides an evidence-based update on anesthetic care for these patients.

PREANESTHETIC EVALUATION AND OPTIMIZATION

The goal of preoperative evaluation is to determine the risk of postoperative morbidity and mortality, and to identify opportunities for risk modification. A number of global risk scores have been developed that can assist in risk stratification and to provide guidance regarding preoperative testing.

The Eurolung risk score was developed from data in the European Society of Thoracic Surgeons (ESTS) database, containing more than 82,000 lung resections. The score is based on patient and surgical variables and can stratify patients with respect to 30-day mortality as well as long-term survival.[1,2]

The Thoracic Revised Cardiac Risk Index (ThRCRI) was developed to address the poor performance of the Revised Cardiac Risk Index (RCRI) in predicting adverse cardiac events in patients within 30 days of lung resection.[3] Compared with the original RCRI, the ThRCRI has been shown to have a greater degree of discrimination (c index 0.72 vs 0.62; $P = .004$).[3]

Further preoperative cardiac assessment is conducted based on the recommendations of the 2014 American College of Cardiology/American Heart Association Guideline on Perioperative Cardiovascular Evaluation and Management of Patients Undergoing Noncardiac Surgery.[4] In general, patients with lung resection with poor (<4 metabolic equivalents [METS]) or unknown functional capacity should undergo functional cardiac testing if the test results will impact perioperative care, otherwise, they should proceed with surgery with goal-directed medical therapy. Recent

The authors have nothing to disclose.
Department of Anesthesia, Critical Care and Pain Management, Massachusetts General Hospital, 55 Fruit Street, Boston, MA 02114, USA
* Corresponding author.
E-mail address: hchitilian@mgh.harvard.edu

studies have shown that the subjective assessment of functional capacity by physicians has low sensitivity for identifying the inability to achieve 4 METS and that the use of the Duke Activity Status Index can be used to identify patients at greater risk for cardiac complications.[5,6]

Preoperative B-type natriuretic peptide concentrations (BNP) and N-terminal fragment of proBNP (NT-proBNP) are independent predictors of postoperative complications.[7–9]

Preoperative pulmonary assessment is conducted based on the guidelines published by the American College of Chest Physicians and the European Respiratory Society/European Society of Thoracic Surgery (ERS/ESTS).[10,11] Both sets of guidelines advocate for further testing for patients with forced expiratory volume in 1 second or diffusing capacity of the lung for carbon monoxide less than 80% predicted; however, they differ with respect to the order in which they prioritize quantitative lung scintigraphy and exercise testing.[10,11]

Prehabilitation

Prehabilitation is a multifaceted approach of improving a patient's functional capacity to allow them to better withstand the stresses associated with the entire perioperative period. In its most advanced and comprehensive iterations, prehabilitation involves (1) personalized strength, flexibility and balance training; (2) dietary modifications designed to favorably modify the balance of catabolism associated with the immediate postoperative period with the anabolism needed for improved recovery; (3) interventions designed to support the patient's resiliency, reduce anxiety, and promote self-efficacy; and (4) cease deleterious habits such as smoking and alcohol abuse. The utilization of such programs is recommended as a component of the current ERAS Society/European Thoracic Surgery guidelines for enhanced recovery after lung surgery with a recommendation grade of "strong" albeit with an evidence level of "low."[12]

A recent meta-analysis identified 10 randomized controlled trials (RCTs) with a total of 676 participants investigated the effects of preoperative exercise training on postoperative pulmonary complications. Pooled data analysis showed a significant reduction in postoperative pulmonary complications (respiratory rate 0.5; 95% confidence interval [CI] 0.39–0.66) and length of stay (LOS) as well as improvements in walking endurance and peak exercise capacity.[13] The quality of evidence was graded as low because of the small number of studies, small sample sizes, and significant risks of bias in the study designs.

Furthermore, the type, frequency, and intensity of the exercise programs varied across the different studies, making it challenging to recommend a specific intervention. In the studies included for meta-analysis, interventions ranged from 1 week to 4 weeks, training sessions ranged from twice daily to 3 to 7 per week, and training programs varied from aerobic training only to aerobic training with some combination of inspiratory muscle training, strength training, and flexibility training. Another potential challenge for interpretation and application of these findings is that the included studies made no distinction between patients undergoing open lung resections and those undergoing thoracoscopic resections. Significant questions remain with respect to the widespread implementations of prehabilitation programs, including the minimum amount of intervention that is necessary, the necessity of hospital-based or clinic-based intervention, as opposed to home-based programs, as well as the specific patient populations for which the programs offer the greatest benefit.[14]

Enhanced Recovery after Surgery for Thoracic Surgery

As in other surgical fields, there is growing interest in enhanced recovery after surgery (ERAS) pathways, which are evidence-based, protocolized pathways aimed at simultaneously improving perioperative outcomes while increasing cost savings. Guidelines for ERAS after lung surgery were published by the ERAS and ESTS in 2019.[12] The suggested pathway spans the entire care continuum, from preadmission through recovery and includes recommendations for 45 items in total, including an assessment of each item's level of supporting evidence and the Society's strength of recommendation. Recommendations unique to the thoracic ERAS include interventions such as using lung protective ventilation while avoiding overly restrictive fluid resuscitation, muscle-sparing and nerve-sparing surgical techniques, and early removal of chest tubes. Emerging data from clinical studies indicate significant benefits of adoption of ERAS protocols for lung resection.[15–18] Some studies show decreased hospital LOS by 1 to 2 days, decreased cardiopulmonary complications, decreased opioid use, and significant cost savings per patient. Interestingly but perhaps unsurprisingly, these benefits are more pronounced in patients undergoing thoracotomy and open lung resection as opposed to video-assisted thoracoscopic surgery (VATS).[12,18] Still, there may be additional benefits that traditional outcome measures fail to capture that are most important from the patient's perspective; that is, patient-reported outcomes that measure elements of a patient's physical and psychological well-being.[18,19]

ANESTHETIC TECHNIQUE

The anesthetic technique used for lung cancer operations is tailored to the nature of the surgical procedure and the patient's comorbidities. The overarching objective is to provide the safest anesthetic while minimizing complications and improving the patient experience.

Regional and Neuraxial Anesthesia

Thoracic epidural analgesia is typically used intraoperatively and postoperatively to manage the pain associated with thoracotomy. Meta-analyses show that thoracic epidurals reduce pulmonary complications, decrease stress responses, and are consequently associated with better short-term outcomes in thoracic surgery.[20,21] Thoracic epidural should be considered for all patients undergoing thoracotomy unless contraindicated, although some studies suggest paravertebral blocks (PVBs) and catheters provide nearly equivalent analgesia.[22–24] A recent Cochrane Review concluded that thoracic epidural and PVB had equivalent survival, LOS, rates of major complications, and treatment of acute perioperative pain, but there were fewer minor complications in patients receiving PVB.[25] However, due to heterogeneity of available studies and local expertise of practice, this issue remains a subject of considerable debate.[26,27]

Minimally invasive procedures such as VATS usually do not require epidural anesthesia, but PVB, intercostal nerve blocks, or other regional techniques can be used effectively, likely with a better margin of safety compared with epidural anesthesia.[28–32] Intercostal nerve blocks significantly decrease postoperative opioid consumption in patients undergoing VATS; however, they may be inferior to PVB with respect to analgesia and the preservation of pulmonary mechanics.[33,34] Serratus anterior plane and erector spinal plane blocks have also been demonstrated to control pain and improve outcomes in thoracic surgery.[35–38] Despite these compelling findings, whether or not regional anesthesia is even necessary in VATS is also a matter of controversy, with one study showing equivalent outcomes in patients managed with epidural or PVBs compared with intravenous analgesics alone.[39]

Multiple different types of local anesthetics have been used in studies of regional anesthesia for thoracic surgery. Liposomal bupivacaine with its slow-release property and the potential for prolonged pain relief has received considerable attention in thoracic surgery. Although initial retrospective studies appeared promising, the beneficial results have not been reproduced in a clinical trial (NCT 01802411).[40,41] A recent meta-analysis of studies also cast doubt about the superiority of liposomal bupivicaine.[42,43]

Nonintubated Thoracic Surgery with Sedation

General anesthesia with endotracheal intubation and lung isolation remains the standard in anesthesia care for lung resection. A secured airway and controlled 1-lung ventilation (OLV) provide ideal surgical conditions. Nevertheless, before the introduction of double lumen tubes and modern anesthetic agents, thoracic surgery had been successfully performed using local and regional anesthesia.[44] The advancement of imaging technology, minimally invasive approaches, and improved monitoring has rekindled interest in the use of this technique. Reports in the literature have described the use of this approach for a wide array of cases from lung biopsy to pneumonectomy, as well as tracheal and carinal resection and reconstruction.[45–47]

Appropriate patient selection is critical to the success of this approach. Contraindications include anticipated difficult airway management, high risk of aspiration, respiratory failure, elevated intracranial pressure, need for contralateral lung isolation to protect from contamination, contralateral phrenic nerve palsy, and obesity.

A variety of regional anesthetic techniques have been used to control afferent nerve input from the chest wall. These include intercostal nerve block (ICB), thoracic PVB, and thoracic epidural, although the optimal approach has yet to be identified. These techniques can provide adequate anesthesia and analgesia for small peripheral lung cancer resections and pleural surgeries. However, the bronchial tree is innervated by the vagus nerve and sympathetic nerves and thus manipulation of the airway may stimulate strong cough reflexes that interfere with the surgical procedure. Intrathoracic vagus nerve block, preemptive lidocaine nebulization, or ipsilateral phrenic nerve block can all be used in attempt to minimize the cough reflex.[48,49]

Although selective lung cancer resections can be performed using regional anesthesia while the patient is fully awake, in practice some level of sedation is frequently required in nonintubated patients to minimize movement, excessive diaphragmatic motion, and mediastinal swing. Multiple sedatives, including midazolam, propofol, dexmedetomidine, fentanyl, and remifentanil have all been used successfully. Target control infusion of propofol titrated to a Bispectral index value 40 to 60 and respiratory rate of 12 to 20 have been advocated by some high-volume centers.[45,50,51] Our own experience favors the use of propofol and remifentanil infusions because of their titratability as well as analgesic and antitussive effects.

Nonintubated VATS poses a unique challenge to anesthesia providers who battle between keeping patients safe and providing an ideal surgical field. With the creation of surgical pneumothorax and OLV, patients frequently require oxygen supplementation with a face mask or venturi mask to correct hypoxia. Interestingly, early studies have demonstrated that nonintubated patients have equal or even improved oxygenation while undergoing VATS compared with intubated patients.[52,53] Intraoperative hypercapnia is also a common phenomenon, with reports of Pa_{CO_2} values as high as 80 mm Hg. However, it seems to be well tolerated by most patients.[49]

Intubation may be necessary if patients become unstable or surgeons encounter significant technical difficulties. Close communication between the anesthesia and surgical teams is imperative. Because patients remain in a lateral position, supraglottic devices can be easily placed to deliver additional oxygen and inhalation agents. If a more secured airway is necessary, video laryngoscopy can be used to intubate patients laterally. Alternatively, patients can be intubated through supraglottic devices with the assistance of a fiberoptic bronchoscope. Lung isolation can be achieved through the insertion of a bronchial blocker either through the endotracheal tube or supraglottic airway device.

To date, the largest RCT to compare nonintubated VATS with intubated VATS enrolled 354 patients with a variety of surgical indications.[54] The study demonstrated a significant reduction in overall postoperative morbidity (6.7% vs 16.7%, $P = .004$) as well as a reduction in respiratory complications (4.2% vs 10.0%, $P = .039$) in patients undergoing nonintubated VATS. In patients undergoing nonintubated VATS, there were 4 adverse effects related to thoracic epidural, including back pain, dizziness, nausea, and vomiting. In the control group, there were 10 minor events attributable to orotracheal intubation.[54] A recent meta-analysis of 14 randomized controlled studies of nonintubated versus intubated VATS demonstrated equal surgical field satisfaction but decreased air leak from operation, better pain control, and decreased hospital stay for 1.4 days in the nonintubated patient.[55] Common issues with the included trials were small sample sizes and the potential for selection bias of nonintubated patients.

Patients undergoing nonintubated VATS tended to have lower body mass index, minimal airway secretions, and preserved cardiopulmonary function at baseline. Furthermore, there was heterogeneity in the type and extent of thoracic diseases. Nonetheless, the use of nonintubated VATS merits further study in the era of enhanced recovery protocols.

Lung Isolation Techniques and Methodology

Surgical procedures for lung cancer often require lung isolation techniques to facilitate surgical exposure and resection. This is achieved most commonly via several strategies, including the use of left-sided or right-sided double lumen tubes (DLTs), a standard endotracheal tube plus bronchial blocker, or specialized endobronchial tubes.[56,57] Each of these methods has unique advantages and disadvantages. For example, DLTs provide excellent lung isolation and can be used to efficiently change from OLV to 2-lung ventilation, but the tubes are large and require additional expertise to place. Moreover, the large diameter of DLTs can make them very challenging to place in patients with history of difficult intubation. Limited evidence suggests that the most effective means of DLT size can be ascertained by measuring tracheal diameter or main bronchus diameter using computed tomography (CT) scan.[58–60] Bronchial blockers, on the other hand, can be placed through standard endotracheal tubes. In small trials, bronchial blockers have also been associated with lower risk of bronchial or tracheal injury and lower incidence of sore throat compared with DLT.[61,62] However, alternating between OLV and 2-lung ventilation can be time-consuming due to their small orifices for gas efflux and associated delay in lung collapse.

Ventilation Strategies

Current ventilation strategies for 1-lung ventilation (OLV) are adapted from the acute respiratory distress syndrome literature and use lung protective ventilation (LPV), usually defined as tidal volume of 6 mL/kg of ideal body weight or less.[57,63] LPV decreases the incidence of ventilator-induced lung injury (VILI) by reducing the mechanical stress on the alveoli and decreasing the local production of cytokines, chemokines, and other inflammatory mediators.[64–67] Although some studies comparing LPV and conventional ventilation for OLV show fewer postoperative pulmonary complications (PPCs) and shorter hospital LOS with LPV, other studies have failed to show a benefit.[68–70] The use of positive end expiratory pressure and/or recruitment maneuvers in conjunction with LPV might be an important factor explaining this discrepancy.[68]

In patients with severe pulmonary disease, complex masses near the heart or major blood vessels, those who have had prior pneumonectomy or other complex comorbidities, lung resection surgery can be performed using extracorporeal life support (ECLS) modalities, such as venovenous or venoarterial extracorporeal membrane oxygenation.[71,72] These techniques can allow procedures to be completed with minimal or no ventilation, while still achieving adequate CO_2 removal and oxygenation, and are an alternative to conventional cardiopulmonary bypass. As with other interventions, the risks and benefits of using ECLS for lung resection must be carefully considered, and local expertise is a critical determinant of favorable outcomes.

Fluid Management

Lung resections, particularly pneumonectomies and multilobar resections, are typically managed with a highly conservative fluid management strategy (about 1 mL/kg per hour intraoperatively), aimed at minimizing capillary hydrostatic pressure and interstitial and alveolar edema.[73–75] This is particularly important because OLV is associated with significant risk of VILI, leading to capillary membrane injury with increased fluid extravasation and pulmonary edema. However, there are a paucity of studies testing the veracity of this dogma. Recent data from retrospective studies of VATS and open thoracotomy suggest that both overly restrictive and liberal fluid management strategies are associated with increased PPCs, favoring a moderately conservative strategy between 2 and 6 mL/kg per hour of crystalloid on an individually managed basis.[76,77] Presumably, a moderately conservative strategy strikes the balance of avoiding fluid overload while minimizing the risk of organ hypoperfusion.

Maintenance of Anesthesia

There is ongoing debate regarding the benefit of propofol-based, total intravenous anesthesia (TIVA) when compared with volatile anesthetics with respect to improved long-term survival in patients undergoing cancer operations.[78,79] One small prospective RCT in lung cancer resection suggests that the use of volatile anesthetics, not TIVA, may be favorable, with more PPCs (28.4% vs 14.0%, odds ratio [OR] 2.44; 95% CI 1.14–5.26) and increased 1-year mortality (12.5% vs 2.3%, OR 5.37; 95% CI 1.23–23.54) in the TIVA group compared with patients receiving volatile anesthesia.[80] A metanalysis of small RCTs comparing TIVA and volatile anesthetics similarly found that volatile anesthetics were associated with shorter LOS, fewer PPCs, and, interestingly, lower levels of the proinflammatory cytokines tumor necrosis factor-alpha, interleukin (IL)-6, and IL-8 during OLV. However, the inhalational anesthetics can interfere with hypoxic pulmonary vasoconstriction during OLV, and patients were found to have lower Pao_2 at 30 minutes after the initiation of OLV compared with patients maintained with TIVA.[81] Additional trials are needed to definitively address the question.

Pain Management

Thoracic surgery, including minimally invasive approaches like VATS and robotic surgeries are considered to cause moderate to severe pain, with a large fraction of patients developing a chronic pain condition known as postthoracotomy pain syndrome.[82] Intrathoracic procedures also negatively alter respiratory mechanics, resulting in atelectasis, decreased functional residual capacity, decreased compliance, and physical trauma and ischemia/reperfusion injury. Inadequate postoperative analgesia further worsens respiratory mechanics, resulting in splinting with reduced tidal volumes, impaired cough and clearance of secretions, and increased risk of postoperative pulmonary complications.[83,84] Severe postoperative pain is related to nociceptive, neuropathic, inflammatory, and ischemic sources, including incisional pain, disruption of chest wall and intercostal muscles, costovertebral joint disruption, intercostal nerve damage related to retraction and trocar insertion, and pleural disruption and inflammation.[85] Multiple neural pathways mediate nociception from the chest wall, including intercostal nerves, long thoracic and thoracic dorsal nerves for somatic pain, and the vagus and phrenic nerves for visceral pain.[86]

Optimal postoperative pain management begins in the preoperative period, and often involves a multidisciplinary approach.[87] Pain management plans that allow for the minimum use of opioid analgesics are preferred due to the avoidance of their deleterious side-effect profiles. Numerous metanalyses and RCTs support the use of opioid-sparing regimens, and these are therefore a major component of ERAS protocols for thoracic surgery.[12,88] Indeed, patients managed with ERAS protocols after lung resection use fewer opioids than those managed with traditional approaches like patient-controlled analgesia.[89,90] Numerous nonopioid analgesics are used as part of multimodal analgesic strategies for thoracic ERAS protocols, including acetaminophen, nonsteroidal anti-inflammatory drugs, ketamine, dexmedetomidine, local anesthetics including nerve blocks (see preceding section on regional anesthesia) and others. A detailed discussion of each analgesic agent is beyond the scope of this review, as this topic has been extensively reviewed elsewhere.[90,91] An underlying principle in multimodal analgesia is the use of multiple agents that target a range of receptors involved in nociceptive transmission. This not only interrupts nociception from multiple pathways but also may decrease potential side effects of each medication, because smaller doses can be used. At a basic level, ideal strategies rely heavily on regional anesthetic interventions including neuraxial anesthesia, because these can theoretically provide total analgesia with complete or near complete avoidance of opioids.

SUMMARY

Increasingly complex procedures are routinely performed using minimally invasive approaches, allowing cancers to be resected with short hospital stays, minimal postsurgical discomfort, and improved odds of cancer-free survival. Along with these changes, the focus of anesthetic management for lung resection surgery has expanded from the provision of ideal surgical conditions and safe intraoperative patient care to include preoperative patient training and optimization and postoperative pain management techniques that can impact pulmonary outcomes as well as patient lengths of stay.

CLINICS CARE POINTS

- Prehabilitation has been shown to improve postoperative outcomes; however, the specific type of program and the frequency and intensity of exercise that is most effective remains to be determined.

- ERAS pathways specific to pulmonary resection have been shown to improve patient outcome and reduce hospital LOS.

- Regional anesthesia techniques such as serratus anterior plane block and erector spinae block can improve postoperative pain control.

REFERENCES

1. Brunelli A, Cicconi S, Decaluwe H, et al. Parsimonious Eurolung risk models to predict cardiopulmonary morbidity and mortality following anatomic lung resections: an updated analysis from the European Society of Thoracic Surgeons database. Eur J Cardio-thorac Surg 2020;57(3): 455–61.

2. Brunelli A, Chaudhuri N, Kefaloyannis M, et al. Eurolung risk score is associated with long-term survival after curative resection for lung cancer. J Thorac Cardiovasc Surg 2021;161(3):776–86.

3. Brunelli A, Varela G, Salati M, et al. Recalibration of the revised cardiac risk index in lung resection candidates. Ann Thorac Surg 2010;90(1):199–203.

4. Fleisher LA, Fleischmann KE, Auerbach AD, et al. 2014 ACC/AHA guideline on perioperative cardiovascular evaluation and management of patients undergoing noncardiac surgery: executive summary: a report of the American College of Cardiology/American Heart Association Task Force on Practice Guidelines. Circulation 2014;130(24):2215–45.

5. Wijeysundera DN, Beattie WS, Hillis GS, et al. Integration of the Duke Activity Status Index into preoperative risk evaluation: a multicentre prospective cohort study. Br J Anaesth 2020;124(3):261–70.

6. Wijeysundera DN, Pearse RM, Shulman MA, et al. Assessment of functional capacity before major non-cardiac surgery: an international, prospective cohort study. Lancet Lond Engl 2018;391(10140): 2631–40.

7. Rodseth RN, Biccard BM, Le Manach Y, et al. The prognostic value of pre-operative and post-operative B-type natriuretic peptides in patients undergoing noncardiac surgery: B-type natriuretic peptide and N-terminal fragment of pro-B-type natriuretic peptide: a systematic review and individual patient data meta-analysis. J Am Coll Cardiol 2014;63(2):170–80.

8. Young DJ, McCall PJ, Kirk A, et al. B-type natriuretic peptide predicts deterioration in functional capacity following lung resection. Interact Cardiovasc Thorac Surg 2019;28(6):945–52.

9. Nojiri T, Inoue M, Shintani Y, et al. B-type natriuretic peptide-guided risk assessment for postoperative complications in lung cancer surgery. World J Surg 2015;39(5):1092–8.

10. Brunelli A, Kim AW, Berger KI, et al. Physiologic evaluation of the patient with lung cancer being considered for resectional surgery: Diagnosis and management of lung cancer, 3rd ed: American College of Chest Physicians evidence-based clinical practice guidelines. Chest 2013;143(5 Suppl): e166S–90S.

11. Brunelli A, Charloux A, Bolliger CT, et al. ERS/ESTS clinical guidelines on fitness for radical therapy in lung cancer patients (surgery and chemo-radio-therapy). Eur Respir J 2009;34(1):17–41.

12. Batchelor TJP, Rasburn NJ, Abdelnour-Berchtold E, et al. Guidelines for enhanced recovery after lung

surgery: recommendations of the Enhanced Recovery After Surgery (ERAS®) Society and the European Society of Thoracic Surgeons (ESTS). Eur J Cardio-thorac Surg 2019;55(1):91–115.

13. Rosero ID, Ramírez-Vélez R, Lucia A, et al. Systematic review and meta-analysis of randomized, controlled trials on preoperative physical exercise interventions in patients with non-small-cell lung cancer. Cancers 2019;11(7):944.

14. Minnella EM, Baldini G, Quang ATL, et al. Prehabilitation in thoracic cancer surgery: from research to standard of care. J Cardiothorac Vasc Anesth 2021. https://doi.org/10.1053/j.jvca.2021.02.049.

15. Van Haren RM, Mehran RJ, Mena GE, et al. Enhanced recovery decreases pulmonary and cardiac complications after thoracotomy for lung cancer. Ann Thorac Surg 2018;106(1):272–9.

16. Wang C, Lai Y, Li P, et al. Influence of enhanced recovery after surgery (ERAS) on patients receiving lung resection: a retrospective study of 1749 cases. BMC Surg 2021;21(1):115.

17. Martin LW, Sarosiek BM, Harrison MA, et al. Implementing a thoracic enhanced recovery program: lessons learned in the first year. Ann Thorac Surg 2018;105(6):1597–604.

18. Medbery RL, Fernandez FG, Khullar OV. ERAS and patient reported outcomes in thoracic surgery: a review of current data. J Thorac Dis 2019;11(S7): S976–86.

19. Khullar OV, Fernandez FG. Patient-reported outcomes in thoracic surgery. Thorac Surg Clin 2017; 27(3):279–90.

20. Wu CL, Sapirstein A, Herbert R, et al. Effect of postoperative epidural analgesia on morbidity and mortality after lung resection in Medicare patients. J Clin Anesth 2006;18(7):515–20.

21. Pöpping DM. Protective effects of epidural analgesia on pulmonary complications after abdominal and thoracic surgery: a meta-analysis. Arch Surg 2008;143(10):990.

22. Bachman SA, Lundberg J, Herrick M. Avoid suboptimal perioperative analgesia during major surgery by enhancing thoracic epidural catheter placement and hemodynamic performance. Reg Anesth Pain Med 2021;46(6):532–4.

23. Ding X, Jin S, Niu X, et al. A comparison of the analgesia efficacy and side effects of paravertebral compared with epidural blockade for thoracotomy: an updated meta-analysis. PLoS ONE 2014;9(5): e96233.

24. Davies RG, Myles PS, Graham JM. A comparison of the analgesic efficacy and side-effects of paravertebral vs epidural blockade for thoracotomy—a systematic review and meta-analysis of randomized trials. Br J Anaesth 2006;96(4):418–26.

25. Yeung JH, Gates S, Naidu BV, et al. Paravertebral block versus thoracic epidural for patients undergoing thoracotomy. Cochrane Anaesthesia Group. Cochrane Database Syst Rev 2016. https://doi.org/10.1002/14651858.CD009121.pub2.

26. Teeter EG, Kumar PA. Pro: Thoracic epidural block is superior to paravertebral blocks for open thoracic surgery. J Cardiothorac Vasc Anesth 2015;29(6): 1717–9.

27. Krakowski JC, Arora H. Con: Thoracic epidural block is not superior to paravertebral blocks for open thoracic surgery. J Cardiothorac Vasc Anesth 2015;29(6):1720–2.

28. Kosiński S, Fryźlewicz E, Wiłkojć M, et al. Comparison of continuous epidural block and continuous paravertebral block in postoperative analgesia after video-assisted thoracoscopic surgery lobectomy: a randomised, non-inferiority trial. Anaesthesiol Intensive Ther 2016;48(5):280–7.

29. Daly DJ, Myles PS. Update on the role of paravertebral blocks for thoracic surgery: are they worth it? Curr Opin Anaesthesiol 2009;22(1):38–43.

30. Tong C, Zhu H, Li B, et al. Impact of paravertebral blockade use in geriatric patients undergoing thoracic surgery on postoperative adverse outcomes. J Thorac Dis 2019;11(12):5169–76.

31. Wu Z, Fang S, Wang Q, et al. Patient-controlled paravertebral block for video-assisted thoracic surgery: a randomized trial. Ann Thorac Surg 2018;106(3): 888–94.

32. Yeap YL, Wolfe JW, Backfish-White KM, et al. Randomized prospective study evaluating single-injection paravertebral block, paravertebral catheter, and thoracic epidural catheter for postoperative regional analgesia after video-assisted thoracoscopic surgery. J Cardiothorac Vasc Anesth 2020;34(7):1870–6.

33. Bolotin G, Lazarovici H, Uretzky G, et al. The efficacy of intraoperative internal intercostal nerve block during video-assisted thoracic surgery on postoperative pain. Ann Thorac Surg 2000;70(6): 1872–5.

34. Matyal R, Montealegre-Gallegos M, Shnider M, et al. Preemptive ultrasound-guided paravertebral block and immediate postoperative lung function. Gen Thorac Cardiovasc Surg 2015;63(1):43–8.

35. Blanco R, Parras T, McDonnell JG, et al. Serratus plane block: a novel ultrasound-guided thoracic wall nerve block. Anaesthesia 2013;68(11):1107–13.

36. Liu X, Song T, Xu H-Y, et al. The serratus anterior plane block for analgesia after thoracic surgery: a meta-analysis of randomized controlled trails. Medicine (Baltimore) 2020;99(21):e20286.

37. Huang J, Liu J-C. Ultrasound-guided erector spinae plane block for postoperative analgesia: a meta-analysis of randomized controlled trials. BMC Anesthesiol 2020;20(1):83.

38. Finnerty DT, McMahon A, McNamara JR, et al. Comparing erector spinae plane block with serratus

anterior plane block for minimally invasive thoracic surgery: a randomised clinical trial. Br J Anaesth 2020;125(5):802–10.

39. Haager B, Schmid D, Eschbach J, et al. Regional versus systemic analgesia in video-assisted thoracoscopic lobectomy: a retrospective analysis. BMC Anesthesiol 2019;19(1):183.

40. Rice DC, Cata JP, Mena GE, et al. Posterior intercostal nerve block with liposomal bupivacaine: an alternative to thoracic epidural analgesia. Ann Thorac Surg 2015;99(6):1953–60.

41. Khalil KG, Boutrous ML, Irani AD, et al. Operative intercostal nerve blocks with long-acting bupivacaine liposome for pain control after thoracotomy. Ann Thorac Surg 2015;100(6):2013–8.

42. Hussain N, Brull R, Sheehy B, et al. Perineural liposomal bupivacaine is not superior to nonliposomal bupivacaine for peripheral nerve block analgesia. Anesthesiology 2021;134(2):147–64.

43. Ilfeld BM, Eisenach JC, Gabriel RA. Clinical effectiveness of liposomal bupivacaine administered by infiltration or peripheral nerve block to treat postoperative pain. Anesthesiology 2021;134(2):283–344.

44. Ossipov BK. Local anesthesia in thoracic surgery: 20 years experience with 3265 cases. Anesth Analg 1960;39:327–32.

45. Hung W-T, hsu H-H, Hung M-H, et al. Nonintubated uniportal thoracoscopic surgery for resection of lung lesions. J Thorac Dis 2016;8(Suppl3):S242–50.

46. Hung W-T, Liao H-C, Cheng Y-J, et al. Nonintubated thoracoscopic pneumonectomy for bullous emphysema. Ann Thorac Surg 2016;102(4):e353–5.

47. Liu J, Li S, Shen J, et al. Non-intubated resection and reconstruction of trachea for the treatment of a mass in the upper trachea. J Thorac Dis 2016;8(3):594–9.

48. Zhao Z-R, Lau RWH, Ng CSH. Non-intubated video-assisted thoracic surgery: the final frontier? Eur J Cardiothorac Surg 2016;50(5):925–6.

49. Liang H, Gonzalez-Rivas D, Zhou Y, et al. Nonintubated anesthesia for tracheal/carinal resection and reconstruction. Thorac Surg Clin 2020;30(1):83–90.

50. Sunaga H, Blasberg JD, Heerdt PM. Anesthesia for nonintubated video-assisted thoracic surgery. Curr Opin Anaesthesiol 2017;30(1):1–6.

51. Yang S-M, Wang M-L, Hung M-H, et al. Tubeless uniportal thoracoscopic wedge resection for peripheral lung nodules. Ann Thorac Surg 2017;103(2):462–8.

52. Tacconi F, Pompeo E. Non-intubated video-assisted thoracic surgery: where does evidence stand? J Thorac Dis 2016;8(S4):S364–75.

53. Wu C-Y, Chen J-S, Lin Y-S, et al. Feasibility and safety of nonintubated thoracoscopic lobectomy for geriatric lung cancer patients. Ann Thorac Surg 2013;95(2):405–11.

54. Liu J, Cui F, Li S, et al. Nonintubated video-assisted thoracoscopic surgery under epidural anesthesia compared with conventional anesthetic option: a randomized control study. Surg Innov 2015;22(2):123–30.

55. Zhang X-X, Song C-T, Gao Z, et al. A comparison of non-intubated video-assisted thoracic surgery with spontaneous ventilation and intubated video-assisted thoracic surgery: a meta-analysis based on 14 randomized controlled trials. J Thorac Dis 2021;13(3):1624–40.

56. Ashok V, Francis J. A practical approach to adult one-lung ventilation. BJA Educ 2018;18(3):69–74.

57. Campos JH, Feider A. Hypoxia during one-lung ventilation-a review and update. J Cardiothorac Vasc Anesth 2018;32(5):2330–8.

58. Pedoto A. How to choose the double-lumen tube size and side. Anesthesiol Clin 2012;30(4):671–81.

59. Brodsky JB, Macario A, Mark JBD. Tracheal diameter predicts double-lumen tube size: a method for selecting left double-lumen tubes. Anesth Analg 1996;82(4):861–4.

60. Jeon Y, Ryu HG, Bahk JH, et al. A new technique to determine the size of double-lumen endobronchial tubes by the two perpendicularly measured bronchial diameters. Anaesth Intensive Care 2005;33(1):59–63.

61. Lu Y, Dai W, Zong Z, et al. Bronchial blocker versus left double-lumen endotracheal tube for one-lung ventilation in right video-assisted thoracoscopic surgery. J Cardiothorac Vasc Anesth 2018;32(1):297–301.

62. Mourisse J, Liesveld J, Verhagen A, et al. Efficiency, efficacy, and safety of EZ-Blocker compared with left-sided double-lumen tube for one-lung ventilation. Anesthesiology 2013;118(3):550–61.

63. Ventilation with lower tidal volumes as compared with traditional tidal volumes for acute lung injury and the acute respiratory distress syndrome. N Engl J Med 2000;342(18):1301–8.

64. Goodman RB, Pugin J, Lee JS, et al. Cytokine-mediated inflammation in acute lung injury. Cytokine Growth Factor Rev 2003;14(6):523–35.

65. Schilling T, Kretzschmar M, Hachenberg T, et al. The immune response to one-lung-ventilation is not affected by repeated alveolar recruitment manoeuvres in pigs. Minerva Anestesiol 2013;79(6):590–603.

66. Michelet P, D'Journo X-B, Roch A, et al. Protective ventilation influences systemic inflammation after esophagectomy. Anesthesiology 2006;105(5):911–9.

67. Michelet P, Roch A, Brousse D, et al. Effects of PEEP on oxygenation and respiratory mechanics during one-lung ventilation. Br J Anaesth 2005;95(2):267–73.

68. Güldner A, Kiss T, Serpa Neto A, et al. Intraoperative protective mechanical ventilation for prevention of

postoperative pulmonary complications. Anesthesiology 2015;123(3):692–713.

69. Serpa Neto A, Hemmes SNT, Barbas CSV, et al. Protective versus conventional ventilation for surgery. Anesthesiology 2015;123(1):66–78.

70. Blank RS, Colquhoun DA, Durieux ME, et al. Management of one-lung ventilation. Anesthesiology 2016;124(6):1286–95.

71. Reeb J, Olland A, Massard G, et al. Extracorporeal life support in thoracic surgery. Eur J Cardiothorac Surg 2018;53(3):489–94.

72. Koryllos A, Lopez-Pastorini A, Galetin T, et al. Use of extracorporeal membrane oxygenation for major cardiopulmonary resections. Thorac Cardiovasc Surg 2021;69(03):231–9.

73. Lohser J, Slinger P. Lung injury after one-lung ventilation: a review of the pathophysiologic mechanisms affecting the ventilated and the collapsed lung. Anesth Analg 2015;121(2):302–18.

74. Chau EHL, Slinger P. Perioperative fluid management for pulmonary resection surgery and esophagectomy. Semin Cardiothorac Vasc Anesth 2014;18(1):36–44.

75. Kutlu CA, Williams EA, Evans TW, et al. Acute lung injury and acute respiratory distress syndrome after pulmonary resection. Ann Thorac Surg 2000;69(2):376–80.

76. Wu Y, Yang R, Xu J, et al. Effects of intraoperative fluid management on postoperative outcomes after lobectomy. Ann Thorac Surg 2019;107(6):1663–9.

77. Kim JA, Ahn HJ, Oh AR, et al. Restrictive intraoperative fluid management was associated with higher incidence of composite complications compared to less restrictive strategies in open thoracotomy: a retrospective cohort study. Sci Rep 2020;10(1):8449.

78. Hong B, Lee S, Kim Y, et al. Anesthetics and long-term survival after cancer surgery—total intravenous versus volatile anesthesia: a retrospective study. BMC Anesthesiol 2019;19(1):233.

79. Oh TK, Kim K, Jheon S, et al. Long-term oncologic outcomes for patients undergoing volatile versus intravenous anesthesia for non-small cell lung cancer surgery: a retrospective propensity matching analysis. Cancer Control 2018;25(1). 107327481877536.

80. de la Gala F, Piñeiro P, Reyes A, et al. Postoperative pulmonary complications, pulmonary and systemic inflammatory responses after lung resection surgery with prolonged one-lung ventilation. Randomized controlled trial comparing intravenous and inhalational anaesthesia. Br J Anaesth 2017;119(4):655–63.

81. Cho YJ, Kim TK, Hong DM, et al. Effect of desflurane-remifentanil vs. Propofol-remifentanil anesthesia on arterial oxygenation during one-lung ventilation for thoracoscopic surgery: a prospective randomized trial. BMC Anesthesiol 2017;17(1):9.

82. Wildgaard K, Ravn J, Kehlet H. Chronic post-thoracotomy pain: a critical review of pathogenic mechanisms and strategies for prevention☆. Eur J Cardiothorac Surg 2009;36(1):170–80.

83. Sabanathan S, Eng J, Mearns AJ. Alterations in respiratory mechanics following thoracotomy. J R Coll Surg Edinb 1990;35(3):144–50.

84. Ballantyne JC, Carr DB, deFerranti S, et al. The comparative effects of postoperative analgesic therapies on pulmonary outcome: cumulative meta-analyses of randomized, controlled trials. Anesth Analg 1998;86(3):598–612.

85. Goto T. What is the best pain control after thoracic surgery? J Thorac Dis 2018;10(3):1335–8.

86. Marshall K, McLaughlin K. Pain management in thoracic surgery. Thorac Surg Clin 2020;30(3):339–46.

87. Memtsoudis SG, Poeran J, zubizarreta, et al. Association of multimodal pain management strategies with perioperative outcomes and resource utilization: a population-based study. Anesthesiology 2018;128(5):891–902.

88. Piccioni F, Segat M, Falini S, Marzia Umari. Enhanced recovery pathways in thoracic surgery from Italian VATS Group: perioperative analgesia protocols. J Thorac Dis 2018;10(Suppl4):S555–63.

89. Rice D, Rodriguez-Restrepo A, Mena G, et al. Matched pairs comparison of an enhanced recovery pathway versus conventional management on opioid exposure and pain control in patients undergoing lung surgery. Ann Surg 2020. https://doi.org/10.1097/SLA.0000000000003587.

90. Thompson C, French DG, Costache I. Pain management within an enhanced recovery program after thoracic surgery. J Thorac Dis 2018;10(S32):S3773–80.

91. Razi SS, Stephens-McDonnough JA, Haq S, et al. Significant reduction of postoperative pain and opioid analgesics requirement with an Enhanced Recovery After Thoracic Surgery protocol. J Thorac Cardiovasc Surg 2021;161(5):1689–701.

Paraneoplastic Syndromes in Lung Cancers
Manifestations of Ectopic Endocrinological Syndromes and Neurologic Syndromes

Farid M. Shamji, MBBS, FRCSC, FACS[a],*, Gilles Beauchamp, MD, FRCSC[b],
Donna E. Maziak, MDCM, MSc, FRCSC, FACS[c], Joel Cooper, MD, FACS, FRCSC[d]

KEYWORDS

- Lung cancer • Paraneoplastic syndromes • Endocrine and neurologic • Hypercalcemia
- Hypertrophic pulmonary osteoarthropathy • Subacute cerebellar degeneration
- Syndrome of inappropriate ADH secretion • Myopathy • Neuropathy

KEY POINTS

- Classification of paraneoplastic endocrine syndromes and paraneoplastic neurologic syndromes.
- Secretion of ectopic hormones and immunoreactivity.

INTRODUCTION
Primary Lung Cancer

Bronchogenic carcinoma is a disease of considerable importance because it is now the commonest fatal cancer, and in the Western world in men aged 45 to 64 years deaths from lung cancer are now equal to deaths from breast, colon, and prostate cancer together. Careful epidemiologic studies have shown that the way is opened to diminish, and perhaps largely obliterate, its incidence. The incidence of this cancer parallels the incidence of cigarette smoking, and that the risk is greatest among the heaviest smokers. Cigarette smoke contains both cancer initiators and cancer promoters. In man the risk of developing lung cancer is increased approximately 30-fold for those smoking 30 cigarettes per day.

THE PARANEOPLASTIC SYNDROMES

The term paraneoplastic syndrome encompasses a variety of nonmetastatic metabolic or neuromuscular manifestations of lung cancer.[1–4] Although such syndromes may occur with all major types of lung cancer, they are most frequently associated with small cell carcinoma, which commonly elaborates ectopic hormones from neurosecretory granules contained within its cells. These peptide hormones are produced in healthy subjects, not only in neural tissue including the hypothalamus and anterior and posterior pituitary, but also in the gut-derived tissues and are therefore sometime referred to as gut–brain peptides. A number of metabolic paraneoplastic syndromes are, however, well-recognized clinically, and these are included in the discussion that follows. The mechanisms by which the paraneoplastic

a University of Ottawa, General Campus, Ottawa Hospital, 501 Smyth Road, Ottawa, Ontario K1H 8L6, Canada; b Thoracic Surgery Unit, Department of Surgery, Maisonneuve-Rosemount Hospital, University of Montreal, 5415 L'Assomption Boulevard, Montreal, Quebec H1T 2M4, Canada; c Surgical Oncology, Division of Thoracic Surgery, Ottawa Hospital - General Division, University of Ottawa, 501 Smyth Road, 6NW-6364, Ottawa, Ontario K1H 8L6, Canada; d Hospital of the University of Pennsylvania, Ravdin 6, 3400 Spruce Street, Philadelphia, PA 19104, USA
* Corresponding author.
E-mail address: faridshamji@hotmail.com

Thorac Surg Clin 31 (2021) 519–537
https://doi.org/10.1016/j.thorsurg.2021.06.001
1547-4127/21/© 2021 Elsevier Inc. All rights reserved.

neuromuscular syndromes arise remain for the most part obscure. These syndromes may antedate the discovery of a neoplasm by months or even years.[5]

Definition of Paraneoplastic Syndromes

Paraneoplastic syndromes are classified as paraneoplastic endocrine syndromes and paraneoplastic neurologic syndromes.[3] In addition to direct, local invasion and metastatic spread, cancers may give rise to distant symptoms and/or signs through 2 main mechanisms:

- An immune response to the malignancy producing antibodies to tumor cells that cross-react with normal cells. In many cases, the antibodies may target normal neurones producing well characterized, complex neurologic presentations.
- Release of cytokines/hormones by malignant cells, such as ectopic adrenocorticotrophic hormone, which may be released by a variety of cancers, including pulmonary carcinomas.

The associated clinical syndromes may precede, follow, or present at the same time as the primary malignancy (**Box 1, Table 1**).

Dermatomyositis

Dermatomyositis is a rare but very disabling complication of lung cancer.[14,15] The patient presents weakness and a characteristic heliotrope rash and erythematous rash on face, neck, chest, back, and shoulders (last of which is known as the shawl sign); the rash may be photosensitive.

Sometimes, the disease presents as a cardiac or pulmonary disease, as well as swallowing difficulty. Muscle weakness usually moves gradually and progressively. Muscle tenderness and aches may be very striking. The inflammation characteristically causes elevations of serum levels of aldolase and creatinine kinase, and alternation of liver function tests. Although most patients respond initially to corticosteroids, cytotoxic drugs are sometimes added when steroid toxicity or refractoriness develops.

This is a disease of adults and about 20% of cases have an associated neoplasm. Occasionally antibodies are formed in the serum which react with tumor extracts and immunoglobulins can be demonstrated in the skin and muscle.

Diagnostic studies
- Laboratory findings
  Elevated serum creatine kinase, aspartate aminotransferase, alanine aminotransferase, lactate dehydrogenase, and aldolase

- Electromyography: increased spontaneous activity with fibrillations, complex repetitive discharges, and positive sharp waves
- Muscle biopsy: perivascular or interfascicular septal inflammation and perifascicular atrophy

Associated cancers
- Ovarian, breast, prostate, lung, colorectal, non-Hodgkin lymphoma, nasopharyngeal

Treatment options
  Most patients respond initially to corticosteroids and cytotoxic drugs is added to minimize steroid toxicity,
- Prednisone 80 to 100 mg/d orally
- Methylprednisolone up to 1 g/d intravenously (IV)
- Azathioprine, up to 25 g/wk orally
- Cyclosporine A, 100 to 150 mg orally twice daily
- Mycophenolate mofetil 2 g/d orally
- Cyclophosphamide 0.5 to 10 g/m^2 IV
- IV immunoglobulinIVIG), 400 to 1000 mg/d to total of 2 to 3 g
- Proximal muscle weakness and pain
- Swallowing and respiratory difficulty

Diagnostic studies and laboratory findings
- Laboratory findings
  Elevated serum creatine kinase, aspartate aminotransferase, alanine aminotransferase, lactate dehydrogenase, and aldolase
- Electromyography: increased spontaneous activity with fibrillations, complex repetitive discharges, and positive sharp waves
- Muscle biopsy: perivascular or interfascicular septal inflammation and perifascicular atrophy

Associated cancers
- Ovarian, breast, prostate, lung*, colorectal, non-Hodgkin lymphoma, nasopharyngeal

Treatment options
  Most patients respond initially to corticosteroids and cytotoxic drugs is added to minimize steroid toxicity,
- Prednisone 80 to 100 mg/d orally
- Methylprednisolone up to 1 g/d IV
- Azathioprine, up to 25 g/wk orally
- Cyclosporine A, 100 to 150 mg orally twice daily
- Mycophenolate mofetil 2 g/d orally
- Cyclophosphamide 0.5 to 10 g/m^2 IV
- IVIG, 400 to 1000 mg/d to total of 2 to 3 g

Box 1
Paraneoplastic dermatologic and rheumatological syndromes

Paraneoplastic dermatologic and rheumatologic syndromes are well-recognized and are classified as:

a. *Polymyositis and dermatomyositis* may be associated with overt or occult malignancy. Dermatomyositis and polymyositis present as gradually progressive muscle weakness predominantly affecting the proximal musculature, coming on over a period of months.[14,16]

Dermatomyositis is a rare but very disabling complication of lung cancer. The patient presents with weakness and a characteristic heliotrope and erythematous rash on the face, neck, chest, back, and shoulders (last of which is known as *shawl sign*); the rash may be photosensitive.

Sometimes the disease presents as a cardiac or pulmonary disease, as well as with swallowing difficulty. Weakness usually moves gradually and progressively. Muscle tenderness and aches may be very striking. The inflammation characteristically causes elevations of serum levels of aldolase and creatinine kinase, and alternation of liver function tests. Although most patients respond initially to corticosteroids, cytotoxic drugs are sometimes added when steroid toxicity or refractoriness develops.

This is a disease of adults and about 20% of cases have an associated neoplasm. Occasionally, antibodies are formed in the serum that react with tumor extracts and immunoglobulins can be demonstrated in the skin and muscle.

Although these disorders are not universally associated with malignancy, patients suffering from them have a greatly increased risk of an underlying neoplasm compared with the general public, and malignancies of the breast, lung, gastrointestinal, and genitourinary tracts should be considered. Thus, dermatomyositis may be the alerting presenting sign of a deep-seated cancer that has yet to declare itself.

b. *Visual ophthalmologic paraneoplastic events,*[5] for example, cancer-associated retinopathy and optic neuritis, occur but are rare, being best documented in lung cancer and lymphoma.

Ophthalmologic paraneoplastic syndromes related to the retina or optic nerves can be seen in lung cancer cases, and particularly in small cell lung cancer. Retinopathy and optic neuropathy may develop and result in visual dysfunctions. Paraneoplastic syndrome in these cases is caused by the development of immune reaction. The antigens associated with paraneoplastic retinopathy are recoverin and alpha-enolase, whereas collapsin response mediator protein 5 is the antigen associated with paraneoplastic optic neuropathy.[5]

Treatment is based primarily on immunosuppressive therapies. However, visual function may not improve despite immunosuppressive therapy and effective treatment of the underlying cancer.

Paraneoplastic neurologic syndromes result from immune cross-reactivity between tumor cells and components of the nervous system. In response to a developing cancer, a patient produces tumor-directed antibodies known as onconeural antibodies. Because of antigenic similarity, these onconeural antibodies and associated onconeural antigens of cases, specific T lymphocytes inadvertently attack components of the nervous system as well. In contrast with paraneoplastic endocrinologic syndromes, paraneoplastic syndromes are detected before cancer is diagnosed in 80% of cases. Because tumor cells themselves do not directly produce the causative agents of paraneoplastic syndromes, and because onconeural antibodies may cause permanent damage, successful cancer treatment does not necessarily result in neurologic improvement. Immunosuppressive therapy is a mainstay of paraneoplastic syndrome treatment.[5]

Paraneoplastic neurologic syndromes can affect the central nervous system (eg, limbic encephalitis and paraneoplastic subacute cerebellar degeneration, the neuromuscular junction (eg, Lambert–Eaton myasthenia syndrome) or the peripheral nervous system (eg, autonomic neuropathy and subacute sensory neuropathy), and retinopathy. Cancer-associated retinopathy, often associated with small cell lung cancer, is associated with a triad of symptoms, namely, photosensitivity, ring scotomatous visual field loss, and attenuated retinal arteriole caliber.

Table 1
Paraneoplastic neurologic syndromes[4–8]

Syndrome	Clinical Features	Antibody	Associated Tumors	Investigations
Retinal degeneration	Painless progressive visual loss	Antiretinal	Small cell carcinoma of lung	Chest radiograph, CT scan of the chest, electroretinogram
Opsoclonus myoclonus	Arrhythmic chaotic rapid eye movements	Anti-RI	Lung cancer, ovarian cancer, neuroblastoma	Chest radiograph, CT scan of the chest, pelvic ultrasound examination, or CT
Limbic encephalitis	Memory loss, progressive dementia, seizures	Anti-Hu	Small cell carcinoma of lung	Chest radiograph, CT scan of the chest, MRI head, CSF (pleocytosis, raised protein)
Sensory neuropathy[9]	Limb pain, parasthesia, distal numbness	Anti-Hu	Small cell carcinoma of lung, Hodgkin's disease	Chest radiograph, CT scan of the chest, nerve conduction studies
Myelitis[9]	Progressive spinal cord lesion (usually cervical cord)	Anti-Hu	Small cell carcinoma of lung	Chest radiograph, CT scan of the chest, MRI of the head and spinal cord
Subacute cerebellar degeneration[10–13]	Progressive ataxia, nystagmus (down-beating), vertigo	Anti-Yo Anti-Hu	Small cell carcinoma of lung, Ovarian cancer, Hodgkin's disease	Chest radiograph, CT scan of the chest, MRI of the head, pelvic ultrasound examination or CT scan, CSF (raised protein, oligoclonal bands)
Subacute motor neuropathy[9]	Subacute, patchy progressive, usually limb weakness and wasting	Anti-Hu	Small cell carcinoma of lung, Hodgkin's disease	Chest radiograph, CT scan of the chest, nerve conduction studies/EMG
Sensorimotor peripheral neuropathy[9]	Mild, nondisabling peripheral; limb numbness and parasthesia	Not known	Small cell carcinoma of lung, breast Another carcinoma	Chest radiograph, CT scan of the chest, nerve conduction studies/EMG
Lambert–Eaton myasthenic syndrome[10–12]	Weakness of proximal limb muscles, fatigue with exertion after initial recovery, areflexia	Anti-Ca^{++} channel	Small cell carcinoma of lung	Chest radiograph, CT scan of the chest, EMG

Dermatomyositis/polymyositis[14,15]	Proximal limb muscle weakness and pain, heliotrope skin rash, Grotten's papules on knuckles	Anti-Jo-1	Lung, breast, ovary	Chest radiograph, CT scan of the chest, Creatine kinase, EMG, muscle biopsy
Guillain–Barré syndrome	Ascending weakness, distal parasthesia	Not known	Hodgkin's disease	Nerve conduction studies/EMG

Abbreviations: CSF, cerebrospinal fluid; CT, computed topography; EMG, electromyography.

Polymyalgia rheumatica

Clinical presentation[14,16]
  Limb girdle pain and stiffness

Laboratory findings
- Elevated serum erythrocyte sedimentation rate (often not as high as in nonparaneoplastic polymyalgia rheumatica)
- And elevated C-reactive protein

Associated cancers
- Leukemia and lymphoma
- Myelodysplastic syndromes
- Cancer of the colon, lung,* renal, prostate, breast

Treatment options
- Prednisone 15 mg/d orally
- Methotrexate 10 mg/wk orally

Acanthosis nigricans

Clinical presentation
- Velvety, hyperpigmented skin (usually on flexural regions)
- Papillomatous changes involving mucous membranes and mucocutaneous junctions
- Rugose changes on palms and dorsal surface of large joints (eg, tripe palms)

Diagnostic studies
- Skin biopsy histology shows hyperkeratosis and papillomatosis

Associated cancers
- Adenocarcinoma of the abdominal organs, especially gastric adenocarcinoma (90% of malignancies in patients with acanthosis nigricans are abdominal)
- Gynecologic cancers

Treatment options
- Topical corticosteroids

Paraneoplastic Metabolic and Endocrinology Syndromes

Hypercalcemia

Malignant disease is the commonest cause of hypercalcemia in the hospital population, accounting for about 60% of cases, hyperparathyroidism being the second most frequent cause (**Table 2**).[19] About 8% of patients with lung cancer will be found to have hypercalcemia, and the majority of these patients will have squamous cell carcinoma.

Pathogenesis Hypercalcemia associated with tumors is most commonly caused by destruction of bone by osteolytic metastases. True ectopic parathyroid hormone production is extremely rare, but substances produced by lung cancers, especially *squamous carcinoma*, do have parathyroid hormone-like effects in that calcium is mobilized from bone at such a fast rate that the kidneys' ability to excrete it is exceeded, in part as a result of increased renal tubular absorption of calcium. A low plasma phosphate may also be found, as is the case in true hyperparathyroidism, in which phosphate excretion is promoted.

Clinical features The effect of hypercalcemia, regardless of whether it results from bony metastases or ectopic parathyroid hormone-like substance, is to produce polyuria, nocturia and thirst that persists resulting in dehydration, hypovolemia, and ultimately renal failure. As this situation develops, the patient may experience malaise, weakness, anorexia, nausea, vomiting, psychotic behavior, and ultimately coma. These symptoms may develop either insidiously or rapidly, so that the patient presents as a medical emergency.

Treatment Treatment should be vigorous if it is felt that the patient would benefit from therapeutic intervention. This may include resection of the tumor to correct the metabolic abnormality if the tumor is found to be operable. The mainstay of medical treatment is to correct associated dehydration with 3 to 6 L of IV saline per day and hypokalemia.

Hypercalcemia occurs in 3 forms
1. Mild: serum Ca++ level 10.5 to 11.9 mg/dL
2. Moderate: serum Ca++ level 12.0 to 13.9 mg/dL
3. Severe: serum Ca++ level ≥14 mg/dL

For severe hypercalcemia, or if plasma calcium level has not decreased significantly in the first 24 hours despite volume repletion, a loop diuretic such as furosemide should be given in addition to IV fluids to force a diuresis. If hypercalcemia persists despite these measures, sodium phosphate 500 mg of elemental phosphorus (1 phosphate Sandoz tablet) every 6 hours orally to inhibit bone resorption should be given for several days. Mithramycin is a cytotoxic antibiotic given intravenously as a single dose of 25 μg/kg in a liter of dextrose infused over 6 hours. Calcitonin subcutaneously or IV has been used alone or in combination with corticosteroids.

Table 2
Paraneoplastic endocrine/metabolic syndrome[1–3,5,6,14]

Syndrome	Clinical Features	Antibody or Hormone Secreted	Associated Tumors	Investigations
Hypercalcemia[15–29]	Polyuria, nocturia, thirst, malaise, weakness, dehydration, hypovolemia, constipation, obtundation, drowsiness, psychotic behavior, renal failure, ultimately coma	PTHrP	Squamous cell carcinoma of lung	Chest radiograph, CT scan of the chest, PET scan Serum Ca^{++} and PO_4 level, Serum PTH level Hypercalcemia occurs in 3 forms: Mild: serum Ca^{++} level 10.5–11.9 mg/dL Moderate: serum Ca^{++} level 12.0–13.9 mg/dL Severe: serum Ca^{++} level $\geq$14 mg/dL
Cushing syndrome[30,31]	Anorexia, mental slowing, psychosis, and muscle weakness, and presence of hypokalemic metabolic alkalosis	Ectopic ACT secretion resulting in production and release of cortisol, corticosterone, and to a lesser extent androgens and estrogens	Small cell lung cancer and bronchial carcinoid tumor	Chest radiograph, CT scan of the chest, MRI of the head, PET scan Elevated plasma cortisol level >29 µg/dL Failure to respond to high-dose dexamethasone suppression

(continued on next page)

Table 2
(continued)

Syndrome	Clinical Features	Antibody or Hormone Secreted	Associated Tumors	Investigations
Bronchial neuroendocrine carcinoid tumor producing carcinoid syndrome and carcinoid crisis[31–37]	Neoplastic enterochromaffin cells have features of Amine content, *Precursor Uptake,* and *Decarboxylation:* (APUD cell) Carcinoid crises	Kultschitzky cells (cells of origin are neoplastic enterochromaffin cells with affinity for silver) Enterochromaffin cells have secretory granules and lysosomes. Secretory granule is the site of biosynthesis, storage, and release of serotonin. Lysosomes are small vesicles containing destructive enzymes – hydrolases such as phosphatase and proteases such as kallikrein	Carcinoid tumors	Chest radiograph, CT scan of the chest, PET scan Liberation of the contents of the lysosome vesicles after protean stimuli, which includes trauma, anoxia, and catecholamines. These stimuli have clinical significance in the operating room where all may converge to initiate a massive release of kallikrein with resultant refractory hypotension and carcinoid crises manifesting with hypotension, severe diarrhea, bronchoconstriction
Galactorrhea[38]	Inappropriate uncontrolled discharge of milk-containing fluid from the	Elevated serum prolactin level above normal level of 9 µg/L	Mucoepidermoid bronchial carcinoma of lung	Chest radiograph, CT scan of the chest, PET scan

	breast which has persisted without stimulation for longer than 6 mo after childbirth			
Syndrome of excessive inappropriate antidiuretic hormone production and secretion (SIADH)[14,16,17,39]	Water intoxication, with anorexia, nausea, and vomiting, accompanied by increasingly severe neurologic complications. Impaired concentration with forgetfulness and confusion. With plasma sodium level of <115 mEq/L, seizures ard coma may occur. Hypo-osmotic hyponatremia. Inappropriately concentrated urine (urine osmolarity >100 mosmol/kg water) Euvolemia	Inappropriate ADH secretion (SIADH)	Small cell carcinoma of lung. Breast carcinoma	Chest radiograph, CT scan of the chest. PET scan. Hyponatremia: Mild: serum Na+ 130–134 mEq/L. Moderate: Serum Na+ 125–129 mEq/L. Severe: <125 mEq/L. Plasma osmolality: <275 mosmol/kg water (normal osmolality 285–295 mosmol/kg water). Inappropriately increased urine osmolality >200 mosmol/kg water
Gynecomastia[37,38]	Precocious puberty and gynecomastia	β-Human chorionic gonadotrophin (β-HCG) secreted by lung cancer: large cell and adenocarcinoma	Ectopic human chorionic gonadotrophin (β-HCG) secretion by lung cancer and germ cell tumors.	Chest radiograph. Chest CT scan. PET scan. Serum β-HCG stimulating testicular estrogen overproduction

(continued on next page)

Table 2
(continued)

Syndrome	Clinical Features	Antibody or Hormone Secreted	Associated Tumors	Investigations
Hypertrophic pulmonary osteoarthropathy[3,4,40]	Often resembles rheumatoid arthritis. Manifest by painful symmetric polyarthritis involving ankles, wrists, and knees Hypertrophic pulmonary osteoarthropathy is due to proliferative periostitis of long bones, often with little or no evidence of clubbing.	Cause is not known and may be due to a humoral agent	Non-small cell lung cancer of the adenocarcinoma cell type. Most patients are female over the age of 50 y. May present without clubbing. Gynecomastia may coexist with hypertrophic pulmonary osteoarthropathy.	Chest radiograph, CT scan of the chest, PET scan, radionuclide bone scans typically showing increased uptake at the distal ends of the affected long bones and evidence of new bone formation on plain films

Abbreviations: ACTH, adrenocorticotrophic hormone; CT, computed tomography; PTH, parathyroid hormone; PTHrP, PTH-related protein.

Syndrome of inappropriate antidiuretic hormone secretion

When significant hyponatremia (plasma sodium <120 mmol/L) occurs in association with lung cancer, it is usually part of the syndrome of inappropriate secretion of antidiuretic hormone. The histologic type involved is nearly always small cell carcinoma, reported in between 5% and 22% of patients.

Diagnostic criteria The syndrome of inappropriate secretion of antidiuretic hormone is characterized by dilutional hyponatremia, so that the plasma sodium is low in the presence of abnormal water retention, resulting in a low plasma osmolality (<260 mosmol/kg water). There is continued urinary loss of sodium but at a level inappropriate for the plasma sodium concentration (always >20 mmol/L and often >50 mmol/L) so that urine osmolality is disproportionately high, being at least twice that of the plasma (normal range of plasma osmolality 285–295 mosmol/kg water). If a plasma immunoassay of antidiuretic hormone is carried out, the level can be shown to be increased.

Clinical features The patient may be asymptomatic or may complain of anorexia, weakness, nausea, vomiting, and headache. As hyponatremia worsens, impaired concentration with forgetfulness and confusion may develop. With the plasma sodium level is less than 115 mmol/L, seizures and coma may occur.

Pathogenesis The syndrome of inappropriate secretion of antidiuretic hormone is rare in lung cancer other than small cell carcinoma. A prominent ultrastructural feature of this tumor group is the presence of neurosecretory granules. These granules may elaborate many different peptide hormones, of which antidiuretic hormone or arginine vasopressin is one. When antidiuretic hormone is produced inappropriately by a small cell carcinoma, its normal physiologic actions are uncontrolled, so that the epithelium of the collecting ducts of nephrons become increasingly permeable to water that is, reabsorbed into the hypertonic renal medullary tissues and thence to the blood, whereas sodium continues to be excreted in the usual manner. Extensive small cell carcinoma is more likely to produce these effects.

Treatment The cornerstone of the syndrome of inappropriate secretion of antidiuretic hormone is water deprivation, 500 mL of fluid being given per day in addition to the previous 24 hours' losses. Treatment of small cell lung cancer, usually with chemotherapy, may produce a prompt response. The antibiotic demeclocycline given orally has proved successful in doses of 900 to 1200 mg/d in divided doses with a maintenance dose of 600 to 900 mg/d. Furosemide at a dose of 40 to 80 mg/d is given to promote a diuresis and allowing unlimited fluids and replacing the electrolytes with 2 to 3 g salt daily.

Ectopic adrenocorticotrophic hormone syndrome

Abnormalities of cortisol metabolism may be found in more than 40% of patients with small cell carcinoma. These usually take the form of a loss of diurnal variation or failure of cortisol to suppress after dexamethasone. Despite this, the clinical syndrome of ectopic adrenocorticotrophic hormone secretion has been found to be present in less than 8% of patients with small cell carcinoma. Patients do not ordinarily develop the signs associated with Cushing's syndrome. The diagnosis is usually made when symptoms such as anorexia, mental slowing, or psychosis and muscle weakness, which may be profound, are associated with the finding of a hypokalemic metabolic alkalosis, owing to the urinary loss of potassium. Confirmation of the diagnosis is made by the (i) finding of an elevated cortisol level with loss of diurnal variation, (ii) failure of the morning cortisol level to suppress after 2 mg dexamethasone given every 6 hours for 2 days, and (iii) elevated levels of plasma adrenocorticotrophic hormone.

The biochemical abnormality responds to treatment of the tumor with chemotherapy, by tumor resection if limited disease, bilateral adrenalectomy, or oral treatment with aminoglutethimide to inhibit steroid synthesis in the adrenal cortex.

Hypertrophic pulmonary osteoarthropathy

Hypertrophic pulmonary osteoarthropathy is a syndrome characterized by periostitis of long bones, most commonly affecting the tibia, fibula, radius, and ulna at their distal ends, so that the patient complains of pain and swelling of the wrists, ankles, and knee joints, which are hot and tender to touch. Clubbing of the digits is found in more than 90% of cases and is often gross.

Pathogenesis Hypertrophic pulmonary osteoarthropathy is most commonly associated with adenocarcinoma of the lung, being found in up to 12% of cases and in other cell types but it is rarely associated with small cell carcinoma. It has been shown that blood flow to the calf and forearm is increased in hypertrophic pulmonary osteoarthropathy, and this hyperemia is directed particularly toward connective tissue and bone. Where finger clubbing is present, the digits and nail beds are also hyperemic and, in both cases, this increased perfusion is likely due to the opening up of fine arteriovenous anastomoses in both the dermis and periosteum. The periostitis results in loosely packed new bone being laid down outside the original cortex, producing the characteristic bony radiographic changes.

Although the mechanism by which cancer produces hypertrophic pulmonary osteoarthropathy is obscure, there is some evidence to support a vagally mediated afferent neural output from the tumor-bearing lung playing a role. It was noted in the 1950s that division of the vagal branches around the hilum by suprahilar vagotomy during unsuccessful attempts to resect lung cancer resulted in symptomatic relief, with regression of pain and swelling in hypertrophic pulmonary osteoarthropathy. Afferent vagal fibers synapse in the medulla of the brain and there is even greater uncertainty regarding subsequent efferent pathways to the target tissues in the limbs.

Investigations When the diagnosis is suspected, radiographs of the lower end of the radius, ulna, tibia, and fibula and the whole hands are indicated. If the knees are painful, the proximal tibia and fibula and distal femoral shaft should also be x-rayed. The characteristic radiographic finding is a 1 to 2 mm line shadow running parallel to the cortex. This parallel line is the lifted periosteum separated from the cortex by a radiolucent zone. The active deposition of new bone along the inner aspect of the periosteum can be demonstrated on nuclear bone scan using technetium-99m pyrophosphate.

Treatment
1. Thoracotomy undertaken for attempted cure by successful removal of tumor for dramatic response.
2. Nonsteroidal anti-inflammatory drug with indomethacin.
3. Corticosteroid may produce relief like indomethacin.

Gynecomastia

This may occasionally occur in association with lung cancer; the histologic types most frequently found are large cell and adenocarcinoma. The mechanism is thought to involve the production and secretion of human chorionic gonadotrophin by tumor cells, this substance resulting in testicular estrogen overproduction. Chorionic somatomammotrophin (also known as human placental lactogen) is another hormone that may be produced by lung cancer and that might cause gynecomastia. Successful surgical resection of the lung cancer deals with this complication.

Somatostatinoma syndrome

Increased hypothalamic hormone somatostatin (also known as growth hormone release-inhibiting factor) levels have been reported in a few patients with small cell lung cancer. It may produce a rare syndrome comprising abdominal pain, vomiting, diarrhea, cholelithiasis, and diabetes mellitus.

Eosinophilia

An association between bronchogenic carcinoma and blood eosinophilia results from increased bone marrow production, prolonged eosinophil survival time or the production of an eosinophilotactic factor. A high total white cell count, neutrophilia, and eosinophilia results. It tends to be associated advanced and rapidly progressive cancer with a risk for eosinophilic endomyocardial disease (Loffler's endocarditis) resulting in cardiac failure.

Carcinoid syndrome and carcinoid crisis

Carcinoid syndrome and carcinoid crisis is due to the oversecretion of 5-hydroxytryptamine and other and vasoactive peptides from neuroendocrine tumors.[31–36] Episodic flushing is the most common feature, which can become a fixed facial erythema after some time. Diarrhea and abdominal colic are also part of the syndrome, as may be bronchospasm. Right heart failure with the murmur of tricuspid regurgitation, owing to endocardial fibrosis, also occurs with time.

Carcinoid tumors Pulmonary carcinoid tumors, typical and atypical types, are rarely associated with carcinoid syndrome and even less commonly with carcinoid crisis. The cell of origin of the tumors, is the granular, chromium-staining cells of the crypt described in the nineteenth century by Kultschitzky and others. Carcinoid tumors are endocrinologically active under certain circumstances. Page and co-workers showed an increase in 5-hydroxyindolacetic acid in the urine of a patient with carcinoid syndrome.

Carcinoid tumors accounts for 1% to 2% of all invasive lung malignancies. The treatment of choice of pulmonary carcinoids is surgical resection. Patients with typical carcinoid have an excellent prognosis and rarely die from their tumors. Five to 10% of typical carcinoids have regional lymph node involvement that does not affect their clinical outcome. Compared with typical carcinoid, atypical carcinoid presents with a larger tumor size, a higher rate of metastases in regional lymph nodes and distant (5%–15% regional lymph node metastases at presentation in typical carcinoid compared with 40%–48% in atypical carcinoid and higher rate of distant metastases in atypical carcinoid at 20% and rare in typical carcinoid), and a significantly lower survival rate at 5 years at 58% in atypical carcinoid and much favorable at 90% to 95% in typical carcinoid.

Pathophysiology of carcinoid syndrome The carcinoid syndrome is an endocrine manifestation of neoplastic enterochromaffin cells. The entero-chromaffin cell belongs to a larger family which has been characterized for sharing the features of *a*mine content, *p*recursor *u*ptake, and *d*ecar-boxylation (hence the mnemonic name APUD).

The enterochromaffin cell has 2 ultrastructural characteristics: secretory granules and lyso-somes. The secretory granule is the site of biosyn-thesis, storage, and release of serotonin. The lysosomes are small vesicles with thin membranes in which are packaged a dangerous array of destructive enzymes, for example, hydrolases such as acid phosphatase and proteases such as kallikrein. Liberation of the contents of these vesicles follows protean stimuli, which include trauma, anoxia, and catecholamines. These stim-uli have clinical significance in the operating room where all may converge to initiate a massive release of kallikrein with resultant refractory hypo-tension and carcinoid crisis.

Serotonin Serotonin is synthesized by the hydrox-ylation of the essential amino acid tryptophane to form 5-hydroxytryptophane and subsequent decarboxylation to 5-hyroxytryptamine (seroto-nin). Most serotonin remains in the secretory gran-ules where it is synthesized. Catabolism occurs by deamination by the ubiquitous monoamine oxi-dase to form 5-hudroxyindoleacetaldehyde, which is then oxidized by aldehyde dehydrogenase to form 5-hydroxyindoleacetic acid, which is excreted in the urine.

Bradykinin The release of kallikrein from carcinoid tumors by adrenergic stimulation, ethanol inges-tion, and other factors, catalyzes the conversion of kininogen to lysyl-bradykinin. In plasma the *N*-terminal lysine is cleaved off by aminopeptidase to liberate bradykinin, one of the most potent va-sodilators. In addition, it is a bronchoconstrictor and a stimulant of intestinal motility. The half-life of bradykinin is brief. It is rapidly catabolized to inactive peptides and amino acids by several kini-nases (**Fig. 1**).

Somatostatin analogues can control carcinoid syndrome or crisis with tumors of gastrointestinal origin. Flushing is a vasomotor sign characterized by a brief paroxysmal pink flush of the face and neck associated with transient drop in blood pres-sure. The flushes are precipitated by ethanol, exer-tion, emotion, and other factors. Bradykinin does

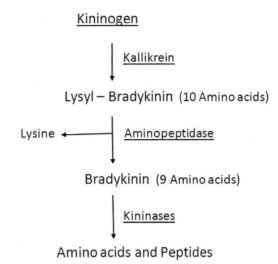

Fig. 1. The role of kallikrein in the activation of bradykinin.

reproduce the symptom from endogenous or exogenous epinephrine stimulation causing the release of kallikrein, which results in activation of bradykinin. Flushing over the face spreads over the chest and arms and eventually telangiectasia may develop. Facial flush may be accompanied by facial edema, and it responds favorably to steroids.

Carcinoid crisis

The responsiveness of carcinoid tumors to regula-tory mediators is of practical importance in the management of fulminant episodes of mediator release that may be associated with anesthesia, surgery, or aggressive chemotherapy.[31–36] Such carcinoid crises may include hypotension, severe diarrhea, and bronchoconstriction. Because cate-cholamines are powerful stimuli for the release of the carcinoid vasodilators, the use of drugs with β-adrenergic actions must be avoided in carcinoid crises.

Somatostatin analogue, in contrast, represents a rational pharmacologic intervention for the treat-ment of the crises associated with massive release of mediators from enterochromaffin-cell neo-plasms. A case report by Riyad Karmy-Jones and Eric Vallieres[32] on the patient with carcinoid crisis after biopsy of a bronchial carcinoid tumor and subsequent safe resection of the functional typical carcinoid tumor after 10 days of preopera-tive preparation with three daily subcutaneous doses of 50-μg octreotide (a somatostatin analogue) and cimetidine 400 mg orally twice daily before right lower lobectomy. Perioperative man-agement of patients with carcinoid tumors in-cludes the avoidance of known precipitating agents, proper hydration, and the use of cimetidine to inhibit histamine release, and the importance of somatostatin. Somatostatin naturally inhibits the release of a variety of peptides, including serotonin, by blocking calcium channels. In carcinoids, it diminishes the synthesis and secretion of serotonin via a second messenger system. Long-acting somatostatin analogues have been used as prophylaxis for and treatment of both carcinoid syndrome and carcinoid crisis. A somatostatin analogue may be life-saving in the rare event of carcinoid crisis associated bronchopulmonary carcinoids. The publication cites the incidence of carcinoid syndrome to be 2% to 12%, and the rarity of the syndrome as well as the carcinoid crisis in the absence of spread.

Biochemical factors The cause of carcinoid syndrome and carcinoid crisis are related to secretion of vasoactive peptides, of which histamine and serotonin are believed to cause the carcinoid syndrome. Carcinoid crisis manifests with severe hypertension, flushing, and acidosis owing to serotonin release or hypotension, diarrhea, and bronchoconstriction attributable to kallikrein or histamine release. Pulmonary carcinoid tumors are rarely associated with carcinoid syndromes and even less commonly with carcinoid crisis. Somatostatin analogues can control carcinoid syndrome or crisis with tumors of gastrointestinal origin.

The carcinoid syndrome typically occurs when degrading enzymatic systems in liver or lung are bypassed or overwhelmed. The incidence of carcinoid syndrome is 2% to 12%, and the syndrome as well as the crisis are rare in the absence of tumor spread.

Pulmonary carcinoid tumors are rarely associated with carcinoid syndromes and even less commonly with carcinoid crisis. Somatostatin analogues can control carcinoid syndrome or crisis owing to tumors of gastrointestinal origin.

PARANEOPLASTIC NEUROLOGIC SYNDROMES

Paraneoplastic neurologic syndromes result from immune cross-reactivity between tumor cells and components of the nervous system.[2,11] In response to a developing cancer, a patient produces tumor-directed antibodies known as onconeural antibodies. Because of antigenic similarity, these onconeural antibodies and associated onconeural antigens of cases, specific T lymphocytes inadvertently attack components of the nervous system as well. In contrast with paraneoplastic endocrinologic syndromes, paraneoplastic syndromes are detected before cancer

is diagnosed in 80% of cases. Because tumor cells themselves do not directly produce the causative agents of paraneoplastic syndromes, and because onconeural antibodies may cause permanent damage, successful cancer treatment does not necessarily result in neurologic improvement. Immunosuppressive therapy is a mainstay of paraneoplastic syndrome treatment.

Paraneoplastic neurologic syndromes can affect the central nervous system (eg, limbic encephalitis and paraneoplastic subacute cerebellar degeneration, the neuromuscular junction (eg, Lambert–Eaton myasthenia syndrome, or the peripheral nervous system (eg, autonomic neuropathy and subacute sensory neuropathy), and retinopathy.

Paraneoplastic Subacute Cerebellar Degeneration

Several early reports showed an association between cerebellar degeneration and malignancy.[10–13,31] Small cell lung cancer in particular is more likely to be associated compared with ovarian cancer, breast cancer, and Hodgkin's lymphoma. Subacute cerebellar degeneration results in a rapidly progressive loss of cerebellar function. Ataxic gait, lack of coordination, vertigo, nystagmus, and dysarthria are the characteristic features. Diffuse degeneration and depletion of Purkinje cells, as well as other degenerative changes, occur in the cerebellum.

Clinical presentation may be quite pronounced with the onset of:

- Cerebellar ataxia with impaired gait and coordination progressing over weeks interfering with walking
- Loss of coordination in the upper and lower extremities
- Dysarthria and nystagmus associated with oscillopsia
- Profound interference with daily living by limiting ambulation, vision, and communication
- Diplopia
- Dysphagia
- Prodrome of dizziness, nausea, vomiting

The pathogenesis of paraneoplastic subacute cerebellar degeneration is thought to be related to an autoimmune phenomenon characterized by destruction of Purkinje cells. In contrast, 2 patients with paraneoplastic subacute cerebellar degeneration with small cell lung cancer had antibodies directed against neuronal nuclear antigens, termed anti-Hu antibodies, which are also commonly associated with paraneoplastic encephalomyelitis. In addition, researchers using specific assays to detect antibodies against Purkinje cell antigens, also termed anti-yo antibodies, reported positive results in patients with gynecologic malignancies and paraneoplastic subacute cerebellar degeneration, but patients with small cell lung cancer and paraneoplastic subacute cerebellar degeneration were frequently negative.

Treatment for paraneoplastic subacute cerebellar degeneration in patients with small cell lung cancer has been disappointing, perhaps because the autoimmune process leads to rapid cerebellar damage that is difficult to ameliorate unless the diagnosis is made relatively quickly. There have been reports in which chemotherapy and irradiation in the treatment of small cell lung cancer stopped the progression of the cerebellar signs and symptoms of paraneoplastic subacute cerebellar degeneration and even reverse these effects in some cases.

Paone and Jeyasingham[13] reported a case of paraneoplastic subacute cerebellar degeneration in a patient with limited small cell lung cancer in whom the cerebellar signs and symptoms resolved after surgery for pneumonectomy.[31,49] IVIG has been reported to be effective in helping slow the progression of paraneoplastic subacute cerebellar degeneration when diagnosed early and even reverse the profound effects while definitive treatment of the tumor is undertaken. Plasmapheresis has been of limited value in the treatment of this disease.

Diagnostic studies
- PET with fluorodeoxyglucose: increased metabolism (early stage) and then decreased metabolism (late stage) in cerebellum
- MRI: cerebellar atrophy (late stage)

Associated cancers
- Small cell lung cancer*
- Hodgkin lymphoma
- Breast cancer
- Gynecologic cancers

Treatment options
- IVIG, 400 to 1000 mg/d to a total of 2 to 3 g
- Methylprednisolone, up to 1 g/d IV
- Plasma exchange
- Cyclophosphamide
- Rituximab, 375 mg/m² IV per dose

The Myasthenic Lambert–Eaton Syndrome

A report was published in 1953 by Anderson and colleagues[10,11] in which a patient with oat cell carcinoma of the lung was noted to have neuromuscular weakness. Subsequently in 1956, Lambert, Eaton, and Rooke published their classic report of "an unusual defect of neuromuscular conduction in patients with malignant tumor in the chest," distinct from that seen in typical myasthenia gravis. The constellation of signs, symptoms, physical findings, and electrophysiologic results noted in patients with small cell lung cancer came to be known as Lambert–Eaton myasthenic syndrome. The patient presents with proximal muscle weakness that, in contrast with myasthenia gravis, improves with repeated effort. These changes are reflected in the electromyographic findings, which show initially small action potentials in affected muscle, increasing in amplitude with repetitive electrical stimulation.

Proximal muscle weakness, hyporeflexia, and autonomic dysfunction (dry mouth, erectile dysfunction, constipation, and blurred vision) characterize Lambert–Eaton myasthenia syndrome. The pathognomonic electromyographic finding is a marked increase of the compound muscle action potential after high rates of nerve stimulation. Similarly, augmentation of strength and reflexes can be demonstrated after maximal contraction of the involved muscle groups.

Clinical manifestations are due to antibodies to P/Q type voltage-gated calcium channels expressed on the presynaptic cholinergic synapses of peripheral nerves that interfere with the release of acetylcholine. These voltage-gated calcium channels also appear on small cell lung cancer cells.

Clinical presentation
- Lower extremity proximal muscle weakness, fatigue
- Diaphragmatic weakness
- Bulbar symptoms (usually milder than in myasthenia gravis) later in the disease course
- Autonomic symptoms (ptosis, impotence, dry mouth) in most patients

Associated antibodies
- Anti-VGCC (P/Q type)

Diagnostic studies
- Electromyography: low compound muscle action potential amplitude: decremental response with low-rate stimulation but incremental response with high rate of stimulation.

Associated cancers
- Small cell lung cancer (3% of patients have Lambert–Eaton myasthenia syndrome)*

- Prostate cancer
- Lymphomas
- Adenocarcinomas

Treatment options
- 3,4-DAP, maximum of 80 mg/d orally – 3,4-di-amino pyridine increases presynaptic calcium influx
- Guanidine, 575 mg/d orally with pyridostigmine
- Pyridostigmine, 240 to 360 mg/d orally (with guanidine) – inhibits acetylcholinesterase
- Prednisolone, 60 to 100 mg orally every other day
- Azathioprine, up to 2.5 mg/kg/d orally
- IVIG, 400 to 1000 mg/d to a total of 2 to 3 g
- Plasma exchange
- Treatment of the underlying tumor: approximately one-third to one-half of patients with Lambert–Eaton myasthenia syndrome improve with treatment of the underlying small cell lung cancer.

Autonomic Neuropathy

Clinical presentation
- Panautonomic neuropathy, often subacute onset (weeks), involving sympathetic, parasympathetic, and enteric systems
- Orthostatic postural hypotension
- Gastrointestinal dysfunction: dry eyes/mouth; bowel/bladder dysfunction; altered pupillary light reflexes; loss of sinus arrhythmia
- Chorionic growth hormone-prolactin (CGP): disturbances of gastrointestinal motility including intestinal pseudo-obstruction, constipation, nausea/vomiting, dysphagia, weight loss, abdominal distension

Associated antibodies
- Anti-Hu
- Anti-CRMP5 (anti-CV2)
- Anti-nAchR
- Anti-amphiphysin

Diagnostic studies
- Abdominal radiography/barium studies/CT scan: gastrointestinal dilatation but no mechanical obstruction (for CGP)
- Esophageal manometry: achalasia or spasms (for CGP)

Associated cancers
- Small cell lung cancer*
- Thymoma

Treatment options
- For orthostatic hypotension: water, salt intake
  Fludrocortisone, 0.1 to 1.0 mg/d orally
  Midodrine, 2.5 to 10 mg orally 3 times daily
- Caffeine, 200 mg/d orally
- For pseudo-obstruction
  Neostigmine, 2 mg IV

Subacute Peripheral Sensory, motor, or Mixed Neuropathy

Clinical presentation
- Paresthesia/pain (typically upper extremities before lower), followed by ataxia[2,4,5,9,11]
- Multifocal/asymmetric distribution.
- All sensory modalities decreased, but especially deep sensation or pseudoarthrosis of hands
- Deep tendon reflexes decreased or absent
- Muscle weakness and wasting with loss of deep tendon reflexes
- Stocking and glove hypoesthesia
- Onset over weeks to months

Associated antibodies
- Anti-Hu
- Anti-CRMP5 (anti-CV2)
- Anti-amphiphysin

Diagnostic studies
- Nerve conduction studies: decreased or absent sensory nerve action potentials
- Cerebrospinal fluid analysis: pleocytosis, high IgG, oligoclonal bands

Associated cancers
- Lung (70%–80%), usually small cell lung cancer*
- Breast
- Ovarian
- Sarcomas
- Hodgkin lymphoma

Treatment options
- Methylprednisolone, up to 1 g/d IV
- Cyclophosphamide 3 mg/kg/d orally
- IVIG, 400 to 1000 mg/d to a total of 2 to 3 g
- Plasma exchange

Limbic Encephalitis

Clinical presentation
- Mood changes
- Hallucinations
- Memory loss
- Seizures

- Less commonly: hypothalamic symptoms (hyperthermia, somnolence, endocrine dysfunction); onset over days to months

Associated antibodies
- Anti-Hu (typically with small cell lung cancer)
- Anti-Ma2 (typically testicular cancer)
- Anti-CRMP5 (anti-CV2)
- Anti-amphiphysin

Diagnostic studies
- Electroencephalography: epileptic foci in temporal lobe(s); focal or generalized slow activity
- PET with fluorodeoxyglucose: increased metabolism in temporal lobe(s)
- MRI: hyperintensity in medial temporal lobe(s)
- Cerebrospinal fluid analysis: pleocytosis, elevated protein, elevated IgG, oligoclonal bands

Associated cancers
- Small cell lung cancer* (40% to 50% of patients with limbic encephalitis)
- Testicular germ cell (20% of patients with limbic encephalitis)
- Breast cancer (8% of patients with limbic encephalitis)
- Thymoma, teratoma, Hodgkin lymphoma

Treatment options
- IVIG, 400 to 1000 mg/d to a total of 2 to 3 g
- Methylprednisolone, up to 1 g/d IV
- Prednisone, 1 mg/kg/d orally
- Plasma exchange
- Cyclophosphamide, 2 mg/kg/d orally
- Rituximab, 375 mg/m^2 IV per dose

Acute Transverse Myelopathy

This paraneoplastic association is very rare and may evolve rapidly, giving rise to a flaccid paraparesis with a sensory level and loss of sphincter control. The condition may be difficult to distinguish from spinal cord metastases or radiation myelopathy.

Progressive Multifocal Leukoencephalopathy

This condition is no longer considered to be a true paraneoplastic syndrome because it is caused by a papova virus infection in the brain of an immunocompromised host. It results in progressive intellectual deterioration with an impaired consciousness level and an advancing motor and sensory deficit, which may include cortical blindness.

SUMMARY

Paraneoplastic syndromes are clinical entities associated with cancers and often overlap with metabolic and endocrine syndromes. The cell types of lung cancer involved are frequently small cell, squamous cell, adenocarcinoma, large cell, and carcinoid tumor.

Management

Management is directed at the primary tumor and the paraneoplastic manifestations. Occasionally, successful therapy of the tumor is associated with improvement of the paraneoplastic syndrome. Some improvement may occur after IV administration of immunoglobulins.

Systemic paraneoplastic manifestations in lung cancer have been described. Besides producing sometimes unexpected symptoms and signs by may of metastases, primary lung cancer can also be responsible for other syndromes for which the presence of tumor cannot be directly implicated. The management is directed at the primary tumor and the paraneoplastic manifestations.

In addition to generalized clinical features that are commonly associated with the presentation of malignant disease, there are a variety of syndromes for which the term paraneoplastic has been used. These syndromes include many that arise as a result of the secretion into the blood of tumor products (usually polypeptide hormones) which produce clinical symptoms and signs as a consequence of their action on target organs remote from the primary tumor.

A number of neurologic paraneoplastic syndromes have been described for which the tumor product remains unknown. These include peripheral neuropathies, a myasthenia-like syndrome, and subacute cerebellar degeneration. Although all of these syndromes may improve with successful treatment of the primary tumor, complete resolution is rare.

Endocrinological syndromes are particularly associated with small cell carcinoma. These include (1) Cushing's syndrome with hyperplasia of the adrenal cortex and (2) inappropriate secretion of antidiuretic hormone, leading to hyponatremia which cannot be attributed to bone metastases.

Neurologic syndromes include a peripheral neuromyopathy and subacute cerebellar degeneration.

Other syndromes include dermatomyositis, hypertrophic pulmonary osteoarthropathy, polymyositis, and thrombophlebitis migrans, and retinopathy.[5]

CLINICS CARE POINTS

- Definition and classification of paraneoplastic syndromes and identification of paraneoplastic dermatological and rheumatological syndromes, paraneoplastic neurological syndromes, polymyalgia rheumatica, paraneoplastic metabolic and endocrinology syndromes, hypercalcemia, Cushing syndrome, Carcinoid syndrome and Carcinoid crisis, syndrome of excessive inappropriate antidiuretic hormone secretion, Hypertrophic pulmonary osteoarthropathy, Paraneoplastic neurologic syndromes, Myasthenic Lambert-Eaton Syndrome.

- Clinical presentation of the paraneoplastic metabolic and hormone syndromes and neurologic syndromes.

- Biochemistry and antibodies markers of syndromes.

- Drugs used in the management.

REFERENCES

1. Maurer LH. Ectopic hormone syndromes in small cell carcinoma of the lung. Clin Oncol 1985;4:67.
2. Posner JB. Non-metastatic effects of cancer on the nervous system. In: Wyngaarden JB, Smith LH, editors. Textbook of medicine. Philadelphia: W.B. Saunders; 1982.
3. Patel AM, Davila DG, Peters SG, et al. Paraneoplastic syndromes associated with lung cancer. Mayo Clin Proc 1993;68:278–87.
4. Ashokakumar MP, Davila DG, Peters SG. Paraneoplastic syndromes associated with lung cancer. Mayo Clin Proc 1993;68(3):278–87.
5. Kanaji N, Watanabe N, Kita N, et al. Paraneoplastic syndromes associated with lung cancer. World J Clin Oncol 2014;5(3):197–223.
6. Le Roux BT. Bronchial carcinoma. London: E. & S. Livingstone LTD; 1968.
7. Editors Deslauriers J, Pearson FG, Shamji FM. Thoracic Surgery Clinics. Lung Cancer, Part I (May 2013); Consulting Editor M. Blair Marshall.
8. Editors Deslauriers J, Pearson FG, Shamji FM. Thoracic Surgery Clinics. Lung Cancer, Part II (August 2013); Consulting Editor M. Blair Marshall.
9. Dalmau J, Graus F, Rosenblum MK. Anti-Hu-associated paraneoplastic encephalomyelitis/sensory neuronopathy: a clinical study of 71 patients. Medicine 1992;71:59–72.
10. Lennon VA, Kryzer TJ, Griesmann GE, et al. Calcium-channel antibodies in the Lambert-Eaton syndrome and other paraneoplastic syndromes. N Engl J Med 1995;332(22):1467–74.
11. Dalmau J, Posner JB. Paraneoplastic syndromes affecting the nervous system. Semin Oncol 1997; 24:318–28.
12. Satoyoshi E, Kowa H, Fukunaga N. Subacute cerebellar degeneration and Eaton-Lambert syndrome with bronchogenic carcinoma. Neurology 1973;23:764.
13. Paone JR, Jeyasingham K. Remission of cerebellar dysfunction after pneumonectomy for bronchogenic carcinoma. New Engl J Med 1980;302:156.
14. Haslett C, Chilvers ER, Hunter JA, et al, editors. Davidson's principles and practice of medicine. 18th edition. Chapter 12. Churchill Livingstone, 1999. p. 801–76.
15. Dalakas MC. Polymyositis and dermatomyositis. Lancet 2003;362:971–82.
16. Hainsworth JD, Workman R, Greco A. Management of the syndrome of inappropriate antidiuretic hormone secretion in small cell lung cancer. Cancer 1983;51:161–5.
17. Tai P, Yu E, Jones K, et al. Syndrome of inappropriate antidiuretic hormone secretion (SIADH) in patients with limited stage small cell lung cancers. Lung Cancer 2006;53:211–5.
18. Bender RA, Hansen H. Hypercalcemia in bronchogenic carcinoma: a prospective study of 200 patients. Ann Intern Med 1974;80:205–8.
19. Burtis WJ. Parathyroid hormone-related protein: structure, function, and measurement. Clin Chem 1986;4:1191–8.
20. Fisken RA, Heath DA, Bold AM. Hypercalcemia – a hospital survey. Q J Med 1980;49:405.
21. Chopra D, Clerkin EP. Hypercalcemia, and malignant disease. Med Clin N Am 1975;59:441.
22. Ralston S, Fogelman I, Gardner MD, et al. Hypercalcemia and metastatic bone disease: is there a causal link? Lancet 1982;2:903.
23. Stevenson JC. Malignant Hypercalcemia. Br Med J 1985;291:421.
24. Ralston S, Fogelman I, Gardner MD, et al. Hypercalcemia of malignancy: evidence for a non-parathyroid humoral agent with an effect on renal tubular handling of calcium. Clin Sci 1984;66:187.
25. Wilkinson R. Treatment of hypercalcemia associated with malignancy. Br Med J 1984;288:812.
26. Mundy GR, Wilkinson R, Heath DA. Comparative study of available medical therapy for hypercalcemia of malignancy. Am J Med 1983;74:421.
27. Suki WN, Yium JJ, von Minden M, et al. Acute treatment of hypercalcemia with furosemide. New Engl J Med 1970;283:836.
28. Mazzaferri EL, O'Dorisio TM, LoBuglio AF. Treatment of hypercalcemia associated with malignancy. Semin Oncol 1978;5:141.
29. Ilias I, Torpy DJ, Pacak K, et al. Cushing's syndrome due to ectopic corticotropin secretion: twenty years'

experience at the National Institutes of Health. J Clin Endocrinol Metab 2005;90:4955–62.

30. Arnaldi G, Angeli A, Atkinson AB, et al. Diagnosis and complications of Cushing's syndrome: a consensus statement. J Clin Endocrinol Metab 2003;88:5593–602.

31. Hunt BM, Horton MP, Vallières E. Bronchogenic carcinoid tumors that are 18F-fluorodeoxyglucose avid on positron emission tomography. Eur J Cardio-Thoracic Surg 2014;45:527–30.

32. Karmy-Jones R, Vallières E. Carcinoid crisis after biopsy of a bronchial carcinoid. Ann Thorac Surg 1993;56:1403–5.

33. Gupta P, Kaur R. Management of bronchial carcinoid: an anesthetic challenge. Indian J Anaesth 2014;58(2):202–5.

34. Oates JA. The Carcinoid Syndrome. N Engl J Med 1986;315(11):702–4.

35. Hughes EW, Hodkinson BP. Carcinoid syndrome: the combined use of ketanserin and octreotide in the management of an acute crisis during anaesthesia. Anaesth Intensive Care 1989;17(3): 367–9.

36. Braunstein GD, Vaitukaitis JL, Carbone PP, et al. Ectopic production of human chorionic gonadotrophin by neoplasms. Ann Int Med 1973;78:39.

37. Rabson AS, Rosen SW, Tashjian AH, et al. production of human chorionic gonadotrophin in vitro by a cell line derived from a carcinoma of the lung. J Nat Cancer Inst 1973;50:669.

38. Rosen SW, Weintraub BD, Vaitukaitis JL, et al. Placental proteins and their subunits as tumor markers. Ann Intern Med 1975;82:71.

39. List AF, Hainsworth JD, Davis BW, et al. The syndrome of inappropriate secretion of anti-diuretic hormone in small cell lung cancer. J Clin Oncol 1986;4: 1191–8.

40. Qian X, Qin J. Hypertrophic pulmonary osteoarthropathy with primary lung cancer. Oncol Lett 2014; 7(6):2079–208.

UNITED STATES POSTAL SERVICE®

Statement of Ownership, Management, and Circulation
(All Periodicals Publications Except Requester Publications)

1. Publication Title	2. Publication Number	3. Filing Date
THORACIC SURGERY CLINICS	013 – 126	9/18/2021

4. Issue Frequency	5. Number of Issues Published Annually	6. Annual Subscription Price
FEB, MAY, AUG, NOV	4	$397.00

7. Complete Mailing Address of Known Office of Publication (Not printer) (Street, city, county, state, and ZIP+4®)

ELSEVIER INC.
230 Park Avenue, Suite 800
New York, NY 10169

Contact Person
Malathi Samayan
Telephone (Include area code)
91-44-4299-4507

8. Complete Mailing Address of Headquarters or General Business Office of Publisher (Not printer)

ELSEVIER INC.
230 Park Avenue, Suite 800
New York, NY 10169

9. Full Names and Complete Mailing Addresses of Publisher, Editor, and Managing Editor (Do not leave blank)

Publisher (Name and complete mailing address)
Dolores Meloni, ELSEVIER INC.
1600 JOHN F KENNEDY BLVD. SUITE 1800
PHILADELPHIA, PA 19103-2899

Editor (Name and complete mailing address)
JOHN VASSALLO, ELSEVIER INC.
1600 JOHN F KENNEDY BLVD. SUITE 1800
PHILADELPHIA, PA 19103-2899

Managing Editor (Name and complete mailing address)
PATRICK MANLEY, ELSEVIER INC.
1600 JOHN F KENNEDY BLVD. SUITE 1800
PHILADELPHIA, PA 19103-2899

10. Owner (Do not leave blank. If the publication is owned by a corporation, give the name and address of the corporation immediately followed by the names and addresses of all stockholders owning or holding 1 percent or more of the total amount of stock. If not owned by a corporation, give the names and addresses of the individual owners. If owned by a partnership or other unincorporated firm, give its name and address as well as those of each individual owner. If the publication is published by a nonprofit organization, give its name and address.)

Full Name	Complete Mailing Address
WHOLLY OWNED SUBSIDIARY OF REED/ELSEVIER US HOLDINGS	1600 JOHN F KENNEDY BLVD, SUITE 1800 PHILADELPHIA, PA 19103-2899

11. Known Bondholders, Mortgagees, and Other Security Holders Owning or Holding 1 Percent or More of Total Amount of Bonds, Mortgages, or Other Securities. If none, check box ► ☐ None

Full Name	Complete Mailing Address
N/A	

12. Tax Status (For completion by nonprofit organizations authorized to mail at nonprofit rates) (Check one)
The purpose, function, and nonprofit status of this organization and the exempt status for federal income tax purposes:
☒ Has Not Changed During Preceding 12 Months
☐ Has Changed During Preceding 12 Months (Publisher must submit explanation of change with this statement)

PS Form 3526, July 2014 [Page 1 of 4 (see instructions page 4)] PSN: 7530-01-000-9931   PRIVACY NOTICE: See our privacy policy on www.usps.com.

---

13. Publication Title			14. Issue Date for Circulation Data Below
THORACIC SURGERY CLINICS			MAY 2021

15. Extent and Nature of Circulation			Average No. Copies Each Issue During Preceding 12 Months	No. Copies of Single Issue Published Nearest to Filing Date
a. Total Number of Copies (Net press run)			223	202
b. Paid Circulation (By Mail and Outside the Mail)	(1)	Mailed Outside-County Paid Subscriptions Stated on PS Form 3541 (Include paid distribution above nominal rate, advertiser's proof copies, and exchange copies)	100	98
	(2)	Mailed In-County Paid Subscriptions Stated on PS Form 3541 (Include paid distribution above nominal rate, advertiser's proof copies, and exchange copies)	0	0
	(3)	Paid Distribution Outside the Mails Including Sales Through Dealers and Carriers, Street Vendors, Counter Sales, and Other Paid Distribution Outside USPS®	77	73
	(4)	Paid Distribution by Other Classes of Mail Through the USPS (e.g., First-Class Mail®)	0	0
c. Total Paid Distribution (Sum of 15b (1), (2), (3), and (4))			177	171
d. Free or Nominal Rate Distribution (By Mail and Outside the Mail)	(1)	Free or Nominal Rate Outside-County Copies included on PS Form 3541	27	16
	(2)	Free or Nominal Rate In-County Copies Included on PS Form 3541	0	0
	(3)	Free or Nominal Rate Copies Mailed at Other Classes Through the USPS (e.g., First-Class Mail)	0	0
	(4)	Free or Nominal Rate Distribution Outside the Mail (Carriers or other means)	0	0
e. Total Free or Nominal Rate Distribution (Sum of 15d (1), (2), (3) and (4))			27	16
f. Total Distribution (Sum of 15c and 15e)			204	187
g. Copies not Distributed (See Instructions to Publishers #4 (page 83))			19	15
h. Total (Sum of 15f and g)			223	202
i. Percent Paid (15c divided by 15f times 100)			86.76%	91.44%

* If you are claiming electronic copies, go to line 16 on page 3. If you are not claiming electronic copies, skip to line 17 on page 3.

16. Electronic Copy Circulation	Average No. Copies Each Issue During Preceding 12 Months	No. Copies of Single Issue Published Nearest to Filing Date
a. Paid Electronic Copies		
b. Total Paid Print Copies (Line 15c) + Paid Electronic Copies (Line 16a)		
c. Total Print Distribution (Line 15f) + Paid Electronic Copies (Line 16a)		
d. Percent Paid (Both Print & Electronic Copies) (16b divided by 16c × 100)		

☒ I certify that 50% of all my distributed copies (electronic and print) are paid above a nominal price.

17. Publication of Statement of Ownership

☒ If the publication is a general publication, publication of this statement is required. Will be printed in the NOVEMBER 2021 issue of this publication.
☐ Publication not required.

18. Signature and Title of Editor, Publisher, Business Manager, or Owner	Date
Malathi Samayan - Distribution Controller *Malathi Samayan*	9/18/2021

I certify that all information furnished on this form is true and complete. I understand that anyone who furnishes false or misleading information on this form or who omits material or information requested on the form may be subject to criminal sanctions (including fines and imprisonment) and/or civil sanctions (including civil penalties).

PS Form 3526, July 2014 (Page 3 of 4)   PRIVACY NOTICE: See our privacy policy on www.usps.com

Moving?

Make sure your subscription moves with you!

To notify us of your new address, find your **Clinics Account Number** (located on your mailing label above your name), and contact customer service at:

Email: journalscustomerservice-usa@elsevier.com

800-654-2452 (subscribers in the U.S. & Canada)
314-447-8871 (subscribers outside of the U.S. & Canada)

Fax number: 314-447-8029

Elsevier Health Sciences Division
Subscription Customer Service
3251 Riverport Lane
Maryland Heights, MO 63043

*To ensure uninterrupted delivery of your subscription, please notify us at least 4 weeks in advance of move.

Printed and bound by CPI Group (UK) Ltd, Croydon, CR0 4YY

08/05/2025

01864697-0018